Nurse
Anesthesia
SECRETS

Nurse Anesthesia SECRETS

MARY KARLET, CRNA, PHD
Director, Nurse Anesthesia Program
Duke University School of Nursing
Durham, North Carolina

SERIES EDITOR
LINDA SCHEETZ, EDD, APRN, BC, CEN
Assistant Professor
College of Nursing
Rutgers, The State University of New Jersey
Rutgers, New Jersey

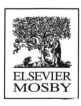

ELSEVIER
MOSBY

ELSEVIER
MOSBY

11830 Westline Industrial Drive
St. Louis, Missouri 63146

Notice

Nurse Anesthesia is an ever-changing field. Standard safety precautions must be followed, but as new research and clinical experience broaden our knowledge, changes in treatment and drug therapy may become necessary or appropriate. Readers are advised to check the most current product information provided by the manufacturer of each drug to be administered to verify the recommended dose, the method and duration of administration, and contraindications. It is the responsibility of the licensed health care provider, relying on experience and knowledge of the patient, to determine dosages and the best treatment for each individual patient. Neither the publisher nor the author assumes any liability for any injury and/or damage to persons or property arising from this publication.

The Publisher

International Standard Book Number 0-323-03144-7

Acquisitions Editor: Sandra Clark Brown
Senior Developmental Editor: Cindi Anderson
Publishing Services Manager: Melissa Lastarria
Senior Project Manager: Joy Moore
Design Project Manager: Bill Drone

Printed in the United States of America.

Last digit is the print number: 9   8   7   6   5   4   3   2   1

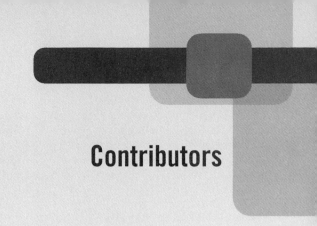

Contributors

STEVE L. ALVES, CRNA, PHD
Coordinator, Nurse Anesthesia Program
Northeastern University
Bouvé College of Health Sciences—
    School of Nursing
Boston, Massachusetts
    20. Neurological Disorders
    38. Neurosurgical Principles

COLLEEN M. BEAUCHAMP, RPH, CRNA, MS
CRNA Education Coordinator
Department of Anesthesia
William Beaumont Hospital
Adjunct Faculty
Beaumont Oakland University Graduate
    Program of Nurse Anesthesia
Royal Oak, Michigan
    16. Diuretics and Antiemetics

KASEY P. BENSKY, CRNA, MSNA
Staff Nurse Anesthetist
Department of Nurse Anesthesia
Presbyterian Hospital
Charlotte, North Carolina
    35. Ear, Nose, and Throat Surgery

MICHAEL BOYTIM, CRNA, MN
Assistant Director
School of Anesthesia
Kaiser Permanente
Pasadena, California
    3. Anesthesia Circuits

CARL S. BROW, III, MS, CRNA
Staff Nurse Anesthetist
Department of Anesthesia
Robert E. Bush Naval Hospital
Twentynine Palms, California
    30. Genitourinary Surgery

JENNIFER BURD, CRNA, MSN
Staff Nurse Anesthetist
Department of Anesthesiology
Duke University Medical Center
Durham, North Carolina
    45. Outpatient Anesthesia

LINDA CALLAHAN, CRNA, PHD
Associate Professor
Department of Nursing
California State University
Long Beach, California
    18. Cardiovascular Disease

KATHLEEN CARL, CRNA, MS
Staff Nurse Anesthetist
Department of Anesthesia
Detroit Medical Center
Detroit, Michigan
    25. Acid-Base Balance

ANTHONY JAMES CHIPAS, CRNA, PHD
Program Director
Nurse Anesthesia
Newman University
Wichita, Kansas
    33. Vascular Surgery

KATHLEEN A. COOK, CRNA, MS
Faculty-Instructor
Wayne State University School of Nurse
  Anesthesia
Director of Anesthesia Services
Sinai Grace Hospital
Detroit, Michigan
  37. Neuroskeletal Surgery

THERESA L. CULPEPPER, CRNA, PHD
Director of Clinical Anesthesia Services
Department of Nurse Anesthesia
Ida V. Moffett School of Nursing
Samford University
Birmingham, Alabama

THOMAS COREY DAVIS, CRNA, MSNA
Department of Nurse Anesthesia
Virginia Commonwealth University
  Health Systems
Medical College of Virginia Hospitals &
  Physicians
Richmond, Virginia
  7. Advanced Hemodynamic Monitoring

MICHAEL P. DOSCH, CRNA, MS
Chairman and Program Director
Department of Nurse Anesthesiology
University of Detroit Mercy
Detroit, Michigan
  2. The Anesthesia Machine

SASS ELISHA, CRNA, MS
Academic Instructor
School of Anesthesia
Kaiser Permanente
Pasadena, California
  10. Induction Drugs
  11. Narcotics and Benzodiazepines

DONNA JEAN FUNKE, CRNA, MS
Staff Nurse Anesthetist
University of California Los Angeles
Kaiser Woodland Hills
Health South Channel Island Surgical
  Center
Los Angeles, California
  40. Obstetrics and Anesthesia

REBECCA L. M. GOMBKOTO, CRNA, MS
Program Director
Minneapolis School of Anesthesia
St. Louis Park, Minnesota
Assistant Professor, Program Director
Saint Mary's University of Minnesota
Minneapolis, Minnesota
  27. Gastrointestinal Disorders

RICK HAND, CRNA, DNSC
Associate Director of Didactic Education
Raleigh School of Nurse Anesthesia
University of North Carolina—
  Greensboro
Raleigh, North Carolina
  53. Pain Management

ANNE B. HARRINGTON, CRNA, MSN
Staff Nurse Anesthetist
Critical Health Systems
Raleigh, North Carolina
  46. Trauma

WILLIAM HARTLAND, JR, PHD, CRNA
Associate Professor
Director of Education
Department of Nurse Anesthesia
School of Allied Health Professions
Virginia Commonwealth University
Richmond, Virginia
  56. Cardiopulmonary Resuscitation

SHARON HAWKS, CRNA
Staff Nurse Anesthetist
Department of Anesthesiology
Duke University and Health Systems
Durham, North Carolina
  34. Cardiac Surgery

DIANNA M. HEIKKILA, CRNA, MSN
Nurse Anesthetist
Boise, Idaho
  44. Anesthesia for the Geriatric Patient

JAMES B. HICKS, CRNA, MSN
Chief Nurse Anesthetist
Department of Anesthesia Services
Nash Health Care Systems
Rocky Mount, North Carolina
  13. *Cholinesterase Inhibitors and
      Anticholinergic Drugs*

ANNE MARIE HRANCHOOK, CRNA, MSN
Nurse Anesthetist
Oakland University
William Beaumont Hospital
Royal Oak, Michigan
  16. *Diuretics and Antiemetics*
  29. *Endocrine Disorders*

CRAIG K. HUARD, MSN, CRNA
Education Coordinator, Simulation
  Technologies
Perioperative Services Education
William Beaumont Hospital
Royal Oak, Michigan
  36. *Noncardiac Thoracic Anesthesia and
      One-Lung Ventilation*

DONNA LANDRISCINA JOHNSON, CRNA,
HSNA
Adjunct Assistant Professor
Assistant Director of Education
Staff Nurse Anesthetist
Department of Nurse Anesthesia
Virginia Commonwealth University
  Health Systems
Richmond, Virginia
  49. *Subarachnoid Block*

JOSEPH ANTHONY JOYCE, CRNA, BS
Department of Anesthesia
Wesley Long Community Hospital
Moses Cone Health System
Greensboro, North Carolina
  47. *Burn Patients*

LYNN H. KARLET, BSJ, MBA, JD
Attorney and Counselor at Law
Brown, Flebotte, Wilson, & Horn, PLLC
Greensboro, North Carolina
  59. *Legal Terminology*

MICHAEL J. KREMER, DNSc, CRNA, FAAN
Associate Professor, Adult Health Nursing
Co-Director, Rush University Simulation
  Labs
Assistant Director, Nurse Anesthesia
  Program
Rush University College of Nursing
Chicago, Illinois
  24. *Fluid Management and Transfusion*

KIRSTIN MICHELLE LAWLER, BSN, MSN,
CRNA
Nurse Anesthetist
Department of Anesthesia
Durham Anesthesia Associates
Durham Regional Hospital
Durham, North Carolina
  39. *Laparoscopic Surgery*

LE-LAN LE, MSN, CRNA
Department of Anesthesia
Kaiser Permanente Medical Center
Oakland, California
  12. *Neuromuscular Blocking Drugs*

LYNN L. LEBECK, CRNA, DNSc
Clinical Assistant Professor
Anesthesia Program Director
University of Michigan–Flint/Hurley
  Medical Center
Flint, Michigan
  58. *History and Organizational
      Structure of the Nurse Anesthesia
      Profession*

ROCHELLE LETHIOT, CRNA, MA
Assistant Director
School of Anesthesia
Kaiser Permanente
Pasadena, California
  4. *Airway Management*

JULIE ANN LOWERY, CRNA, MS
Staff Nurse Anesthetist/Clinical
  Instructor
Department of Anesthesia
University of North Carolina, Chapel Hill
Chapel Hill, North Carolina
  1. *The Operating Room*

KAREN E. LUCISANO, CRNA, MSN
Director Nurse Anesthesia Program
Carolinas Health Care System
Charlotte, North Carolina
   5. ECG Monitoring

JOHN P. MAYE, CRNA, PHD
Director of Research
Orofacial Pain Research Center
National Naval Dental Center
Bethesda, Maryland
   30. Genitourinary Surgery

DEBRA ROSE MERRITT, MSN, CRNA
Staff Nurse Anesthetist
Anesthesia Department
Moses Cone Health System
Greensboro, North Carolina
Member Board of Directors
Malignant Hyperthermia Association of
   the United States
Bethesda, Maryland
   21. Neuromuscular and Musculoskeletal
   Diseases

MEREDITH L. MUNCY, CRNA, MS
Staff Nurse Anesthetist
Department of Anesthesia
Duke University Medical Center
Durham, North Carolina
   31. Ophthalmic Surgery

TIMOTHY L. MURRY, CRNA, MSN
Adjunct Associate Professor
University of North Carolina at Charlotte
Charlotte, North Carolina
   9. Inhalational Anesthetics

JOHN NAGELHOUT, PHD, CRNA
Director
School of Anesthesia
Kaiser Permanente
California State University, Fullerton
Pasadena, California
   15. Local Anesthetics

ERICA D. NELSON, BSN, MSN, CRNA
Staff Nurse Anesthetist
Pitt County Memorial Hospital
Greenville, North Carolina
   8. Patient Positioning

RICHARD G. OUELLETTE, CRNA, MED
Staff Nurse Anesthetist
Wesley Long Community Hospital
Greensboro, North Carolina
   23. Coagulation and Hematologic
   Disorders

SANDRA M. OUELLETTE, CRNA, MED,
FAAN
Director, Nurse Anesthesia Program
Wake Forest University Baptist Medical
   Center
Instructor in Nurse Anesthesia
Wake Forest University School of
   Medicine
Winston-Salem, North Carolina
   23. Coagulation and Hematologic
   Disorders
   26. Renal Disease

SHERRY H. OWENS, CRNA, MSN
Assistant Director
Nurse Anesthesia Program
Wake Forest University Baptist Medical
   Center
Winston-Salem, North Carolina
   43. Pediatric Anesthesia

TIM PALMER, MS, CRNA
Perioperative Services Education
Beaumont Hospital
Royal Oak, Michigan
   14. Inotropic and Vasoactive Drugs
   28. Liver Disease

JOANNE PEARSON, CRNA, MSN
Staff Nurse Anesthetist
Forsythe Medical Center
Winston-Salem, North Carolina
   41. High-Risk Obstetrical Anesthesia

JOSEPH E. PELLEGRINI, CRNA, DNSc
Director of Research
Navy Nurse Corps Anesthesia Program
Naval Medical Education and Training
    Command
Bethesda, Maryland
    50. Epidural Anesthesia and Analgesia

MAUREEN REILLY, PhD, CRNA, MSN,
MHS
Associate Professor
Acute Care Nursing
University of Texas Health Science Center
San Antonio, Texas
    54. Latex Allergy

KAREN F. RICKER, RRT, MSN, CRNA
Clinical Preceptor
Department of Anesthesia
Durham Anesthesia Associates
Davis Ambulatory Surgery Center
Durham, North Carolina
    19. Respiratory Disease

MICHAEL RIEKER, ND, CRNA
Clinical Instructor and Lecturer
Nurse Anesthesia Program
Wake Forest University Baptist Medical
    Center
Winston-Salem, North Carolina
    6. Standard Patient Monitors

CHRISTOPHER G. RUTLEDGE, CRNA, MS
Staff Nurse Anesthetist
Department of Anesthesiology
University of Rochester/Strong Memorial
    Hospital
Rochester, New York
    22. Fluid and Electrolyte Disturbances

ELIZABETH MONTI SEIBERT, MSN, CRNA
Director of Clinical Education/Associate
    Professor
Department of Nurse Anesthesia
School of Allied Health Professions
Virginia Commonwealth University
Richmond, Virginia
    *57. Devices for Managing Cardiac
    Arrhythmias*

GRACE A. SIMPSON CRNA, MSN
Preceptor/Chief Nurse Anesthetist
Department of Anesthesiology
Duke University Medical Center
Durham, North Carolina
    48. Obesity

LISA J. THIEMANN, CRNA, MNA
Associate Director,
Nurse Anesthesia Program
Duke University
Durham, North Carolina
    32. Orthopedic Surgery

J. FRANK TITCH, MSNA, CRNA
Staff Nurse Anesthetist
Department of Anesthesiology
Durham VA Medical Center
Durham, North Carolina
    51. Intravenous Regional Anesthesia
    52. Peripheral Nerve Blocks

SUSAN KATHLEEN TOMSO, CRNA, MSN
Department of Anesthesiology
Duke University Hospital
Durham, North Carolina
    42. Neonatal Anesthesia

DENNIS HUGH WOODS, JR, BSN, MSN,
CRNA
Department of Anesthesia
Anesthesia and Pain Medicine
Augusta, Georgia
    55. Temperature Disturbances

KAREN ZAGLANICZNY, PhD, CRNA, FAAN
Director, Oakland Beaumont Graduate
    Program
Department of Nurse Anesthesia
William Beaumont Hospital—Royal Oak
Oakland University
Royal Oak, Michigan
    17. Herbal Products

REVIEWER

Theresa L. Culpepper, CRNA, PhD
Director of Clinical Anesthesia Services
Department of Nurse Anesthesia
Ida V. Moffett School of Nursing
Samford University
Birmingham, Alabama

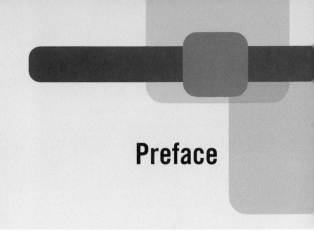

Preface

Nurse Anesthesia Secrets is intended for the nurse anesthesia student or nurse anesthetist practitioner to supplement her or his knowledge of nurse anesthesia practice. Topics are presented in a question and answer format for quick reference in accessing clinical information. Common questions that students or CRNAs may be asked in clinical practice are presented. Controversial topics are highlighted in select chapters, and key points are summarized at the end of each chapter. Internet sites and the bibliography are intended to provide the reader with key resources for exploring the topics in greater detail.

The book is divided into seven sections. The first section provides a guide to anesthesia equipment and common monitors used in anesthesia practice. Section II outlines anesthesia drugs used for general and regional anesthesia. A chapter on herbal agents provides some of the anesthesia implications associated with these products. The physiology and pathophysiology associated with various disease states is presented in Section III. The fourth section describes surgical procedures and associated anesthesia management implications. Questions and answers regarding specific patient groups, including obstetric, neonatal, geriatric, and pediatric patients, are presented in Section V. Commonly used regional techniques and pain management issues are delineated in Section VI. Finally, Section VII outlines various topics that are important to anesthesia practice, including latex allergy, temperature disturbances, cardiopulmonary resuscitation, and key points regarding the history of our professional organization.

The "top secrets" for nurse anesthesia practice are not really secrets at all and serve as a reminder that clinicians should share their professional "secrets" with others to improve the practice of nurse anesthesia and the care of our patients.

Contents

VI   REGIONAL ANESTHESIA AND PAIN MANAGEMENT, 449

VII   SPECIAL CONSIDERATIONS, 499

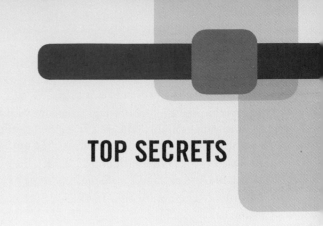

TOP SECRETS

- The most common preventable equipment-related cause of mishaps is a disconnection in the circuit. The most common site of disconnection is the Y-piece.
- The only completely ringed cartilage surrounding the larynx is the cricoid cartilage.
- The specific point on the ECG where most cardiac monitors perform ST-segment quantitative analysis is 80 msec past the J point.
- Chronic anemia produces an increase in 2,3-DPG, which shifts the oxyhemoglobin dissociation curve to the right. For a given PaO_2, the saturation is lower with anemia.
- Pulmonary artery diastolic pressure is considered a reliable indicator of PCWP. CVP is not considered a reliable indicator of PCWP.
- A decreased SvO_2 may be observed with conditions that decrease oxygen delivery, such as decreased cardiac output, decreased arterial oxygen saturation, or decreased oxygen carrying capacity.
- The four peripheral nerves or nerve bundles most commonly injured by improper positioning are the ulnar, brachial plexus, radial, and common peroneal.
- Anesthetic volatile agent uptake depends on blood gas partition coefficient, cardiac output, and anesthetic uptake by tissue.
- MAC is the amount, or concentration, of inhaled anesthetic needed to provide immobility in 50% of patients exposed to surgical stimulation.
- Propofol, ketamine, and all inhalational agents have bronchodilating effects, making them good choices for bronchospasm-susceptible patients. Ketamine is the induction agent of choice in actively wheezing asthmatic patients.
- Benzodiazepines produce their sedative-hypnotic effects through stimulation of GABA receptors.
- Side effects of succinylcholine may include bradycardia, myalgia, hyperkalemia, increased gastric pressure, increased intraocular pressure, increased intracranial pressure, and malignant hyperthermia.
- Central anticholinergic syndrome is characterized by flushing, central nervous system stimulation, severe dryness in the respiratory tract, increased body temperature, and impaired vision.
- Local anesthetics exert their action by blocking neuronal sodium channels.

- True allergy to local anesthetics is rare.
- The addition of epinephrine and attendant vasoconstriction reduces the speed of local anesthetic absorption away from the injection site area, reducing blood levels and toxicity and prolonging duration of action.
- Risk factors for PONV include age, gender, history of PONV, type and duration of anesthesia, use of opioid analgesics, and type of surgical procedure.
- Obstructive respiratory disorders include chronic bronchitis, emphysema, and asthma.
- Autonomic hyperreflexia is an unbridled SNS response below the level of a spinal cord transection.
- Subarachnoid block has been associated with worsening of symptoms in the patient with multiple sclerosis.
- Hyperkalemia is considered a medical emergency at levels greater than 7 mEq/L.
- High serum Mg^{2+} levels may enhance and prolong the effects of nondepolarizing muscle relaxants.
- The PT measures the extrinsic and common coagulation pathways. The APTT measures the intrinsic and common coagulation pathways.
- Dilutional thrombocytopenia is the most common intraoperative coagulation disturbance.
- One unit of platelet concentrate increases the recipient's platelet count by 5,000 to 10,000/mm^3 in an adult.
- Hemolytic transfusion reactions are most likely due to blood incompatibility from clerical errors.
- General and regional anesthesia reduce hepatic perfusion. Abdominal surgery, especially liver surgery, profoundly reduces hepatic perfusion.
- Recurrent laryngeal nerve injury is a potential complication of neck surgery. Unilateral recurrent laryngeal nerve injury causes hoarseness or may be asymptomatic. Bilateral recurrent laryngeal nerve paralysis causes stridor, aphonia, or complete airway obstruction.
- All open radical genitourinary procedures share two major concerns: the potential for significant hemorrhage and positioning.
- Intraocular pressure may increase with coughing, laryngoscopy, vomiting, glaucoma, direct pressure on the eye, hypercarbia, and hypoxia.
- Risk factors for DVT include low cardiac output, prolonged immobilization, obesity, prior DVT or pulmonary embolism, advanced age, and malignancy.
- High pulmonary artery pressure, abnormal pH, local infection, hypothermia, and inhaled anesthetics inhibit hypoxic pulmonary vasoconstriction.
- Burn patients are sensitive to depolarizing muscle relaxants and are at risk for hyperkalemia if depolarizing muscle relaxants are administered.
- Onset of a SAB shows an initial sympathetic blockade, followed by a sensory blockade, and finally motor blockade.

- The crests of the ileum correspond with the L4-5 vertebral level in most patients.
- The epidural space is a potential space that lies just outside of the subarachnoid space and extends from the base of the skull to the sacral hiatus.
- Premature release of the local anesthetic into the systemic circulation is the greatest complication associated with intravenous regional anesthesia.
- The four Ps mnemonic for "push, pull, pinch, pinch" provides a quick assessment tool for adequacy of axillary block.
- The body loses heat from radiation, evaporation, convection, and conduction.
- A rapid-sequence induction is required for general anesthesia in a pregnant patient.
- Capillary engorgement of the mucosa causes swelling of the nasal and oral pharynx, larynx, and trachea in the parturient, increasing the risk of bleeding when manipulating the airway.
- HELLP syndrome in the parturient is associated with hemolysis, elevated serum liver enzymes, and low platelet counts.
- Six diagnoses signal potential maternal hemorrhage: placenta previa; placental abruption; placenta accrete, increta, or precreta; uterine rupture; retained placenta; and uterine atony.
- Hypoxia should be considered first with unexplained bradycardia in the newborn.
- Nurse anesthesia is the oldest nursing specialty.

Section I

Anesthesia Equipment and Monitors

The Operating Room

Julie Ann Lowery

1. **Describe the difference between a nonliquefied compressed gas and a liquefied compressed gas, and give one example of each.**

   A *nonliquefied compressed gas* is one that does not become a liquid or liquefy at an ordinary temperature or under pressures up to 2000 to 2500 psi. An example of a nonliquefied gas is oxygen. Oxygen becomes a liquid at a low temperature, but commonly is stored in its gaseous form. A *liquefied compressed gas* is a gas that becomes a liquid in a container and at pressures of 25 to 2500 psi. A common liquefied compressed gas used in anesthesia is nitrous oxide.

2. **State the principle governing how oxygen is stored as a liquid.**

   Oxygen can be liquefied only if stored below its critical temperature of −119° C. This is governed by the principle stating that gases can be liquefied only if stored below their critical temperature.

3. **Name two methods in which medical gases are supplied to the operating room.**
   - The hospital piping system
   - The E cylinders mounted on the anesthesia machine

4. **What is the pressure of a medical gas being delivered to the operating room via the hospital pipeline system?**

   Medical gases exit the hospital pipeline system at approximately 50 psi.

5. **Explain the only reliable way to determine the volume of nitrous oxide in a tank and why.**

   Any cylinder, such as an E cylinder, containing a gas in its liquid form shows a constant pressure on the gauge as long as there is liquid in the cylinder. Nitrous oxide is stored as a liquid because its critical temperature is 36.5° C—well above room temperature of 20° C. As long as it is kept at a constant temperature, nitrous oxide vaporizes at an equal rate as it is consumed. This results in a constant pressure of 745 psi in the cylinder until the liquid becomes exhausted. When the pressure gauge on a tank of nitrous oxide begins to fall, there is only about

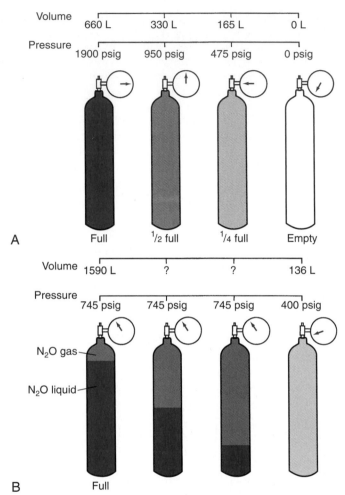

A, Oxygen remains a gas under high pressure. The pressure falls linearly as the gas flows from the cylinder; in contrast to nitrous oxide, the pressure remaining always reflects the amount of gas remaining in the cylinder. **B,** At ambient temperature (20° C), nitrous oxide liquefies under high pressure, and the pressure of the gas above the liquid remains constant *independent* of how much liquid remains in the cylinder. Only when all the liquid has evaporated does the pressure start to fall, then it does so rapidly as the residual gas flows from the cylinder. *(From Ehrenworth J, Eisenkraft JB: Anesthesia equipment principles and applications, St. Louis, 1993, Mosby.)*

250 L of gas left in the tank (see figure above). The only reliable method of determining how much volume of nitrous oxide is present is to weigh the cylinder.

6. **Several devices in the operating room safeguard the delivery of medical gases. Describe three key safety devices.**
   • One of the most visible delivery safety mechanisms is the *color coding* of the hoses that deliver medical gases to the operating room from the hospital piping

system. It is standardized that green is for oxygen, blue is for nitrous oxide, and yellow is for air. This color coding correlates with the color of each gas cylinder.

- A second safety device is the *diameter index safety system (DISS)*. This consists of quick connection mechanisms that connect one end of the medical gas hose to the anesthesia machine and the other end to the appropriate gas outlet on the wall. These connections are noninterchangeable to prevent a gas hose from being hooked up to the wrong gas source.
- A third safety device is the *pin index system* (see the following figure). Any E cylinder has two holes on its cylinder valve that match up with corresponding pins on the anesthesia machine. The positioning of these pins is unique for each gas. This system is designed to prevent the incorrect attachment of a gas cylinder to the outlet on the anesthesia machine. Unless the pins and holes are aligned, the port does not fit correctly against the yoke washer.

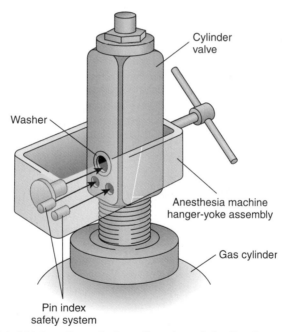

Pin index safety system interlink between the anesthesia machine and gas cylinder. *(From Morgan GE, Mikhail MS, Murray MJ: Clinical anesthesiology, ed 3, New York, 2002, Lange Medical Books/McGraw Hill.)*

7. The operating room is designed to be well ventilated using high airflow exchange air rates, which decrease the potential for contamination of the surgical site. Why is there a separate mechanism for the disposal of anesthetic waste gases?

Although high airflow rates are used in the operating room, the airflow is a combination of fresh air and recirculated air already present in the operating room. This airflow conserves energy and cost. The Occupational Safety and

Health Administration (OSHA) and the National Institute for Occupational Safety and Health (NIOSH) set guidelines for employee exposure to harmful substances in the workplace. These organizations recommend 25 air changes with a minimum of 5 fresh air exchanges per hour. Because air in the operating room is being recirculated, this would recirculate the anesthetic waste gases, resulting in more than one person being anesthetized in the operating room! Each anesthesia machine must have a scavenging system for the disposal of anesthetic waste gases. It is estimated that an efficient scavenging system lowers the ambient concentration of waste gases by 90%.

8. The use of electrical equipment in the operating room is extensive. What is the principle that explains how an electrical shock is received?

An individual can receive an electrical shock when he or she comes in contact with two materials conducting electricity at different voltages, creating a circuit. An example is coming in contact with either a 110 or 240 live volt electrical source, with the second conductor being a ground contact.

9. It is normal for electrical equipment to have electrical current leakage due to inadequate insulation or cross current between internal electrical components. Normally, this leakage is minute and averages less than 1 mA. In the operating room, what is the maximal amount of current leakage allowed?

The maximal amount of current leakage allowed in the operating room is 10 mcA.

10. Why is it crucial in the operating room to keep the allowable current leakage below a maximal level?

The skin offers high resistance to electrical current, and electrical current in this small amount is not detectable to touch. If an electrical current bypasses the insulating effects of the skin, however, it can be conducted directly through the heart. Electrical current as low as 100 mcA applied directly to the heart can induce ventricular fibrillation. For this reason, the maximal amount of allowable current leakage is set well below 100 mcA.

11. What is an isolation transformer?

Ungrounded power is supplied to an operating room via an isolation transformer. In this delivery system, electrical current is supplied to the operating room via two live ungrounded wires. An electrical circuit exists between the two wires, but not between either of the wires and the ground. This is an important safety feature because the chance of receiving an electrical shock is minimized to the patient and to operating room personnel. If one of the wires is touched accidentally, a shock does not occur because a circuit has not been created. With this system, both electrical wires from the isolation transformer would have to be contacted to receive an electrical shock.

12. What is a line isolation monitor?

A line isolation monitor in the operating room monitors the integrity of the isolated power system. If a faulty piece of electrical equipment is plugged into an outlet and subsequently makes contact with one of the two wires, the system is changed back to a standard grounded system. Contact with the other line can complete a circuit via a grounded patient. The line isolation monitor measures the amount of isolation between the two power lines and the ground. It does not indicate how much current is flowing, but it specifies the amount of current that could flow if a fault in the system were to occur. An alarm sounds if an unacceptable level of high electrical current flow to ground is detected, usually at 2 to 5 mA.

13. If the isolation line monitor alarm sounds during a case in the operating room, what action(s) should be taken?

If the line isolation monitor alarm sounds, it does not absolutely indicate that there is a dangerous situation at hand. It does indicate or signal that the isolation power system no longer is isolated from the ground and that one fault has occurred on one of the power lines. The second line would have to fault for a shock to occur because the two lines would create a circuit with the ground. If the line isolation monitor alarm sounds, the last piece of equipment that was plugged in should be identified and removed from service for repair. Even though faulty, this piece of equipment would continue to operate. It could be used safely if it were necessary for the patient's care, until replacement equipment could be secured.

14. What is the purpose of placing a grounding pad on the patient?

The grounding pad acts as a return electrode or exit pathway for electrical current generated through the cautery tip.

15. Why is the proper placement of the grounding pad essential for patient protection?

If the return electrode or grounding pad is not placed properly, has inadequate contact with the patient, or malfunctions, the electrical current generated by the cautery exits the patient in another location, resulting in a burn to the patient. Caution always should be taken to ensure that the grounding pad has good contact on the patient's skin and is not placed over bony prominences.

16. Discuss any special precautions that should be taken if a patient has a pacemaker.

As mentioned in a prior question, electrical current can be conducted through the heart, and this can cause pacemaker malfunction. If a patient has a pacemaker, it is recommended that the grounding pad be placed as close to the surgical site as possible and as far away from the heart as able. A magnet should be available to place over the pacemaker if the electrocautery is causing pacemaker inhibition.

17. Identify some combustible sources found in the operating room.

Main sources of combustion in the operating room are the *anesthetic gases oxygen* and *nitrous oxide.* Anesthetic equipment that may be combustible includes endotracheal tubes, oxygen catheters, surgical drapes, petroleum-based ointments, and skin preparation solutions, especially those containing alcohol.

Key Points

- A nonliquefied compressed gas is one that does not become a liquid or liquefy at an ordinary temperature or under pressures of 2000 to 2500 psi (e.g., oxygen).
- A liquefied compressed gas is a gas that becomes a liquid in a container and at pressures of 25 to 2500 psi (e.g., nitrous oxide).
- Oxygen can be liquefied only if stored below its critical temperature of –119° C.
- Gases are supplied to the operating room via the hospital piping system or E cylinders mounted on the anesthesia machine.
- Medical gases exit the hospital pipeline system at approximately 50 psi.
- The only reliable method of determining how much volume of nitrous oxide is present in an E cylinder is to weigh the cylinder.
- The Occupational Safety and Health Administration and the National Institute for Occupational Safety and Health set guidelines for employee exposure to harmful substances in the workplace.
- Each anesthesia machine must have a scavenging system for the disposal of anesthetic waste gases. It is estimated that an efficient scavenging system lowers the ambient concentration of waste gases by 90%.
- An individual can receive an electrical shock when he or she comes in contact with two materials conducting electricity at different voltages, creating a circuit.
- The maximal amount of current leakage allowed in the operating room is 10 mcA.
- Electrical current of 100 mcA applied directly to the heart can induce ventricular fibrillation.
- Ungrounded power is supplied to an operating room via an isolation transformer.
- If the line isolation monitor alarms, the last piece of equipment that was plugged in should be identified and removed from service for repair.
- If a patient has a pacemaker, it is recommended that the grounding pad be placed as close to the surgical site as possible and as far away from the heart as able.
- Main sources of combustion in the operating room are the anesthetic gases oxygen and nitrous oxide. Anesthetic equipment that may be combustible includes endotracheal tubes, oxygen catheters, surgical drapes, and petroleum-based ointments and skin preparation solutions, especially those containing alcohol.

Internet Resources

The Anesthesia Gas Machine:
http://www.udmercy.edu/crna/agm/index.htm.

GASNet Anesthesiology: Anesthesia Equipment in the MRI Suite:
http://gasnet.med.yale.edu/mri/about/about-mri3.php.

Virtual Anaesthesia Textbook:
http://asevet.com/resources/cgs.htm.

Bibliography

Barash PG, Cullen BF, Stoelting, RK: *Clinical anesthesia*, ed 4, Philadelphia, 2001, Lippincott Williams & Wilkins.

Dorsch JA, Dorsch SE: *Understanding anesthesia equipment*, ed 4, Baltimore, 1999, Lippincott Williams & Wilkins.

Ehrenworth J, Eisenkraft JB: *Anesthesia equipment principles and applications*, St. Louis, 1993, Mosby.

Faust RJ, Cucchiara RF: *Anesthesiology review*, ed 3, New York, 2001, Churchill Livingstone.

Morgan GE, Mikhail MS, Murray MJ: *Clinical anesthesiology*, ed 3, New York, 2002, Lange Medical Books/McGraw Hill.

The Anesthesia Machine

Michael P. Dosch

1. **How should a Certified Registered Nurse Anesthetist (CRNA) calibrate the oxygen analyzer?**

   There are two types of oxygen analyzers: the *galvanic-type sensor* (an older "plug in" type), and the *paramagnetic,* which is built into aspiration-type monitors. The *galvanic oxygen sensor* should be calibrated to room air. The time to 90% response is 15 to 20 seconds; if it takes longer than 40 to 60 seconds to read 21%, the sensor should be changed. Next, the sensor should be exposed to 100% oxygen, and the CRNA should ensure that it reads close to 100%. The practitioner may recalibrate at 100%, but it is not necessary with all monitors. Newer *paramagnetic sensors* use internal calibration routines, and they need only periodic (every 3 to 6 months) exposure to calibration gas. Oxygen analyzer alarms always should be "on" during an anesthetic.

2. **What can the CRNA do to fix an oxygen analyzer that is reading a fraction of inspired oxygen (Fio_2) of 0.16 (and declining) during a general anesthetic?**

   - Attention should not be directed toward "fixing" the monitor—the anesthetist *must* trust the monitor until it is proven wrong.
   - Call for help.
   - Turn on the emergency oxygen cylinder, and disconnect the pipeline from the wall.
   - If the inspired oxygen concentration does not increase with these measures and with adequate fresh gas flow, the anesthetist should ventilate the lungs manually with a breathing bag and room air (or preferably oxygen if a portable tank is available).
   - If patient oxygen desaturation is noted, proper endotracheal tube placement should be checked by noting bilateral midaxillary breath sounds.

3. **Can the anesthetist give an anesthetic when there is no connection for hoses, or if a cylinder is missing?**

   The hanger yoke orients cylinders, provides unidirectional flow, and ensures a gas-tight seal. The check valve in the cylinder yoke functions to minimize trans-filling, allow change of cylinders during use, and minimize leaks to atmosphere if a yoke is empty. There is a check valve in each pipeline inlet as well. The CRNA can give an anesthetic even when there is no connection to the hospital pipeline or if a tank is missing.

4. **What is the first device that informs the CRNA of a "crossover" or nonoxygen gas in the oxygen pipeline? Is it the fail-safe mechanism? Is it the hypoxic guard?**

The first device likely to inform the CRNA of a crossover is the *oxygen analyzer*. The second monitor to respond to a crossover, especially if the first monitor is ignored, might be the *pulse oximeter*.

The *fail-safe mechanism* guards against decreased oxygen *pressure*, not against *crossovers* or *mislabeled contents*. As long as there is any pressure in the oxygen line, nitrous oxide or any other gases mistakenly flowing in the oxygen line continue flowing. If oxygen pressure is lost, the fail-safe mechanism shuts off the flow of all other gases.

The *hypoxic guard system* works by detecting oxygen pressure as well. It controls the ratio of oxygen and nitrous oxide so that there is a minimum of 25% oxygen. It does not *analyze* the oxygen pipeline for the presence of oxygen.

5. **Name two actions that *must* be taken for suspected crossover.**

- Open the oxygen cylinder fully.
- Disconnect oxygen supply source at the wall.

If the practitioner does *not* disconnect the pipeline supply hose at the wall, the pipeline pressure exerted on the oxygen cylinder regulator diaphragm (downstream side) keeps the cylinder gas from flowing because the pipeline is maintained at a slightly higher pressure (50 psi) than the cylinder regulator (45 psi).

6. **What should the anesthetist do if oxygen pipeline pressure is lost?**

- Open the oxygen cylinder fully
- Disconnect the oxygen pipeline connection at the wall.
- An alarm indicates that something is *wrong* with the oxygen pipeline pressure. The supply problem may evolve into a nonoxygen gas in the oxygen pipeline. If so, that gas flows (pipeline pressure 50 psi) rather than the oxygen cylinder source (down-regulated to 45 psi).
- If the oxygen analyzer does not warn of the crossover, the pulse oximeter will— but only *after* the oxygen has been washed out (by ventilation) from the patient's functional residual capacity and vessel-rich group.

7. **The pipeline supply of oxygen has failed. How can the anesthetist make an emergency E tank oxygen supply last as long as possible?**

Driving a ventilator with cylinders causes their rapid depletion. Under such conditions, a full E cylinder can be used up within 1 hour. To prolong cylinder use, the patient should be ventilated manually, with assisted spontaneous ventilation implemented if possible. Use of low flows and the incorporation of air or nitrous oxide with oxygen also prolong cylinder use.

8. **The oxygen pipeline supply fails, and the oxygen cylinder gauge shows 1000 psi. How long will the emergency oxygen supply last?**

The following calculation may be made:

$$\text{Cylinder content (L)} \div \text{gauge pressure (psi)} = \\ \text{capacity (L)} \div \text{service pressure (psi)}$$

Example: 1000 psi shows on the cylinder gauge when the pipeline fails, and the oxygen flow is 2 L/min. Calculate "x" (L)/1000 psi = 660 L/1900 psi. The tank contains 347 L. If the oxygen flow is 2 L/min, the tank will last 173.5 minutes. For compressed gases, which are stored as liquids (nitrous oxide, carbon dioxide), the relationship between pressure and contents is not proportional, so this calculation cannot be made.

9. **Name the only two circumstances when a cylinder valve should be open.**

The cylinder should be turned off except (1) when checking pressure contents, and (2) when the pipeline is unavailable. Otherwise, silent depletion may occur. Pipeline pressure may decrease to less than 45 psi with flushing or ventilator use. If it does, oxygen flows from an opened cylinder. Enough oxygen may be lost over days or weeks to empty the tank, leaving no reserve available if the pipeline supply fails.

10. **List the circumstances that can permit a hypoxic mixture even when the hypoxic guard system is employed.**
    - Wrong supply gas in oxygen pipeline or cylinder
    - Defective pneumatics or mechanics (i.e., the hypoxic guard system is broken)
    - Leaks downstream of flowmeter control valves
    - Inert gas administration (a third gas, such as helium)

The hypoxic guard system connects only oxygen and nitrous oxide. The Datex-Ohmeda Anesthesia Delivery Unit (ADU) also takes desflurane into account. Because desflurane is given in higher concentration than the other agents, it is possible to create a hypoxic mixture with desflurane administered in air. Traditional machines (e.g., Ohmeda Modulus, Dräger Narkomed) and newer gas machines (e.g., ADU) permit this, but both give visible and audible alarms for low inspired oxygen.

11. **What is the most common preventable equipment-related cause of mishaps?**

Disconnection is the most common preventable equipment-related cause of mishaps. The anesthetist must maintain high vigilance, as follows:
- Consistently use a precordial or esophageal stethoscope to monitor breath sounds.

- Visually monitor chest movement with ventilation.
- If the ventilator is temporarily turned off (e.g., for an x-ray), a finger should be kept on the "on/off" switch, as a reminder to turn the machine back on.
- Apnea alarms always should be on. They should never be silenced.
- Extreme care should be exercised after initiating ventilation or whenever ventilation is interrupted. The anesthetist should *never* take for granted that flipping the switches initiates lung ventilation.

12. **What is the most common site of disconnection of the breathing circuit? What is the most important monitor for disconnection?**

The most common site for breathing circuit disconnection is the *Y-piece*. Monitors for disconnection ("apnea alarms") can be based on gas flow (tidal volume), circuit pressure (if the peak inspiratory pressure is below a set threshold, an alarm rings), chemistry (carbon dioxide detection), or acoustics (sound of the precordial or normal sounds of the ventilator cycle). The most important monitor for circuit disconnection is the anesthetist's *precordial* or *esophageal stethoscope*. Capnography is considered to be more important by some. The precordial is stated as the most important monitor in many references because it is inexpensive, it is reliable (cannot break or fail), and its "alarms" cannot be silenced.

13. **Explain the difference between ascending ("standing") and descending ("hanging") bellows?**

Standing bellows rise as the patient exhales; hanging bellows descend as they fill with the patient's exhaled gases. To determine if a bellows is ascending (standing) or descending (hanging), the bellows should be examined during expiration (*remember*: ascend and descend have *e*'s in them). Most modern types of bellows are ascending.

The *disadvantages* of the descending bellows are as follows:
- Unrecognized disconnection (owing to their design, they may fill even when disconnected from the patient)
- Collection of exhaled humidity in the bellows (risking infection and lessening delivered tidal volume)

Only one current anesthesia machine, the Dräger Julian, uses a hanging bellows, but it incorporates capnography and sensors to detect failure of the bellows to fill, both of which may lessen unrecognized disconnections.

14. **Every ventilator is activated differently. What is the best way to initiate mechanical ventilation so that steps are not forgotten?**

Different ventilators have different controls, but with all, mechanical ventilation can be initiated by doing the following:
- Switch the bag/vent switch to vent ("auto").

- Turn the ventilator power switch "on." Mode, volume or pressure, and rate settings should be noted.
- Check for chest expansion with the initial breathing cycles.

15. An emergency, life-threatening case is brought to the operating room. The anesthetist has not checked the machine. What must be checked even when time is at a premium?

A minimum safety test can be done even when time is critically short, as follows:
- A high-pressure test of the breathing circuit ensures that no leaks are present distal to common gas outlet.
- Observing or palpating the breathing bag for fluctuation during the preoxygenation period ensures adequate gas flow, good mask fit, and a breathing patient.
- A functioning suction should be immediately available.

16. Summarize the best way to preoxygenate a patient.

- Fresh gas flow 4 to 6 L/min
- Adjustable pressure-limiting (APL) valve open fully
- Tight mask fit
- 3 to 5 minutes of tidal breathing, or four to eight vital capacity breaths

A tight mask fit is the most significant factor when preoxygenating a patient. Lack of a tight fit cannot be compensated for by increasing the preoxygenation period.

17. In the middle of a case, the soda lime becomes exhausted. Should it be changed?

In a traditional anesthesia machine (Modulus or Excel), no. Increasing the fresh gas flow to 5 to 8 L/min for an adult (1 to 1.5 times minute ventilation) should prevent carbon dioxide rebreathing. Soda lime can be changed more easily in the ADU, without interrupting ventilation.

18. How can the practitioner determine if the patient is in respiratory acidosis from rebreathing carbon dioxide?

Failure of inspiratory or expiratory unidirectional valves and problems with carbon dioxide–absorbent granules (e.g., indicator failure, channeling, exhaustion) are the principal causes of rebreathing. Although most instances should be detected by noting the increase in inspired carbon dioxide on the capnograph, it still is worthwhile to review periodically the clinical signs of respiratory acidosis:
- Increase (and later a decrease) in heart rate and blood pressure
- Hyperpnea
- Signs of sympathetic nervous system activation
- Increased bleeding at the surgical site

Dark blood is not a sign of acidosis.

19. How should an open scavenging interface be set?

The indicator float should be kept between the lines. An audible suction sound is an indication that the interface is functioning properly. This is in contrast to the closed interface, in which a hiss indicates that waste gas is escaping into the room. The open interface is safer for the patient. It is open to the atmosphere, so there is no chance of excess positive or negative pressure being transmitted to the breathing circuit. It is less safe for a caregiver unfamiliar with its use because of potential waste gas exposure.

20. The anesthetist smells isoflurane during a case. What may be the cause?

The smell of gas during a case is abnormal, and the cause should be sought. Possible causes include the following:
- Poor mask fit
- An unscavenged technique, such as insufflation
- Flow from the breathing system into the room air (e.g., a volatile agent turned on before the mask is on)
- Anesthetics exhaled into the room at the end of a case
- Spilled liquid agent
- Uncuffed tracheal tube or leaks around a laryngeal mask airway cuff
- Machine leak
- Scavenger system leak (e.g., open interface with no suction on, closed interface without enough suction, obstructed gas disposal tubing)

The threshold for smelling volatile agents has been estimated to be 5 to 300 ppm. If the practitioner smells *any* gas, the concentration is above the National Institute for Occupational Safety and Health (NIOSH) standards. These guidelines state that no worker should be exposed to concentrations of waste anesthetic gases greater than 2 ppm of any halogenated anesthetic agent.

Nitrous oxide exposure may be more insidious because it cannot be smelled. Nitrous oxide exposure has proven to have ill effects on the reproductive systems of men and women. NIOSH guidelines state that no practitioner should be exposed to an 8-hour time-weighted average concentration of nitrous oxide greater than 25 ppm.

Practitioners concerned about waste gas exposure may consider disconnecting the gas machine nitrous oxide hose from the wall pipeline outlet at the beginning or the end of the day. This junction is a prominent cause of leaks. The gas analysis system should be scavenged. Volatile agent exposure may be limited by filling vaporizers at the end of the day rather than the beginning.

21. To fill a vaporizer properly, should the practitioner hold up the keyed filler until it stops bubbling?

No. The practitioner can overfill with this method if the keyed filler is faulty or the vaporizer dial is "on." It is better to fill vaporizers only to the top etched line within the sight glass. Overfilling is dangerous because discharge of liquid anesthetic distal to the vaporizers causes overdose.

There are two filling mechanisms: (1) the funnel "screw-cap filler" and (2) the agent-specific keyed filler (notches on the neck of the bottle of agent fit a special pouring device, which is keyed to prevent misfilling). The filler port used with the keyed device is low to prevent overfilling.

22. Relate the checkout procedure for the Tec 6 desflurane vaporizer.

- Press and hold the mute button until all lights and alarms are activated.
- Turn on to at least 1% and unplug the electrical connection. A "no output" alarm should ring within seconds; this tests the battery power for the alarms. This step is crucial in relation to the quick emergence characteristics of this agent. Any interruption in its supply must be noted and responded to at once.

23. Discuss the hazards of contemporary vaporizers.

- Filling with an incorrect agent
- Overfilling
- Tipping

If a vaporizer is tipped more than 45 degrees from vertical, liquid agent can obstruct the control mechanisms, with the risk of overdose on subsequent use. A typical treatment is to flush the vaporizer for 20 to 30 minutes at high flow rates with a low concentration set on the dial. The operating manual for the particular vaporizer should be checked because the correct procedure differs for each model. Only two modern vaporizers can be tipped: the Aladin cassettes in the Datex-Ohmeda S/5 ADU, and the Dräger Vapor 2000 (if the dial is set to "T").

 Key Points

- Oxygen monitoring via oxygen analyzer and pulse oximetry are standard care and always should be used to detect hypoxic mixtures of supply gas or gases delivered to patients.
- When a "crossover" is suspected, open the oxygen cylinder fully and disconnect the source at the wall outlet.
- When central oxygen supply fails, use the E cylinders efficiently. Discontinue ventilator use, and manually ventilate with lower flow rates and assisted spontaneous ventilation if possible.
- The most common preventable equipment-related cause of mishaps is a disconnection in the circuit. The most common site of disconnection is the Y-piece.

Continued

Key Points   *continued*

- Most modern ventilators have ascending bellows.
- A complete anesthesia machine check should be done at the beginning of the day. Follow the complete check with a high-pressure test of the breathing circuit to ensure that no leaks are present distal to common gas outlet.
- When soda lime becomes exhausted in the middle of a case, increase the fresh gas flow rates to prevent rebreathing. Change immediately after the case is completed.
- All waste gases should be scavenged.
- An open scavenging system is safer for the patient, preventing excessive positive or negative pressures being transmitted to the breathing circuit.
- When the CRNA smells a volatile agent, causes need to determined.
- Do not overfill vaporizers. Fill only to top etched line within the sight glass.
- Three hazards of contemporary vaporizers are filling with incorrect agent, overfilling, and tipping.

Internet Resources

U.S. Department of Labor: Occupational Safety & Health Administration Safety and Health Topics: Waste Anesthetic Gases:
http://www.osha_slc.gov/SLTC/wasteanestheticgases

Anesthesia Nursing & Medicine Web Site:
www.anesthesia-nursing.com

The Virtual Anesthesia Machine:
www.vam.anest.ufl.edu/

The Walter Reed Army Medical Center: Anesthesiology: Equipment checkout guidelines
http://www.wramc.amedd.army.mil/departments/surgery/Anesthesiology/checkout.htm

American Society of Anesthesiologists: Guidelines For Determining Anesthesia Machine Obsolescence:
www.asahq.org/publicationsAndServices/machineobsolescense.pdf

Bibliography

Benumof JL: Preoxygenation: best method for both efficacy and efficiency? *Anesthesiology* 91:603-605, 1999.

Dosch MP: Anesthesia equipment. In Nagelhout J, Zaglaniczny K, editors. *Nurse anesthesia,* ed 2, Philadelphia, 2001, WB Saunders, pp 245-286.

Dorsch J, Dorsch S: *Understanding anesthesia equipment,* ed 4, Baltimore, 1999, Williams & Wilkins.

Ehrenwerth J, Eisenkraft J, editors: *Anesthesia equipment: principles and applications,* St. Louis, 1993, Mosby.

Waste Anesthetic Gases. http://www.osha_slc.gov/SLTC/wasteanestheticgases. Accessed December 24, 2002.

Anesthesia Circuits

Michael Boytim

1. What is an anesthesia circuit?

An anesthesia circuit delivers anesthetic gases and oxygen from the anesthetic gas machine to the patient. The circuit also removes carbon dioxide, prevents entrainment of room air, and preserves temperature and humidity. In clinical practice, the anesthesia circuit physically extends from the point of the fresh gas inlet to the point at which gas is scavenged from the system.

2. What is the significance of resistance in anesthesia circuits?

Resistance imparted by anesthesia circuits imposes increased work of breathing. Endotracheal tubes usually are the source of more resistance and a more important factor in overall work of breathing than the anesthesia circuit. Replacing angle connectors with straight connectors and using tubes and tube connectors with the largest possible lumens help minimize resistance.

3. Define rebreathing.

Rebreathing occurs when the patient inhales previously exhaled gases. The amount of rebreathing may depend on the amount of fresh gas flow, the mechanical dead space, and the design of the anesthesia circuit. Mechanical dead space is the space in the anesthesia circuit that does not participate in gas exchange. Decreasing dead space in the anesthesia circuit by using the shortest length of tubing possible and increasing fresh gas flows may help prevent rebreathing of carbon dioxide.

4. How are anesthesia circuits classified?

Anesthesia breathing circuits are classified as *open, semiopen, semiclosed,* and *closed*. Classification is based on the presence or absence of the following:
- A reservoir bag
- Rebreathing of exhaled gases
- Chemical neutralization of exhaled carbon dioxide
- Unidirectional valves

Commonly used anesthesia breathing circuits are the Mapleson F, Bain, and Circle systems (see the following table).

Classification of Anesthesia Breathing Systems

System	Reservoir Bag	Rebreathing of Exhaled Gases	Chemical Neutralization of CO_2	Unidirectional Valves	Fresh Gas Inflow Rate*
Open					
Insufflation	No	No	No	No	Unknown
Semiopen					
Bain	Yes	No[†]	No	One	High
Mapleson F	Yes	No[†]	No	One	High
Semiclosed					
Circle	Yes	Partial	Yes	Three	Moderate
Closed					
Circle	Yes	Total	Yes	Three	Low

* High, > 6 L/min; moderate, 3 to 6 L/min; low, 0.3 to 0.5 L/min.
[†] No rebreathing of exhaled gases if fresh gas inflow is adequate.
From Stoelting RK, Miller RD: Basics of anesthesia, ed 4, Philadelphia, 2000, Churchill Livingstone.

In an *open* system, patients inhale only the gases delivered by the anesthesia gas machine. There is no apparatus to absorb carbon dioxide. Exhaled gases are released into the atmosphere.

With a *semiopen* system, exhaled gases flow out of the system and back to the inspiratory limb of the apparatus. There is no apparatus to absorb carbon dioxide, and rebreathing of exhaled gases depends on the amount of fresh gas flow. The amount of rebreathing is inversely related to the total amount of fresh gas flow used. If the amount of fresh gas flow supplied per minute is equal to or greater than the patient's minute volume, no rebreathing occurs as long as exhalation is not impeded. A reservoir bag and unidirectional valves may be present.

In a *semiclosed* system, part of the exhaled gases is scavenged to the atmosphere, and part mixes with the fresh gases to be rebreathed. An apparatus to absorb carbon dioxide, unidirectional valves, and a reservoir bag are present.

In a *closed* system, complete rebreathing of expired gas occurs. An apparatus to absorb carbon dioxide, unidirectional valves, and a reservoir bag are present.

5. Describe a Mapleson F anesthesia breathing system.

The Mapleson F anesthesia circuit, also known as the Jackson-Rees modification, has a common fresh gas inlet, corrugated tubing, an adjustable pressure limiting (APL) valve, and a reservoir bag (see the following figure). The amount

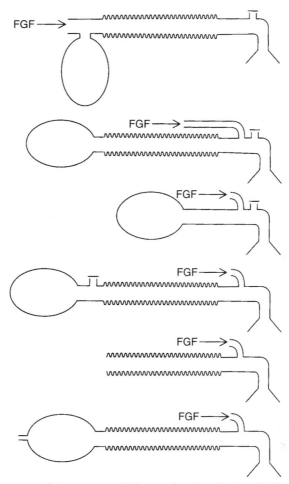

Anesthetic breathing systems classified as semiopen. FGF, fresh gas flow. *(From Stoelting RK, Miller RD: Basics of anesthesia, ed 4, Philadelphia, 2000, Churchill Livingstone, pp 136-147.)*

of rebreathing of exhaled gases in this system is determined by the type of ventilation (spontaneous versus controlled) and the amount of gas that is released into the atmosphere from the APL valve. To minimize rebreathing, it is recommended that the amount of fresh gas flow be twice the patient's minute ventilation.

The Mapleson F system commonly is used during transportation of intubated patients using controlled ventilation. This system was popular in pediatric anesthesia because it minimizes dead space and has low resistance. The Mapleson F system may be used with tracheal tubes or facemasks. Disadvantages of this system include the need for high fresh gas flows to prevent rebreathing, lack of humidification, and heat loss from patients.

6. Describe a Bain system.

A Bain anesthesia system is an adaptation of the Mapleson system in which the fresh gas flow enters through a narrow inner tube incorporated into an outer corrugated expiratory tube (see the following figure). The amount of fresh gas flow that enters through the inner tubing that is necessary to prevent rebreathing is 200 to 300 mL/kg/min for spontaneous breathing and 70 mL/kg/min for controlled ventilation. Advantages of the Bain system over a Mapleson F system include warming of fresh gas inflow from surrounding gases in the expiratory limb of the system, ease of scavenging, the ability to attach an anesthesia mechanical ventilator, light weight, and disposability (sterility). The outer expiratory tube is transparent, which allows visual inspection of the inner tube for possible kinks or disconnections.

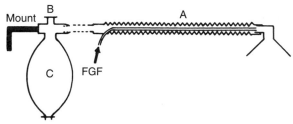

Schematic diagram of the Bain system showing fresh gas flow (FGF) entering a narrow tube within the larger corrugated expiratory limb (*A*). The only valve in the system (*B*) is an adjustable pressure-limiting (overflow) valve located near the FGF inlet and reservoir bag (*C*). *(From Stoelting RK, Miller RD: Basics of anesthesia, ed 4, Philadelphia, 2000, Churchill Livingstone, pp 136-147.)*

7. Describe a Circle system.

The Circle system is the most common circuit used for delivery of anesthetic gases. Two corrugated tubes serve as the conduits for delivery of anesthetic gases and oxygen to the patient (figure on page 25). These corrugated tubes have a large diameter (22 mm) and provide minimal resistance to breathing. Depending on the amount of fresh gas flow and the use of the APL valve, the circle system may be classified as semiopen, semiclosed, or closed. Chemical neutralization of carbon dioxide via an absorber permits partial rebreathing of exhaled gases. Partial rebreathing aids in the conservation of heat and moisture. Unidirectional check valves ensure the flow of gas in one direction. This arrangement prevents the inhalation of exhaled gases until they have passed through a carbon dioxide absorber and have been replenished with a fresh gas supply. Because the absorber eliminates carbon dioxide from the system, fresh gas inflow can be less than the patient's minute ventilation.

The reservoir bag maintains a reserve volume of gas to aid in manual pulmonary ventilation. The APL valve in the breathing system ensures that adequate airway pressures and gas volumes are delivered to the patient.

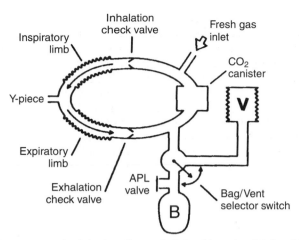

Schematic diagram of the components of a circle absorption anesthetic breathing system. Rotation of the bag/vent selector switch permits substitution of an anesthesia machine ventilator (V) for the reservoir bag (B). The volume of the reservoir bag is determined by fresh gas inflow and adjustment of the adjustable pressure limiting (APL) valve. *(From Stoelting RK, Miller RD: Basics of anesthesia, ed 4, Philadelphia, 2000, Churchill Livingstone, pp 136-147.)*

8. How is carbon dioxide eliminated from anesthesia breathing systems?

Carbon dioxide may be eliminated from the anesthesia breathing system by *venting* all of the exhaled gases to the atmosphere (open and semiopen systems) or through *chemical neutralization* (semiclosed and closed systems). Chemical neutralization is achieved by passing exhaled gases through absorbent materials, such as soda lime or barium hydroxide lime.

The neutralization process begins when carbon dioxide reacts with water to form carbonic acid. Carbonic acid reacts with a base (e.g., sodium hydroxide [NaOH], potassium hydroxide [KOH], calcium hydroxide [CaOH], or barium hydroxide [BaOH]) in the absorbent material to form carbonates, water, and heat.

Soda lime granules consist of CaOH plus smaller amounts of NaOH and KOH. Barium hydroxide lime consists of BaOH and CaOH.

 Key Points

- Rebreathing occurs when the patient inhales previously exhaled gases. It can be influenced by fresh gas flow, mechanical dead space, and design of the circuit.
- Anesthesia circuits are classified as open, semiopen, semiclosed, and closed. Classification is based on the presence or absence of a reservoir bag, rebreathing of exhaled gases, chemical neutralization of exhaled carbon dioxide, and unidirectional valves.

Continued

Key Points　*continued*

- The Mapleson F circuit is a nonrebreathing system. Commonly used for transport of intubated patients, the system's proper function is based on use of gas flow twice the patient's minute volume.
- The Bain breathing system is a coaxial (tube inside a tube) version of the Mapleson D system in which fresh gas flow enters through the inner tube and is exhaled via the outer corrugated tube. Fresh gas flow rate required for spontaneous ventilation is 200 to 300 mL/kg/min. For controlled ventilation, the requirement is 70 mL/kg/min.
- The Circle system is a soda lime canister with two unidirectional valves attached to inspiratory and expiratory tubings. An APL valve and a reservoir bag are connected to the canister. It is an efficient system that uses low fresh gas flows and reduces pollution.
- Soda lime absorbs the exhaled carbon dioxide and produces water and heat (humidifies and warms inspired gases).

Internet Resources

Anesthesia Breathing Systems: An In-Depth Review:
http://www.capnography.com/Circuits/breathingcircuits1.html

Vioworks.com:
http://www.vioworks.com

Nurse-Anesthesia.com: Review Topics, Anesthesia Breathing Systems:
www.nurse-anesthesia.com/review,breathingsystems.htm

The Anesthesia Gas Machine:
http://www.udmercy.edu/crna/agm/06.htm

Bibliography

Dorsch JA, Dorsch SE: *Understanding anesthesia equipment,* ed 4, Baltimore, 1999, Williams & Wilkins, pp 183-205.

Dosch MP: Anesthesia equipment. In Nagelhout J, Zaglaniczny K, editors: *Nurse anesthesia,* ed 2, Philadelphia, 2001, WB Saunders, pp 263-269.

Ehrenwerth J, Eisenkraft JB: *Anesthesia equipment: principles and applications,* ed 2, St. Louis, 1993, Mosby, pp 3-26.

Fisher DM: Anesthesia equipment for pediatrics. In Gregory GA, editor: *Pediatric anesthesia,* ed 4, Philadelphia, 2002, Churchill Livingstone, pp 191-205.

Stoelting RK, Miller RD: *Basics of anesthesia,* ed 4, Philadelphia, 2000, Churchill Livingstone, pp 136-147.

Airway Management

Rochelle Lethiot

1. Where is the larynx located?

The larynx is located in the middle region of the throat at C4 to C6.

2. Name the three paired and three unpaired cartilages of the larynx.

The three *paired* cartilages are arytenoids, conciliate, and cuneiform. The three *unpaired* cartilages are thyroid, cricoid, and epiglottis.

3. Name the only completely ringed cartilage surrounding the larynx.

The only completely ringed cartilage is the cricoid cartilage.

4. Which cartilages are usually visualized during laryngoscopy and intubation?

The arytenoid cartilages usually are visualized during laryngoscopy and intubation.

5. What nerves innervate the larynx?

The nerves that innervate the larynx are the *superior laryngeal* and *recurrent laryngeal nerves*; both are branches of the vagus nerves. The superior laryngeal nerve divides into an internal and an external branch. The internal branch provides sensory innervation to the larynx above the vocal cords. The external branch provides motor innervation to the cricothyroid muscle (tenses the vocal cords). The recurrent laryngeal nerve provides sensory innervation below the vocal cords and motor innervation of the posterior cricoarytenoid muscles, an abductor of the vocal cords. Cranial nerve IX, the glossopharyngeal nerve, provides sensory innervation to the vallecula.

6. Which blade is the best to use for intubation, the straight blade or the curve blade?

Opinions are divided regarding blade preference. Each type has its own features.

The *curved blade* (e.g., MacIntosh) fits into the vallecula. The practitioner keeps this blade midline during visualization and intubation. The curved blade may not always provide full visualization of the vocal cords, especially in patients with a large epiglottis.

The *straight blade* (e.g., Miller) is used to lift the epiglottis during vocal cord visualization. The straight blade does not help the provider determine midline. If visualization is not good, exterior pressure or displacement of the larynx may aid visualization.

7. What can be done to prevent mask airway leaks?

- Gently increase the amount of air in the mask to assist with the facemask seal.
- Gently decrease the amount of air in the mask to allow a softer fit.
- Place both hands on the facemask and ask an assistant to ventilate the patient.
- If the patient's nose is too large to allow a proper fit, turn the mask upside down, placing the wider portion across the nose and the narrower portion below the mouth.
- If the patient's facial hair is preventing a proper fit, it can be hard to mask ventilate, and a laryngeal mask airway (LMA) or intubation may be necessary.

8. What are recommended endotracheal tube (ETT) sizes for adults?

The ideal ETT size for adults is determined primarily by the age and sex of the patient (see the table below).

Endotracheal Tube Sizes		
	Size of ETT	Insertion Length
Women	7.0–8.0	19–21 cm at lip
Male	7.5–8.5	20–23 cm at lip

ETT, endotracheal tube.

9. What are appropriate LMA sizes and cuff volumes for different patient groups?

Appropriate LMA sizes and cuff volumes are presented in the table on page 29.

10. Can an LMA be used in a patient with a "full stomach"?

The LMA only partially protects the larynx from pharyngeal secretions and does not protect against gastric regurgitation. As a general rule, patients with a full stomach should be intubated. The primary exception to this rule is use of the LMA to ventilate temporarily an anesthetized patient who cannot be intubated. In this situation, the LMA can be used to facilitate insertion of an ETT either blindly through the LMA or in conjunction with a fiberoptic bronchoscope.

Laryngeal Mask Airway Sizes

LMA Size	Patient Size	Weight (kg)	Cuff Volume (mL)	ETT Size Able to Insert into LMA
1	Neonates/infants	5	4	3.5
1.5	Infants	5–10	7	4
2	Child	10–20	10	4.5
2.5	Child	20–30	14	5
3	Small adult	>30	20	6
4	Normal adult	—	30	6
5	Large adult	—	40	7
Fastrach				
3	Small	—	≤20 mL	7
4	Medium		≤30 mL	7.5
5	Large		≤40 mL	8

ETT, endotracheal tube; LMA, laryngeal mask airway.

11. **Summarize criteria that may help identify a possible difficult airway during preoperative evaluation.**

LOOK
- Assess the neck. A patient with a short, thick neck may be difficult to intubate. Cervical spine limitations or instability signals a difficult airway.
- Look at the patient's tongue. Patients with thick tongues are more difficult to intubate.
- Look at the patient's teeth.
  - Loose, large, or protruding teeth should be assessed carefully during intubation and extubation.
  - Loose teeth are an aspiration hazard. Check and count loose teeth before and after intubation.
  - Consider using a teeth protecter during intubation and a 4 × 4 gauze wrapped in a tongue blade instead of an oral airway.

LISTEN
- Listen to the patient's voice. Patients with a hoarse, raspy, or whispered voice may have airway tumors, vocal cord paralysis, edema, or arthritis.
- Listen to the patient. Ask the patient if he or she has had intubation problems in the past or surgeries of the head or neck that may cause airway difficulties. Review the chart for past intubation documentation.

FEEL
- Feel the patient's larynx. A stiff, unmovable larynx may make intubation more difficult. The larynx should be palpated in midline.

12. Define the Mallampati classification.

Mallampati is a classification obtained by observing oral structures in a sitting patient with the mouth wide open and tongue extended. It is used as a guide to estimate ease of intubation.
- Class I visualizes the palate, uvula, fauces, and pillars.
- Class II visualizes the soft palate, uvula, and fauces.
- Class III visualizes only the soft palate and base of the uvula.
- Class IV visualizes only the hard palate.

The Mallampati classification is of maximal benefit if it is used in conjunction with assessment of mouth opening, measurement of the thyromental distance, and observation of neck flexion and extension. An adult patient's mouth opening should be at least 4 cm. The thyromental distance is the distance between the thyroid notch and the lower mandibular border, while the neck is fully extended. If this distance is shorter than 6 cm or three fingerbreadths, it can indicate a difficult intubation.

The Mallampati class does not correlate with the ease or difficulty of LMA insertion. A difficult intubation could be an easy LMA insertion.

13. List equipment that should be available for an anticipated difficult intubation.
- Suction
- Difficult airway cart in the room with LMAs and a fiberoptic intubating scope ready
- Several different blade styles and sizes
- Several different sizes of ETTs with stylets
- Eschmann stylet gum bougie

14. Describe the optimal patient position for intubation.

An ideal alignment for intubation requires that the pharyngeal axis, oral axis, and laryngeal axis be in an almost straight line. The head should be in a sniffing position, placed on a pillow or bath blankets. The figures on page 31 show head positions: (1) a neutral position where all three axes are widely apart, (2) a sniffing position where the oral axis is still out of alignment, and (3) a sniffing position with head extension where the three axes are almost in complete alignment and ready for intubation.

15. Describe the use of the fiberoptic bronchoscope for performing intubation in an awake patient.

Fiberoptic-guided intubation can be performed expeditiously if the following preparatory steps are done in the preoperative hold area:
- Use a tongue blade to pull the tongue forward gently, and spray the throat with local anesthetic (Cetacaine aerosol).
- Spray the throat with 4% lidocaine spray (bitter tasting); spray left to right, then down the back of the throat.

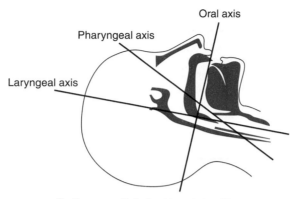

The three axes with the head in neutral position.

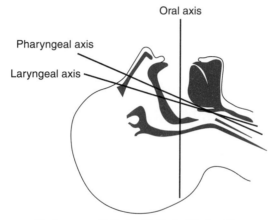

The three axes with the head in the "sniffing" position.

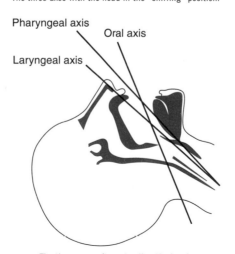

The three axes after extending the head.

- Allow the patient to gargle and spit out the liquid. Swallowing the local anesthetic solution may cause nausea.
- For a nasal intubation, apply phenylephrine (Neo-Synephrine) spray to both nares to decrease bleeding. Place nasal airways, well lubricated with lidocaine jelly, in each nostril (start small and work up to the ETT size being used).
- After each spray, tap the back of the tongue with a tongue blade to determine if the patient still has a gag reflex. Intravenous glycopyrrolate may be used as an antisialogue.

16. What is retrograde intubation?

A retrograde technique may be used to intubate complex airways. The practitioner begins by inserting a wire through the cricothyroid membrane and passing the wire cephalad through the vocal cords into the mouth. An ETT is threaded over the wire into the trachea.

17. What is a percutaneous cricothyrotomy?

A percutaneous cricothyrotomy is an emergency method of establishing a temporary airway.
- The provider inserts a 14-gauge intravenous catheter through the cricothyroid membrane.
- The barrel of a 3-mL syringe is connected to the proximal end of the plastic catheter.
- The connector from a 7.0-mm ETT is attached to the syringe barrel to allow for ventilation support.

Many anesthesia carts carry the 14-gauge intravenous catheter, 3-mL syringe barrel, and 7.0-mm ETT connector preassembled in a sealed clear bag.

18. What is a gum bougie, and how is it used?

A gum bougie is a simple tool to assist with intubation when there is little or no visualization of the vocal cords. The gum bougie first was used as a urology dilator and was adapted to anesthesia needs by an alert anesthesiologist.
- The intubating blade is introduced normally, and the epiglottis is visualized.
- The epiglottis is lifted, and the bougie is introduced gently and slowly in the direction of the vocal cords.
- If the bougie can be advanced without forcing, an ETT is threaded over the bougie into the trachea.

19. Describe other popular methods of intubating a difficult airway.

LMA-FASTRACH
The LMA-Fastrach contains a rigid curved airway tube that is wide enough to accommodate a cuffed 8-mm ETT. After insertion, the patient may be ventilated through the LMA-Fastrach or intubated through the airway using either a fiberoptic intubating scope or blind insertion of an ETT.

INTUBATING LIGHT WAND

The light wand uses a light that can be seen on the neck tissue to identify vocal cord location.

BULLARD FIBEROPTIC LARYNGOSCOPE

The Bullard scope may be considered for patients with a limited ability to open the mouth, congenital airway problems, or an unstable cervical spine. The hockey stick–shaped blade follows the contour of the oral pharynx and allows visualization of the larynx and intubation with minimal mouth opening and with the patient's head in a neutral position.

20. What is laryngospasm, and how is it treated?

Laryngospasm is a partial or complete obstruction of the larynx due to an involuntary spasm of the laryngeal musculature. Common causes include laryngoscopy, extubation, or other airway manipulation; airway secretions; and airway suctioning. If laryngospasm is partial, the patient may present with a crowing sound or stridor. A complete laryngospasm precludes ventilation. Oxygen saturations decline, and breath sounds are absent.

The provider must react to a laryngospasm immediately, as follows:
- Application of positive-pressure ventilation with 100% oxygen often "breaks" the spasm.
- If the laryngospasm is not relieved with positive pressure, intravenous succinylcholine should be given. Dosage may be judged by the patient's status and extent of airway compromise. Some practitioners administer subclinical doses of 0.1 mg/kg, whereas others administer full intubating doses of 1 mg/kg.
- Intravenous lidocaine, 1 to 1.5 mg/kg, may be used to blunt airway reflexes.

 Key Points

- The larynx is located in the middle region of the throat at C4-6.
- The three paired cartilages are arytenoids, conciliate, and cuneiform. The three unpaired cartilages are thyroid, cricoid, and epiglottis.
- The only completely ringed cartilage surrounding the larynx is the cricoid cartilage.
- The cartilages usually visualized during laryngoscopy and intubation are the arytenoid cartilages.
- The nerves that innervate the larynx are the superior laryngeal and recurrent laryngeal nerves, both branches of the vagus nerves.
- A curved (MacIntosh) or straight (Miller) blade is used for intubation of the trachea.
- Generally an adult female trachea can accept a 7.5 to 8.0 mm ETT, and an adult male trachea can accept an 7.5 to 8.5 mm ETT (see table in Question 8).
- Generally an adult can accommodate a size 4 or 5 LMA. A child can accommodate a size 2 to 2.5 LMA (see table in Question 9).

Continued

Key Points   *continued*

- Mallampati is a classification used as a guide to estimate ease of intubation.
- Mallampati class I visualizes the palate, uvula, fauces, and pillars.
- Mallampati class II visualizes the soft palate, uvula, and fauces.
- Mallampati class III visualizes only the soft palate and base of the uvula.
- Mallampati class IV visualizes only the hard palate.
- The Mallampati class does not correlate with the ease or difficulty of LMA insertion.
- An ideal alignment for intubation requires that the pharyngeal axis, oral axis, and laryngeal axis be in an almost straight line. The head should be in a sniffing position, placed on a pillow or bath blankets.
- A percutaneous cricothyrotomy is performed by inserting a 14-gauge intravenous catheter through the cricothyroid membrane.
- A gum bougie is a simple tool to assist with intubation when there is little or no visualization of the vocal cords.
- Laryngospasm must be treated immediately. Positive-pressure ventilation with 100% oxygen, succinylcholine, or lidocaine can be used.

Internet Resources

GASNet Anesthesiology: Management of the Difficult Airway:
http://www.gasnet.org/airway/index.php

GASNet Video Library:
http://www.gasnet.org/videos/index.php

University of Virginia Health System: Airway Management/Induction of Anesthesia:
http://www.healthsystem.virginia.edu/internet/anesthesiology/Dept-Info/Education/Lectures/introair.cfm

Virtual Anaesthesia Textbook:
http://www.virtual-anaesthesia-textbook.com/

Nurse-Anesthesia.com:
http://www.nurse-anesthesia.com/

Update in Anaesthesia: Cumulative Index Arranged by Issue:
http://www.nda.ox.ac.uk/wfsa/html/pages/up_issu.htm#1

Bibliography

Benumof JL: Laryngeal mask airway and the ASA difficult airway algorithm, *Anesthesiology* 84:686, 1996.

Cappello C, Weisbrod J: Airway management. In Nagelhout JJ, Zaglaniczny KL, editors: *Nurse anesthesia,* ed 2, Philadelphia, 2001, WB Saunders, pp 382-395.

Deem S, Bishop M: Evaluation and management of the difficult airway, *Crit Care Clin* 11:1-27, 1995.

Hall S: Respiratory anatomy, physiology, and pathophysiology. In Nagelhout JJ, Zaglaniczny KL, editors: *Nurse anesthesia,* ed 2, Philadelphia, 2001, WB Saunders, pp 504-544.

Mallampati SR: Clinical signs to predict difficult tracheal intubation (hypothesis), *Can Anaesth Soc J* 30:316, 1983.

McIntyre JWR: Laryngoscope design and the difficult adult tracheal intubation, *Can J Anaesthesiol* 36:94, 1989.

Morgan GE Jr, Mikhail MS, Murray MJ: *Clinical anesthesiology,* ed 3, New York, 2002, McGraw-Hill, pp 59-85.

Watson CB: Prediction of a difficult intubation: methods for successful intubation, *Respir Care* 44:777, 1999.

Whitten C: *Anyone can intubate,* ed 4, San Diego, 1997, KW Publications.

ECG Monitoring

Karen E. Lucisano

1. In what three electrocardiogram (ECG) leads can most cardiac ischemia be detected?

In a study by London et al, 100 patients with known coronary artery disease were monitored for ischemia during surgery. The study found that a combination of leads V_4 and V_5 detected 85% of ischemic events and that V_5 was the most sensitive lead. Of the frontal plane leads, lead II was the most sensitive in determining ischemic events (approximately 33%). Additionally, all major anatomic areas of the myocardium are assessed by these two leads. Lead V_5 detects events in the anterior and lateral wall, and lead II detects events in the inferior wall. However, optimal sensitivity is attained when combining all three of these leads (96%). Monitoring in *leads II, V_4 and V_5* provides the greatest sensitivity to detect coronary ischemia (see the following figure).

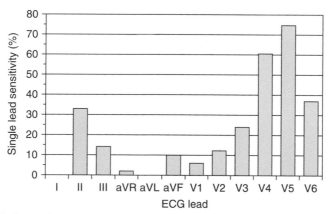

The distribution of ischemic ST-segment changes in each of the 12 leads considered individually.

The advent of invasive interventional cardiac therapy has allowed researchers to correlate single-vessel ischemia (caused by balloon inflation during percutaneous transluminal coronary angioplasty) with real-time ECG changes. A study by Mizutani et al concluded that the most sensitive leads to monitor for ischemia varied by vessel occluded. Occlusion of the left anterior descending coronary artery resulted in ECG changes in leads III, V_3, and V_5; occlusion of the right coronary and left circumflex artery resulted in ECG changes in leads III,

V_2, and V_5. This study suggested that the best option for detection of ischemia originating from any one of the three major coronary vessels is the combination of *leads III and V_5 with either V_2 or V_3.*

2. Identify ECG changes most suggestive of myocardial ischemia.

The most frequent ECG changes that occur as a result of coronary ischemia are *ST-segment deviations*, either depression or elevation.

ST-SEGMENT DEPRESSION

The quality and quantity of ST-segment depression are important determinants of coronary ischemia.

- *Quality of ST-segment depression.* ST-segment depression can be described as upsloping, horizontal, or downsloping (see the figure below). This characteristic of ST-segment depression is assessed immediately after the J point. The least sensitive ST-segment change in regards to coronary ischemia is upsloping ST-segment depression. Horizontal ST-segment depression is intermediate to sensitivity to ischemia. The ST-segment change most suggestive of coronary ischemia is downsloping.
- *Quantity of ST-segment depression.* ST-segment depression characteristic of ischemia is at least 1 mm below the isoelectric baseline, at 0.08 seconds past the J point.

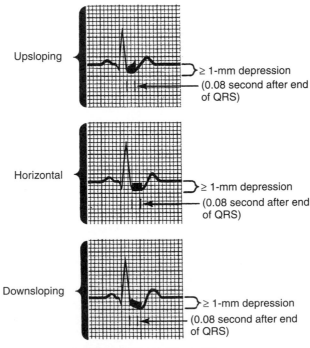

Types of ST-segment depressions.

ST-SEGMENT ELEVATION

Any degree of ST-segment elevation, assuming other causes are ruled out (see Question 6), suggests ischemia. ST-segment elevation that occurs as a result of coronary artery disease may indicate an acute myocardial infarction or transmural ischemia.

3. **Identify the specific points on the ECG where most cardiac monitors perform ST-segment quantitative analysis.**

   The two specific points are the *J point* and *isoelectric baseline*.
   - J point is the transition point between the QRS complex and the ST segment. Typically the ST-segment deviation is measured 80 msec from this point.
   - Isoelectric baseline is the point of reference against which the ST segment is measured (See the following figure).

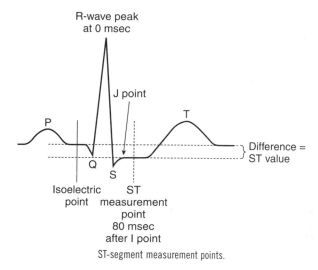

ST-segment measurement points.

4. **Correlate each lead of the standard 12-lead ECG with the specific anatomic area of the myocardium assessed.**

   The table below shows the correlation of leads with specific anatomic areas of the myocardium.

Standard Leads and Their Anatomic Correlates

Area of Myocardium	Corresponding Leads
Inferior	II, III, aVF
Lateral	I, aVL, V5, V6
Anterior	V1-V4
Posterior	V1 (mirror)

5. **Name the three main coronary arteries and the areas of the myocardium they perfuse.**

The following table presents the three main coronary arteries and the areas of the myocardium they perfuse.

Coronary Arteries and Their Coronary Arterial Distributions

Coronary Artery	Anatomic Area of Flow Distribution
Left anterior descending	Anterior
Left circumflex	Lateral, possibly posterior (left dominant)
Right coronary artery	Inferior, possibly posterior (right dominant)

6. **List conditions other than coronary artery disease that can cause ST-segment deviations.**

Conditions that can cause ST-segment deviations include the following:
Elevation
- Acute pericarditis
- Ventricular aneurysm
- Early repolarization

Depression
- Ventricular hypertrophy
- Intraventricular conduction defects
- Drug effects
- Nonspecific causes

7. **Identify the normal cardiac electrical conduction sequence.**

Sinoatrial node → atrioventricular node → bundle of His → right and left bundle branches → Purkinje fibers

8. **Identify and note the significance of each waveform and interval in the normal cardiac conduction cycle (see the figure on page 41).**

Waves

P wave	Atrial depolarization
QRS complex	Ventricular depolarization (<0.12 second)
T wave	Ventricular repolarization

Intervals

P-R interval	The time it takes for an impulse to travel from the sinoatrial node through the conduction system to the ventricular muscle (0.08 to 0.12 second)

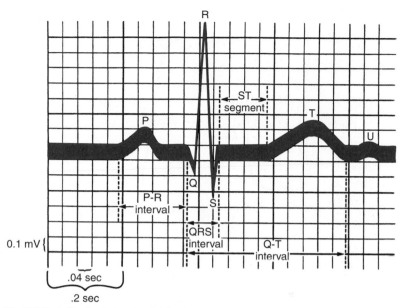

Diagram of the ECG illustrating the designation of deflections and the ECG intervals of the cardiac cycle on the standard grid format used for measuring the amplitude of deflections and the duration of the intervals. The paper speed is 25 mm/sec.

| ST segment | The time between completion of depolarization of the ventricles and the onset of repolarization of the ventricles |
| Q-T interval | The time it takes for complete depolarization and repolarization of the ventricles |

9. Discuss how electrical events lead to mechanical events within the myocardium.

When an action potential arrives at a cardiac cell, it allows the positively charged ions (primarily Na^+ and Ca^{2+}) to move into the cell, causing cell membrane depolarization. Increased intracellular Ca^{2+} initiates mechanical contraction by promoting the movement of actin and myosin contractile proteins within the myocardial cells. Synchronization of this action in the atria and ventricles leads to a contractile state called *systole*. Muscle contraction continues until the positively charged ions are pumped out of the cells. This ionic movement causes repolarization of the cell and initiates *diastole* or relaxation. When the muscle cell has returned to its normal resting state, it is capable of reactivation when the next electrical impulse arrives.

10. Describe the phases of the cardiac action potential (see the figure on page 42).

| Phase 0 | Rapid depolarization; generated by movement of sodium ions into the cell |
| Phase 1 | Brief phase of initial rapid repolarization; the result of inactivation of the sodium channels and transient increase in potassium permeability |

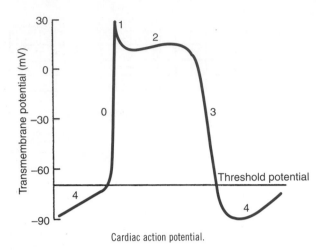

Cardiac action potential.

Phase 2	Plateau phase; sodium channels close, calcium channels open, and calcium diffuses into the cell
Phase 3	Final repolarization phase; calcium channels close; potassium continues to diffuse to the extracellular space
Phase 4	Return of normal sodium and potassium permeability and a normal resting transmembrane potential

11. Identify the proper lead placement for ECG monitors with five-electrode monitoring capability. What leads are available for monitoring with this type of ECG monitor configuration?

PROPER LEAD PLACEMENT
- RA—near right shoulder
- LA—near left shoulder
- RL—right lower abdomen
- LL—left lower abdomen
- V—location specific for precordial lead you wish to monitor; V5 is placed at the intersection of a line drawn parallel to the fifth intercostal space and the anterior axillary line

Leads available for monitoring include I, II, III, aVR, aVL, aVF, and V (lead available for monitoring depends on placement of the precordial electrode).

12. Determine the polarity for the bipolar frontal plane leads I, II, and III based on the Einthoven triangle.

Einthoven was a Dutch physician who invented the ECG in the 1900s. Refer to the following table and figure to answer this question.

Polarity of the Bipolar Frontal Plane Limb Leads

Lead	Negative Electrode	Positive Electrode
I	Right arm	Left arm
II	Right arm	Left leg
III	Left arm	Left leg

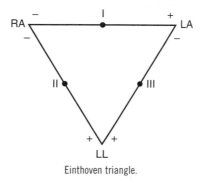

Einthoven triangle.

Key Points

- To detect ischemia originating in any one of the three major coronary vessels, leads III and V_5 with either V_2 or V_3 are the best options.

- The most frequent ECG changes that occur as a result of coronary ischemia are ST-segment deviations, either depression or elevation.

- The quality and quantity of ST-segment depression are important determinants of coronary ischemia.

- Any amount of ST-segment elevation, assuming other causes are ruled out, suggests ischemia. ST-segment elevation that occurs as a result of coronary artery disease may indicate an acute myocardial infarction or transmural ischemia.

- The specific point on the ECG where most cardiac monitors perform ST-segment quantitative analysis is 80 msec past the J point.

- The areas of the myocardium are assessed in the following lead configurations: inferior, leads II, III, aVF; lateral, leads I, aVL, V_5, V_6; anterior, leads I through IV; and posterior, lead V_1.

- The ECG waveform is composed of P wave, QRS complex, and T wave. The intervals are the P-R interval, ST segment, and Q-T interval.

- The cardiac action potential has five phases: rapid depolarization, initial rapid repolarization, plateau phase, final repolarization phase, and return to normal transmembrane potential.

Internet Resources

Nurse-Anesthesia.com: Basic EKG Interpretation, Part I:
www.nurse-anesthesia.com/basicekg.htm

A Guide to Reading and Understanding the EKG:
http://endeavor.med.nyu.edu/student-org/erclub/ekgguide.pdf

Introduction to ECG Interpretation:
http://www.fammed.wisc.edu/pcc/ecg/ecg.html

Basic Electrocardiography:
http://www.sh.lsuhsc.edu/fammed/OutpatientManual/BasicECG.htm

A "Method" of ECG Interpretation:
http://medlib.med.utah.edu/kw/ecg/ecg_outline/Lesson2/index.html

EKG Quizzer 1: Basic EKG Features:
http://www.gwc.maricopa.edu/class/bio202/cyberheart/ekgqzr.htm

Bibliography

Dubin D: *Rapid interpretation of EKG's*, ed 6, Tampa, 2000, COVER Inc.

Foster DB: *Twelve lead electrocardiography for ACLS providers*, Philadelphia, 1996, WB Saunders.

London MJ, Hollenberg M, Wong MG, et al: Intraoperative myocardial ischemia: localization by continuous 12- lead electrocardiography, *Anesthesiology* 69:232-241, 1988.

Mizutani M, Freedman SB, et al: ST monitoring for myocardial ischemia during and after coronary angioplasty, *Am J Cardiol* 66:389-393, 1990.

Scheidt SS, Erlebacher JA: *Basic electrocardiography ECG,* West Caldwell, CIBA-GEIGY Pharmaceuticals, 1986.

Silverman ME, Myerburg JM, Hurst JW: *Electrocardiography basic concepts and clinical application,* New York, 1983, McGraw-Hill.

Wagner GS: *Marriott's practical electrocardiography,* ed 10, Philadelphia, 2001, Lippincott Williams & Wilkins.

Waugaman WT, Foster SD, Rigor BM: *Principles and practice of nurse anesthesia*, ed 3, Stamford, Appleton & Lange, 1999.

Standard Patient Monitors

Michael Rieker

1. How do methylene blue and other dyes affect the pulse oximeter reading?

Although the onset, peak, and duration of the effect are variable, these dyes can produce an erroneous SpO_2 reading. The pulse oximeter determines the percentage of saturated hemoglobin (Hb) by comparing the ratio of absorption of red (660 nm) to infrared (940 nm) light that passes through the body part under the sensor. The ratio is compared with known values that correspond with various saturation levels. When the oxygen saturation is 85%, the ratio of absorption of the two wavelengths is 1.0. Injectable dyes, dark nail polish, and methemoglobin absorb both wavelengths of light, bringing the absorption ratio closer to 1.0 and the saturation reading toward 85%. This effect causes the reading to be falsely low (or falsely high, if the patient's actual saturation is <85%).

2. How does anemia affect the pulse oximeter reading?

Anemia does not affect the oximeter reading directly until plasma Hb declines to extremely low levels. Researchers have observed accurate oximeter readings with Hb levels approaching 2 g/dL. Anemia does affect some correlates of SpO_2, however. Chronic anemia produces an increase in 2,3-diphosphoglycerate (2,3-DPG), which shifts the oxyhemoglobin dissociation curve to the right. For a given PaO_2, the SpO_2 is lower with anemia.

An important consideration regarding SpO_2 interpretation with anemia is the associated arterial oxygen content (CaO_2). CaO_2 (mL/dL) is calculated from the equation: (Hb $\times$ 1.34 $\times$ SaO_2%) + (PaO_2 $\times$ 0.003). Despite a high oxygen saturation, a low Hb value significantly affects the total amount of oxygen that is present in the blood. This relationship can be seen in the figure on page 46, which shows an oxyhemoglobin curve with a Hb of 15 and a rightward-shifted curve with a Hb of 8. Notice the large difference in oxygen content due to the lower Hb in the right-shifted curve.

3. Are there specific considerations when using a pulse oximeter on a neonate?

A pulse oximeter is accurate on a neonate because fetal Hb has a similar absorption spectrum as adult Hb. Frequently oximeters are placed on the toes of pediatric patients to minimize movement and removal by the patient. The user

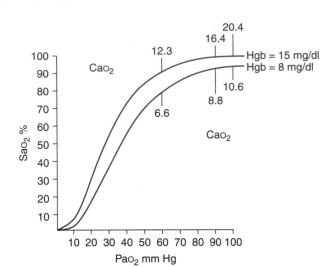

Two oxygen-hemoglobin dissociation curves: a curve on the left with a hemoglobin level of 15 mg/dL and a rightward-shifted curve with a hemoglobin level of 8 mg/dL. The oxygen content values for each curve are embedded in the figure for Pao_2 values of 60 mm Hg, 80 mm Hg, and 100 mm Hg.

might consider, however, that the response time for detection of hypoxemia may be 30 to 60 seconds longer when the probe is placed on the foot compared with finger placement. The response time is shortest when the probe is placed on the ear or cheek.

In the perinatal period or other times when the ductus arteriosus is patent, deoxygenated blood may mix with arterial blood traveling to the left subclavian artery and the descending aorta. Oximetry measurement should be carried out on the right hand, which represents "preductal" blood. Saturation readings in the feet or left arm are lower in the presence of right-to-left shunting, and the discrepancy from preductal readings can be used to estimate the degree of shunt.

4. How can the anesthetist identify spontaneous respiration, rebreathing, or a circuit leak on a capnogram?

To troubleshoot abnormal capnogram waveforms, the Certified Registered Nurse Anesthetist (CRNA) first must understand the normal waveform (see the following figure).

- *1 to 2* indicates inspiration. The measured carbon dioxide (CO_2) is 0 because there is no CO_2 in the inspired gas.
- 2 to 3 is the beginning of expiration. Following dead-space gas, the CO_2 increases quickly.
- *3 to 4* is the expiratory plateau, where varying CO_2 concentrations from different lung regions mix and reach their highest reading at 4, the end-tidal CO_2 ($ETco_2$).

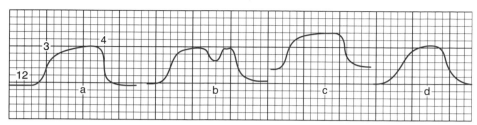

Four capnogram waveforms. **a,** Normal waveform. **b,** Spontaneous respiration. **c,** Rebreathing. **d,** Circuit leak.

- *4 to 5* indicates inspiration. The CO_2 decreases quickly as fresh gas passes the sampling site.
- *B* shows so-called curare clefts (before the advent of nerve stimulators, an indication that the curare was wearing off). The CO_2 dips as the patient attempts to take a breath during the ventilator's expiratory phase. Fresh gas drawn from the inspiratory limb registers a decrease in CO_2 on the capnogram.
- *C* shows rebreathing. When the inspiratory phase does not decrease to 0, this indicates rebreathing of CO_2. The most common cause of rebreathing within a Circle system is malfunctioning valves or exhausted CO_2 absorbent. In a semiopen (Mapleson) system, inadequate fresh gas flow also leads to rebreathing of CO_2.
- *D* indicates a circuit leak. Failure to deliver an adequate breath and failure to sample the complete exhalation cause loss of the crisp waveform, particularly the alveolar plateau.

5. Is ETco$_2$ monitoring accurate in a neonate?

In general, $ETCO_2$ monitoring is accurate, but some neonatal conditions can diminish the accuracy significantly. $ETCO_2$ underestimates $PaCO_2$ in infants with cyanotic heart defects because the right-to-left shunt causes dead space ventilation. A more common problem involves the high rates of sampling with side-stream monitors compared with the small tidal volumes of the neonate. Fresh gas from the inspiratory limb may be entrained toward the end of expiration, leading to loss of the expiratory plateau and a falsely low $ETCO_2$. The ability to reduce the sampling rate can eliminate this problem, but also increases the response time of the monitor.

6. What is the relationship between ETco$_2$ and PAco$_2$?

The $ETCO_2$ is normally 5 to 10 mm Hg lower than the $PaCO_2$. Factors that increase dead-space ventilation, such as pulmonary embolus or lung hypoperfusion, widen the $P(a\ ET)CO_2$ gradient. In contrast, shunting has minimal effect on the $P(a\text{-}ET)CO_2$ difference.

7. What is the correct point to measure the ST segment?

ST-segment deviations from the baseline can indicate myocardial ischemia or injury. To be significant, the deviation must be at least 1 mm (0.1 mV) from the isoelectric line, with other criteria based on the morphology of the wave. Measurement points of 60 msec and 80 msec after the J point have been validated (see the following figure).

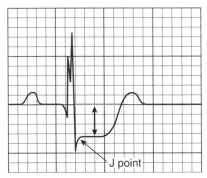

ST-segment depression. The ST segment measured 0.06 second after the J point was depressed 3 mm below the isoelectric line (indicated by dotted line).

8. How can the CRNA monitor anterior electrocardiogram (ECG) leads with a three-wire system?

The *anterior leads, particularly* V_1, can be useful in diagnosing bundle-branch blocks and in differentiating supraventricular tachycardia with aberrancy from ventricular tachycardia. Some ECG monitors use only three lead wires, however, and provide the selection of only leads I, II, or III. In these cases, the anesthetist can monitor *modified chest lead 1*. This is a slightly inferior but reasonable substitute for V_1. It is monitored by (1) setting the ECG lead selector to lead I, (2) placing the positive left arm lead (usually black) on the fourth intercostal space at the right sternal border, and (3) placing the negative right arm lead (usually white) under the outer third of the left clavicle. The ground left leg lead (usually red) can be placed in its usual position.

9. What are the normal ECG intervals?

ECG intervals and the heart rate can be measured by knowing that every small block on the ECG paper represents 0.04 second (at the standard 25 mm/sec speed). With five small blocks within each large block, the large blocks represent 0.2 second. The figure on page 49 shows the correct measurement points for the P-R, QRS, and Q-T intervals.

The normal *P-R interval* is 0.08 to 0.12 second. Prolongation more than 0.20 second indicates a first-degree atrioventricular block. The *QRS duration* should

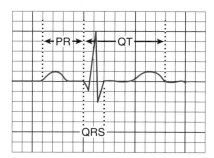

Electrocardiogram intervals. Dotted lines delineating a P-R interval of 0.16 second, a QRS interval of 0.08 second, and a Q-T interval of 0.32 second.

be less than 0.12 second. A QRS duration 0.12 second or greater indicates a ventricular ectopic beat, a bundle-branch block, or an aberrantly conducted supraventricular beat. The *Q-T interval* should be evaluated based on the heart rate. A rate-corrected Q-T (QT$_c$) is determined by dividing the Q-T interval by the square root of the R-to-R interval. The QT$_c$ should be less than 0.44 second.

10. Differentiate usage of the train-of-four (TOF) count and the TOF ratio.

The TOF mode of neuromuscular monitoring can be used in two ways, depending on the degree of neuromuscular block present. The *TOF count* is used to monitor surgical relaxation when at least 75% of acetylcholine receptors are blocked. Eliciting 3 of 4 twitches corresponds with 80% receptor blockade; 2 of 4 corresponds with 85%; 1 of 4 corresponds with 90%, and 0 of 4 indicates greater than 92% receptor blockade.

When the level of blockade is less than 75%, the TOF indicates 4 of 4 twitches, regardless of whether there is 70% receptor blockade or 10%. The *TOF ratio (T4/T1)* is a quantitative measurement of fade, used to evaluate levels of blockade less than 75%. The T4/T1 is the height of the fourth twitch compared with the height of the first twitch. Used to distinguish small levels of residual relaxation, this mode is most helpful in preparing for extubation. A T4/T1 greater than 0.9 correlates with adequate muscle strength for extubation if no other contraindications are present.

11. Are there important differences between anatomical sites when monitoring neuromuscular function?

Because of differences in nerve fibers and stimulation rates, the degree of neuromuscular block assessed at one site does not equal the degree of block at another site. The *pharmacokinetics* (speed of onset and recovery) and the *pharmacodynamics* (specific effect at receptors) differ between monitoring sites and between specific agents. The following figure outlines relaxant effects on the diaphragm, facial nerve, and ulnar nerve.

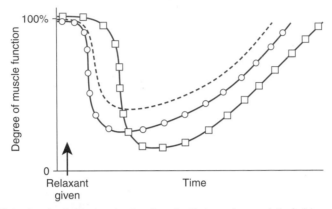

Time course and effects of nondepolarizing muscle relaxants on the diaphragm (–o–o–o–), the facial nerve (– – – –), and the ulnar nerve (–□–□–□–). These curves are theoretical renditions because the actual values vary among individual drugs and with the speed of administration.

Blockade at the *ulnar nerve* occurs later and more intensely than blockade at the diaphragm. This may explain why surgeons may note that patients are "tight" while the nerve stimulator shows 0 of 4 twitches at the hand.

Blockade at the *facial nerve* follows the time course of blockade at the diaphragm better than the ulnar nerve does. The facial nerve is a better site to monitor for onset of block because the larynx also mimics the response of the diaphragm.

Because the *ulnar nerve* is more sensitive to relaxants than the diaphragm, it is a useful site to monitor for recovery. The diaphragm is likely to have more function than what is evident at the ulnar nerve.

12. **True or false? If a patient has 0 of 4 twitches, there should be no need for additional muscle relaxant.**

   False. The results obtained from one monitoring site (e.g., the ulnar nerve) do not correlate precisely with the degree of blockade at another site (e.g., the diaphragm or larynx). For abdominal surgery, the CRNA might need to administer additional relaxant even if the ulnar nerve shows 0 of 4 twitches.

13. **How can the CRNA determine the depth of neuromuscular blockade when the TOF shows 0/4?**

   The posttetanic count (PTC) can be used to determine the relative level of blockade when the TOF shows 0 twitches. The PTC is performed by administering a continuous tetanic stimulation for 5 seconds, waiting 2 seconds, and administering a repetitive single twitch at 1 Hz (1 stimulus/sec). The number of motor responses elicited varies inversely with the depth of neuromuscular blockade. One posttetanic response indicates return of single twitch response in 10 minutes with intermediate-acting muscle relaxants (vecuronium) and in 30 minutes with long-acting relaxants (pancuronium). Ten posttetanic responses indicate imminent return of a single twitch response with intermediate agents and return in 10 minutes with long-acting agents. By estimating the time to return of a single twitch, PTC can help predict when the patient will be reversible.

14. How is double-burst stimulation (DBS) used?

The DBS pattern was developed to add accuracy to the TOF ratio measurement. Research has shown that human observers have low accuracy in quantitatively measuring the T4/T1. This low accuracy is because of the difficulty in perceiving subtle levels of fade and because of the distracting effect of the intervening second and third twitches. DBS improves accuracy over the T4/T1 by using a stronger pattern of stimulation and eliminating the second and third twitches. Adequate recovery using DBS is assessed by finding the second twitch to be at least 70% of the height of the first twitch. In practice, any manually detectable fade in the second twitch of the DBS probably indicates a significant amount of residual relaxation.

15. How is posttetanic potentiation helpful in determining the degree of neuromuscular blockade?

Posttetanic potentiation is the increased twitch response observed after a tetanic stimulation. It results from an accumulation of calcium in the nerve terminal, which increases the quantal release of acetylcholine with subsequent stimuli. Posttetanic potentiation is helpful by producing the posttetanic count, the test that elicits twitches when the TOF is 0 of 4. However, the increase in acetylcholine release lasts about 5 minutes after a tetanic stimulation. When the CRNA assesses the response to tetany or PTC, any other test (e.g., TOF) performed within 5 minutes at that site shows an exaggerated result.

16. What is the most accurate place to monitor body temperature?

The *tympanic membrane* closely reflects brain temperature, it responds quickly to changes, and it is not subject to environmental influences. Monitoring this site carries the risk of membrane puncture, however. A nasopharyngeal probe or a lower esophageal thermometer provides the excellent combination of accuracy, economy, and safety.

17. Where should the precordial stethoscope be placed?

The precordial stethoscope should be placed on an area that provides good sound quality while not interfering with surgical exposure. Given the propensity for a main stem intubation to occur on the right side as opposed to the left, precordial placement on the left chest serves as an early indication of this complication.

18. What bispectral index level should be maintained during general anesthesia?

A bispectral index value less than 60 indicates a low probability of recall or consciousness. During general anesthesia, the bispectral index should be maintained at less than 60. A value less than 40 is indicated when a deep hypnotic state is desired.

Key Points

- Pulse oximeter readings are affected by injectable dyes, dark nail polish, and methemoglobin. The readings usually are falsely low.

- Anemia does not affect the oximeter reading directly until plasma Hb declines to extremely low levels. Chronic anemia produces an increase in 2,3-DPG, which shifts the oxyhemoglobin dissociation curve to the right. For a given Pao_2, the saturation is lower with anemia.

- An abnormal capnogram waveform can identify spontaneous respiration, rebreathing of CO_2, or a circuit leak.

- Two factors influence the accuracy of $ETco_2$ monitoring in the neonate: infants with cyanotic heart disease and the high rates of sampling with side stream monitors.

- The anterior myocardium can be monitored with a three-wire system by placing the leads as follows: set monitor on lead I, LA on fourth intercostal space at right sternal border, RA under outer third of left clavicle, and LL in usual position.

- TOF count is used to monitor neuromuscular block when 75% of acetylcholine receptors are blocked. T4/T1 is a quantitative measurement of fade, used to evaluate levels of blockade less than 75%.

- Posttetanic potentiation is the increased twitch response observed after a tetanic stimulation. Posttetanic potentiation is helpful by producing the PTC, the test that elicits twitches when the TOF is 0 of 4.

- The tympanic membrane closely reflects brain temperature, it responds quickly to changes, and it is not subject to environmental influences.

- A bispectral index value less than 60 indicates a low probability of recall or consciousness.

Internet Resources

Walter Reed Army Medical Center: Anesthesiology:
http://www.wramc.amedd.army.mil/departments/surgery/Anesthesiology/monitors.htm

Update in Anaesthesia Issue 5 (1995) Article 2: Pulse Oximetry:
http://www.nda.ox.ac.uk/wfsa/html/u05/u05_003.htm

Virtual Anaesthesia Textbook: Standard monitors:
http://www.virtual-anaesthesia-textbook.com/vat/monitoring.html#standard

Respiratory Care, April 2003 Vol 48 No 4: Neonatal and Pediatric Pulse Oximetry:
http://www.rcjournal.com/contents/04.03/04.03.0386.pdf

Capnography.com: An educational website dedicated to patient safety:
http://www.capnography.com/index.html

Capnography Quiz:
http://www.nepeanicu.org/Capno.htm

Scanlon Bibliography: Capnography (End-Tidal CO2 Monitoring):
http://www.umdnj.edu/rspthweb/bibs/capnogph.htm

Bibliography

Connelly N, Silverman D: *Review of clinical anesthesia*, ed 3, Philadelphia, 2001, Lippincott Williams & Wilkins.

Crawford MH, et al: ACC/AHA guidelines for ambulatory electrocardiography, *J Am Coll Cardiol* 34:912-948, 1999.

Engbaek J, Ostergaard D, Viby-Morgensen J: Double burst stimulation (DBS): a new pattern of nerve stimulation to identify residual neuromuscular block, *Br J Anaesth* 62:274-278, 1989.

Gravenstein D, Goldman JM, Souders JE: Respiratory monitoring. In Kirby R, Gravenstein N, Lobato E, Gravenstein J, editors: *Clinical anesthesia practice,* ed 2, Philadelphia, 2002, WB Saunders, pp 361-383.

Gregory G: *Pediatric anesthesia,* New York, 2002, Churchill Livingstone, pp 250-261.

Jay GD, Hughes L, Renzi FP: Pulse oximetry is accurate in acute anemia from hemorrhage, *Ann Emerg Med* 24:32-35 1994.

Kossick MA: Clinical monitoring in anesthesia. In Nagelhout J, Zaglaniczny K, editors: *Nurse anesthesia,* ed 2, Philadelphia, 2001, WB Saunders, pp 287-307.

Tavel ME, Shaar C: Relationship between the electrocardiographic stress test and degree and location of myocardial ischemia, *Am J Cardiol* 84:119-124, 1999.

Advanced Hemodynamic Monitoring

Thomas Corey Davis

1. What are the indications for intraarterial blood pressure monitoring?

Intraarterial blood pressure monitoring is required for "beat-to-beat" blood pressure readings. Conditions requiring intraarterial monitoring include the following:
- Anticipated cardiovascular instability (e.g., massive fluid shifts, trauma, recent myocardial infarction, extreme age)
- Deliberate hypotension
- Inability to measure blood pressure accurately by noninvasive means (e.g., morbid obesity)
- Need for frequent arterial blood sampling

2. List the contraindications for intraarterial blood pressure monitoring.

Relative contraindications include the following:
- Infection at the monitoring site
- Coagulopathies (choose more peripheral, easily compressible sites)
- Reynaud's syndrome (avoid peripheral sites in extremities)

Any proximal arterial obstruction, as with thoracic outlet syndrome, is an *absolute contraindication* to arterial cannulation of the upper extremities.

3. Explain what is meant by an "overdamped" system. What is meant by an "underdamped" system?

In an *overdamped pressure-transducer system,* the waveform does not oscillate after a high-pressure flush, slowly returning to the 0 baseline. An overdamped system underestimates systolic blood pressure and overestimates diastolic blood pressure. Overdamping usually is a result of air bubbles in the tubing, a kinked catheter, or a thrombus within the catheter or vessel. Removal of any of these factors improves the accuracy of the waveform.

In an *underdamped pressure-transducer system,* the waveform oscillates three to four times before settling back to a 0 baseline. An underdamped system overestimates systolic blood pressure and underestimates diastolic blood pressure. Most systems are underdamped, usually because of the length and flexibility of tubing. Underdamping usually is a result of long connecting tubing, small tubing or catheter diameter, or the occlusion of the vessel by a catheter that is too large.

4. What is the phlebostatic axis?

The accuracy of hemodynamic monitoring depends on proper alignment and calibration of the transducer at the desired point of reference. For most adult patients in the supine position, this point of reference is the heart and is referred to as the *phlebostatic axis* (literally, "phlebo"—vein or blood; "stasis"—standing still). The phlebostatic axis refers to a standard reference point on the body used to calibrate pressure transducer systems to atmospheric pressure (*zeroing*). This point is the approximate location of the right ventricle of the heart, located at the midaxillary line, fifth intercostal space.

5. Where is the systolic blood pressure highest in the body?

The *dorsalis pedis pulse* reflects the highest systolic blood pressure in the body. As the arterial pulse leaves the heart, pulse pressure increases due to decreasing arterial lumen size and the reflection of the blood pressure wave as it moves toward the periphery. This reflection causes an additive effect for systolic blood pressure.

6. Describe various techniques for arterial cannulation.

- *Seldinger technique—catheter-over-wire technique:* Dorsiflex wrist over a small towel roll, advancing needle at a 30- to 45-degree angle. On blood flash, lower angle to 10 degrees, and advance 1 to 2 mm before advancing guidewire. Advance guidewire into artery, and advance catheter over guidewire with needle stationary.
- *Direct cannulation— catheter-over-needle technique:* Use a standard 20-gauge catheter-over-needle intravenous catheter. Follow Seldinger technique without use of guidewire.
- *Transfixation—catheter-over-wire or catheter-over-needle technique:* Advance needle through artery. Withdraw needle slowly until blood flash, then advance guidewire or catheter.

7. Describe the characteristics of the arterial waveform (see the following figure).

- *Anacrotic limb— initial "upsweep":* Reflects contractility. A steep upstroke indicates strong left ventricular function. A slow rise indicates delayed ejection, as seen in aortic stenosis or outflow obstruction.
- *Dicrotic limb—"downstroke":* Reflects systemic vascular resistance (SVR). A steep downstroke with a low dicrotic notch indicates rapid diastolic runoff and a low SVR.
- *Dicrotic notch—"groove" noted in dicrotic limb:* Reflects closure of the aortic valve during diastole. As left ventricular pressure decreases to less than aortic root pressure, the aortic valve snaps shut, resulting in a brief upstroke on the

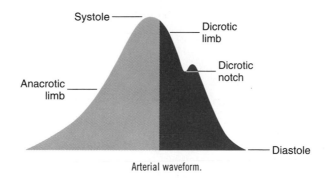

Arterial waveform.

waveform due to a pressure increase as blood rushes back against a closed valve. This notch marks the beginning of diastole and may not be distinct with aortic valve regurgitation/insufficiency.

8. Describes the indications and contraindications for central venous pressure (CVP) monitoring.

Indications for right heart pressure monitoring, commonly referred to as CVP monitoring, include anticipated large fluid shifts in a patient without cardiovascular or pulmonary disease or situations in which urine output is not available or an unreliable method of determining fluid status. CVP monitoring also is indicated to monitor indirectly the filling pressures of the left heart (when pulmonary status is normal) and for access to the central venous system for infusion of hemodynamic agents.

Superior vena cava syndrome is an *absolute contraindication* for CVP placement in the upper thorax, although femoral placement is acceptable. Relative contraindications include infection at the insertion site, coagulopathy, or the presence of newly inserted pacemaker leads.

9. Detail the components of the CVP waveform (see the figure on page 58).

- *a wave—due to atrial contraction:* Follows P wave on electrocardiogram (ECG), positive deflection, most prominent wave, absent in atrial fibrillation, exaggerated in junctional rhythms
- *c wave—due to the bulging of a closed tricuspid valve into the atrium during isovolumetric contraction of the ventricle:* Positive deflection, follows QRS on ECG
- *x wave—negative deflection; origin unknown ("X files"?):* Possibly due to systolic collapse in atrial pressure resulting in a downward displacement of the tricuspid valve
- *v wave—due to venous filling of the right atrium against a closed tricuspid valve:* Positive deflection, follows T wave on ECG
- *y wave—negative deflection, origin unknown ("whY is it there?"):* possibly due to diastolic collapse in atrial pressure with opening of tricuspid valve and filling of the right ventricle.

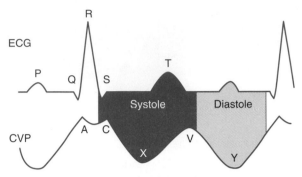

EKG tracing and CVP waveform.

10. Name some uses for pulmonary artery (PA) catheters.

Functional uses of a PA catheter include assessment of volume status, measurement of cardiac function (e.g., cardiac output), and derivation of hemodynamic parameters (SVR and pulmonary vascular resistance). Measurement of mixed venous oxygen saturation may be obtained by blood sampling from the distal (PA) port or continuous monitoring with an appropriate catheter.

11. Name contraindications for PA catheter insertion.

Absolute contraindications to PA catheter insertion are tricuspid or pulmonic valve stenosis, tetralogy of Fallot (uncorrected), and masses in the right heart (atrial or ventricular). *Relative contraindications* are severe dysrhythmias, coagulopathies, and newly inserted pacemaker leads.

12. Does PA monitoring improve outcome in critically ill patients?

CONTROVERSIAL
Reports in the early 1980s and a study by Conners et al in 1996 suggested that PA catheters may be associated with increased morbidity and mortality in patients who receive them. The results are difficult to interpret because patients who receive PA catheters by definition are more prone to an increased morbidity and mortality from their clinical condition. Today's trend is toward more discriminant monitoring in select patients.

13. Describe the placement of a PA catheter and the changes noted in the pressure waveform.

- After placement of the balloon-tipped catheter beyond the tip of the introducing catheter (about 20 cm), the balloon is inflated to facilitate placement and prevent intravascular injury (thus the term, "floating the Swan").
- The pressure waveform is observed as the catheter is advanced (see the figure on page 59).

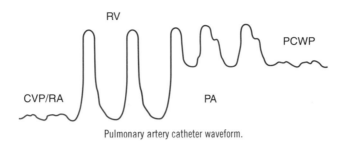

Pulmonary artery catheter waveform.

- The initial waveform is the CVP waveform. This changes to the right ventricular waveform when the catheter passes through the tricuspid valve, at approximately 30 cm. Although diastolic pressure remains similar to the CVP waveform, the systolic pressure increases sharply. Ventricular ectopy may occur as the tip of the catheter irritates the walls of the ventricle.
- The pulmonary valve is encountered at approximately 45 cm, and the waveform changes, reflecting PA pressures. The systolic PA pressure remains similar to the right ventricular pressure, and that diastolic pressure increases sharply. A prominent dicrotic notch is present in patients with a competent pulmonary valve. If the PA waveform is not encountered by 60 cm of catheter placement, the catheter is likely to be coiling in the right ventricle. In this event, the balloon is deflated and the catheter is withdrawn gently back to a CVP waveform, the balloon is reinflated, and placement is reattempted.
- Advancing slowly and gently, the pulmonary capillary wedge pressure (PCWP) is elicited as the balloon occludes the PA. The balloon tip is deflated, noting a return of the PA waveform.

14. What is "zone III" of the lung, and how does it affect PA pressure monitoring?

To assess most closely the function and volume status of the left heart, the PA catheter must rest in a static column of blood that is unobstructed and unaffected by other pressures within the lungs. West et al in 1964 described three "zones" of the lung by comparing vascular and alveolar pressure relationships. In *zone I*, alveolar pressures exceed arterial pressures. In *zone II*, alveolar pressures exceed venous pressures. Only in *zone III* do arterial and venous pressures exceed alveolar pressures, ensuring continuous, unobstructed blood flow. Most of the lung enters zone III when the patient is in the supine position.

15. Is the PA diastolic pressure a reliable indicator of PCWP?

Because of the increased risk of PA rupture during "wedging" of the balloon tip, many practitioners use the PA diastolic pressure as an estimate of PCWP. In the absence of factors that increase pulmonary vascular resistance (e.g., respiratory failure, chronic obstructive pulmonary disease, pulmonary edema, hypoxia, hypothermia), PA diastolic pressure is considered a reliable indicator of PCWP.

16. Is CVP a reliable indicator of PCWP?

CVP is not considered a reliable indicator of PCWP.

17. State the normal PA pressure ranges, and list factors that cause derangement of these values.

NORMAL VALUES IN AVERAGE ADULTS

CVP/right atrial	5 mm Hg (mean)
Right ventricular	25/4 mm Hg
PA	25/12 mm Hg
PCWP	10 mm Hg (mean)

Factors that cause derangement of these values include the following:
- Increased PA systolic—increased pulmonary vascular resistance
- Increased PA diastolic or PCWP—volume overload, left heart dysfunction or failure, mitral stenosis or regurgitation/insufficiency, decreased left ventricular compliance, cardiac tamponade
- Decreased PA systolic, PA diastolic, or PCWP—hypovolemia

18. What is mixed venous oxygen saturation (Svo_2), and why is it measured?

Svo_2 reflects the oxygen content of venous blood returning to the lungs. Its measurement is a useful indicator of the balance between oxygen delivery and oxygen consumption.

19. Name possible causes of a decreased Svo_2?

A decreased Svo_2 may be observed with conditions that decrease oxygen delivery, such as a decreased cardiac output, decreased arterial oxygen saturation, or decreased oxygen carrying capacity (e.g., decreased hemoglobin). A decreased Svo_2 also may be seen with conditions that increase oxygen consumption, such as sepsis, burns, or hyperthermia.

20. Name possible causes of an increased Svo_2.

An increased Svo_2 is most often the result of a permanently "wedged" PA catheter. It also may be due to conditions that result in an increased cardiac output (e.g., sepsis, burns, left-to-right shunts, inotropic excess, hepatitis, pancreatitis), or a decreased rate of oxygen consumption (e.g., cyanide toxicity, carbon monoxide poisoning, increased methemoglobin, hypothermia).

Key Points

- Intraarterial monitoring should be considered when there is anticipated cardiovascular instability, deliberate hypotension, inability to measure blood pressure accurately by noninvasive means, and need for frequent arterial blood sampling.

- Relative contraindications to intraarterial monitoring include infection at the monitoring site, coagulopathies, or Raynaud's syndrome. Any proximal arterial obstruction, as with thoracic outlet syndrome, is an absolute contraindication to arterial cannulation of the upper extremities.

- The "phlebostatic" axis refers to a standard reference point on the body used to calibrate pressure transducer systems to atmospheric pressure.

- The three most common techniques for arterial cannulation are Seldinger (catheter over wire), direct cannulation (catheter over needle), and transfixation.

- The arterial waveform has three components—anacrotic limb, dicrotic limb, and dicrotic notch (see the figure in Question 7).

- The CVP waveform has five distinct parts: the A wave, C wave, X wave, V wave, and Y wave (see figure in Question 9).

- Functional uses of a PA catheter include assessment of volume status, measurement of cardiac function, and derivation of hemodynamic parameters.

- Tricuspid or pulmonic valve stenosis, tetralogy of Fallot (uncorrected), and masses in the right heart are absolute contraindications to PA catheter insertion. Severe dysrhythmias, coagulopathies, and newly inserted pacemaker leads are relative contraindications.

- Pulmonary artery diastolic pressure is considered a reliable indicator of PCWP. CVP is not considered a reliable indicator of PCWP.

- Normal PA pressure ranges in the average adult are as follows:
  - CVP/right atrium: 5 mm Hg (mean)
  - Right ventricle: 25/4 mm Hg
  - PA: 25/12 mm Hg
  - PCWP: 10 mm Hg (mean)

- Sv_{O_2} reflects the oxygen content of venous blood returning to the lungs.

- A decreased Sv_{O_2} may be observed with conditions that decrease oxygen delivery, such as a decreased cardiac output, decreased arterial oxygen saturation, or decreased oxygen carrying capacity.

Internet Resources

Hemodynamic Monitoring:
http://www.lhsc.on.ca/resptherapy/students/lectures/hemodyn.htm

GASNet Search: Hemodynamic Monitoring:
http://www.gasnet.org/about/search.php?p1=hemodynamic+monitoring

Virtual Anaesthesia Textbook:
http://www.virtual-anaesthesia-textbook.com/

Monitoring in Anaesthesia:
http://www.anaesthetist.com/anaes/monitor/index.htm

Bibliography

Afessa B, et al: Association of pulmonary artery catheter use with in-hospital mortality, *Crit Care Med* 29:1145-1148, 2001.

Benumof JL: *Clinical procedures in anesthesia and intensive care,* Philadelphia, 1992, Lippincott.

Connors AF Jr: Pitfalls in estimating the effect of interventions in the critically ill using observational study designs, *Crit Care Med* 29:1283-1284, 2001.

Connors AF Jr, et al: The effectiveness of right heart catheterization in the initial care of critically ill patients, *JAMA* 276:889-897, 1996.

Cruz K, Franklin C: The pulmonary artery catheter: Uses and controversies, *Crit Care Clin* 17:271-289, 2001.

Daily EK: Hemodynamic waveform analysis, *J Cardiovasc Nurs* 15:6-22, 2001.

Dalen JE, Bone RC: Is it time to pull the pulmonary artery catheter? *JAMA* 276:916-918 (editorial), 1996.

Ivanov R, et al: The incidence of major morbidity in critically ill patients managed with pulmonary artery catheters: a meta-analysis, *Crit Care Med* 28:615-619, 2000.

Lake CL: *Clinical monitoring for anesthesia and critical care,* ed 2, Philadelphia, 1994, WB Saunders.

Morgan EG Jr, Mikhail MS, Murray MJ: *Clinical anesthesiology,* ed 3, New York, 2001, Lange Medical Books/McGraw-Hill.

Murdoch SD, et al: Pulmonary artery catheterization and mortality in critically ill patients, *Br J Anaesth* 85:611-615, 2000.

Prentice D, Ahrens T: Controversies in the uses of the pulmonary artery catheter, *J Cardiovasc Nurs* 15:1-4, 2001.

Sakka SG, et al: Is the placement of a pulmonary artery catheter still justified solely for the measurement of cardiac output? *J Cardiothorac Vasc Anesth* 14:119-124, 2000.

Seldinger SI: Catheter replacement of the needle in percutaneous arteriography, *Acta Radiol* 39:368-376, 1953.

Soni N: Swan song for the Swan-Ganz catheter? *BMJ* 313:763-764 (editorial), 1996.

Spodick DH: Pulmonary artery catheterization in the ICU/critical care unit: indications and contraindications remain objectively undefined, *Chest* 119:999-1000 (editorial), 2001.

Stocking JE, Lake CL: The role of the pulmonary artery catheter in the year 2000 and beyond, *J Cardiothorac Vasc Anesth* 14:111-112 (editorial), 2000.

Swan HSC, Ganz W, Forrester J, et al: Cardiac catheterization of the heart in man with the use of a flow directed balloon tipped catheter, *N Engl J Med* 283:447-451, 1970.

Swann DG: The utility of pulmonary artery catheterization, *Br J Anaesth* 85:501-503 (editorial), 2000.

West JB, Dollery CT, Naimark A: Distribution of blood flow in isolated lung: relation to vascular and alveolar pressures, *J Appl Physiol* 19:713-724, 1964.

Chapter 8

Patient Positioning

Erica D. Nelson

1. Who is responsible for patient positioning during surgery?

Although positioning patients for and during surgery is largely the anesthetist's responsibility, it is a team effort shared by the anesthetist, surgeon, and operating room nurses. The patient initially must be placed in a position that maximizes exposure without causing injury. During the operation, the anesthetist must monitor vigilantly for any changes in position, while documenting accurately the position used and the use of pillows, padding, and other equipment.

2. List risk factors for injury secondary to positioning.

Patient risk factors that increase the probability of injury secondary to positioning include the following:
- Concurrent cardiac or respiratory disease
- Musculoskeletal diseases, such as osteoarthritis or rheumatoid arthritis
- Diabetes
- Extremes of age
- Obesity
- Dehydration
- Debilitation
- Renal failure
- Peripheral neuropathies
- Paraplegia/quadriplegia
- Malnourishment
- Prolonged surgery

3. Describe the most common physiological outcome of positioning.

The most common physiological outcome of positioning is *postural hypotension*. This frequent event can be minimized or avoided by maintaining a light level of anesthesia, preventing sudden position changes, and keeping the patient well hydrated. A patient's position should be reversed if the patient becomes hemodynamically unstable.

4. Which four peripheral nerves are commonly injured by improper positioning?

Peripheral nerve injury is a common, often debilitating problem. Although most nerve injuries resolve within 6 to 12 weeks, some can endure for months to years.

- The *ulnar nerve* is the most commonly injured nerve. Risk factors for this injury include a hospital stay longer than 14 days, male gender, and a extremely thin or obese body type. The anatomy of the ulnar nerve as it traverses the elbow makes it vulnerable to injury because there is little tissue or fat to protect the nerve from external compression. Injury to the ulnar nerve may occur when the elbow is flexed greater than 90 degrees for an extended time or by compression against the posterior aspect of the humerus by the armboard or side of the bed.
- The *brachial plexus* is the second most commonly injured nerve bundle. This nerve bundle often is injured because of stretch and compression and is associated with extremes of age and prolonged surgery. The brachial plexus may be injured by extreme arm abduction, extension, or external rotation. Damage also may occur in the lateral decubitus position due to improper placement of the axillary roll. Mechanisms to avoid brachial plexus injury include avoiding arm abduction greater than 60 degrees, steep Trendelenburg position, and downward pressure on the clavicle or head of the humerus.
- *Radial nerve* injury may be associated with nerve entrapment against the spiral groove of the humerus. Potential causes include improperly securing the arm, compressing the nerve against the operating table or anesthesia screen, or excessive cycling of an automatic blood pressure cuff.
- Common *peroneal nerve* injuries may occur in the lithotomy position if the legs are compressed against the stirrups or placed in the stirrups improperly or if the patient is in the lithotomy position for more than 2 hours. This nerve is the most commonly injured nerve of the lower extremities. Proper padding of the stirrups decreases the occurrence of common peroneal nerve injury.

5. **List procedures that may use the supine, prone, lithotomy, sitting, and lateral decubitus positions.**

    See the following table.

Procedures That May Use Supine, Prone, Lithotomy, Sitting, and Lateral Decubitus Positions				
Supine	**Prone**	**Lithotomy**	**Sitting**	**Lateral Decubitus**
Procedures of the abdomen, chest, head, neck, or extremities	Procedures of the spinal cord and some intracranial procedures	Procedures that require access to perineal structures	Procedures of the posterior fossa and cervical spine, shoulder arthroplasty/arthroscopy, breast reconstruction, and mammoplasty	Procedures of the thorax, kidney, and shoulder

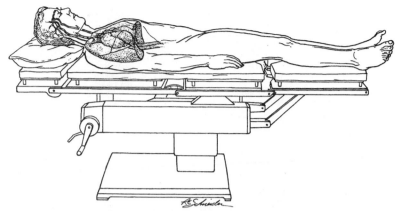

Supine adult with minimal gradients in the horizontal vascular axis. Pulmonary blood volume is greatest dorsally. Viscera displace the dorsal diaphragm cephalad. Cerebral circulation is slightly above heart level if the head is on a small pillow.

6. Discuss specific considerations of the supine position.

When employing the supine position (see the figure above), the anesthetist must maintain the head in a neutral position or in a position favored by the awake patient. A pillow or pad may be placed under the head to avoid alopecia and to ease the stress on the neck and lumbar spine. It is important to monitor for heel breakdown and ensure that the legs are uncrossed to avoid compression of blood vessels in the lower legs. Placing a pillow under the patient's knees increases the patient's level of comfort postoperatively, as does placing a wedge under the back to reduce the incidence of backache. The patient's arms may be tucked at the sides or extended on padded arm boards at less than a 90-degree angle. Padding the elbow and supinating the forearm may help avoid ulnar nerve damage. Bony prominences, such as the occiput, scapula, sacrum, and calcaneus areas, are prone to pressure-related injuries and should be padded and monitored.

7. Describe potentially detrimental cardiac and respiratory effects that can occur in the supine position.

The supine position produces minimal effects on circulation and ventilation. Functional residual capacity decreases secondary to the abdominal contents impinging on the diaphragm. Volatile anesthetics, muscle relaxants, and obesity further decrease functional residual capacity.

8. Discuss the physiologic changes associated with the Trendelenburg positioning.

The Trendelenburg position (see the figure on page 68) is a head-down variation of the supine position. Cephalad movement of the abdominal viscera pushes the diaphragm up, diminishing pulmonary compliance and functional residual capacity. Myocardial workload may increase, the result of increased preload and

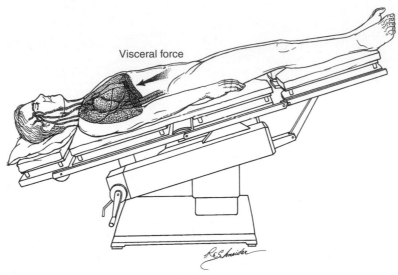

Visceral force

Head-down tilt aids blood return from lower extremities but encourages reflex vasodilation, congests vessels in the poorly ventilated lung apices, and increases intracranial blood volume.

stroke volume. Conversely, decreased cardiac output may be the result of heart compression and activation of baroreceptors.

This position may be detrimental to patients with increased intracranial or intraocular pressure (e.g., glaucoma). Other potential adverse effects include facial edema, retinal detachment, and gastric regurgitation. Although this position traditionally has been used to correct hypotension, most studies reveal either no hemodynamic benefit or unchanged blood pressure when used as a treatment for hypotension.

9. Name the advantages of the lawn-chair position.

A variation of the supine position, the lawn-chair position adds slight flexion to the hips and knees. This position facilitates venous return by optimizing perfusion and blood return from the lower extremities and abdomen. Joints are placed in a more neutral and comfortable position, resulting in less discomfort postoperatively.

10. How should patients be positioned properly in the prone position?

When using the prone position (see the figures on page 69), the anesthetist must maintain alignment of the head and neck and support the head in a neutral position with a pillow or head-holding device. Extreme lateral rotation of the neck may compromise cerebral blood flow and impair cerebral venous drainage. Hyperextension of the arms is avoided by tucking the arms against the body or extending them less than 90 degrees alongside the head on armboards. The eyes

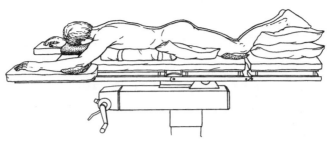

The classic prone position. Flat table with relaxed arms extended alongside patient's head. Parallel chest rolls extend from just caudad of clavicle to just beyond inguinal area, with pillow over pelvic end. Elbows and knees are padded, and legs are bent at the knees. Head is turned onto a C-shaped foam sponge that frees the down-side eye and ear from compression.

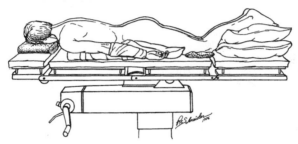

The classic prone position with arms snugly retained alongside torso.

should be protected with eye pads and free of pressure. Firm rolls may be placed under the patient's sides to relieve abdominal compression by the mattress. Compression stockings on the legs minimize pooling of blood. Intraoperatively the anesthetist should examine the patient's ears, eyes, chin, nose, shoulder, breasts, and genitalia frequently for areas of pressure. Because the anesthetist does not have access to the airway in the prone position, the endotracheal tube must be taped securely in place.

11. Discuss important considerations when positioning the patient in the lateral decubitus position.

When using the lateral decubitus position (see the figure on page 70), a roll should be placed under the thorax just below the axilla to avoid compression of the dependent neurovascular bundle in the axilla. The radial pulse on the dependent arm should be checked regularly to help ensure the absence of neurovascular compression. Pillows or padding beneath the head minimizes stretch on the dependent brachial plexus. The nurse anesthetist should ensure the spine is in an anatomically correct position. Pillows should be placed between the knees. The dependent leg should be flexed at the hip to decrease stretch on nerves in the lower extremities. Finally the dependent eye, ear, and breast should be examined closely to eliminate any pressure complications.

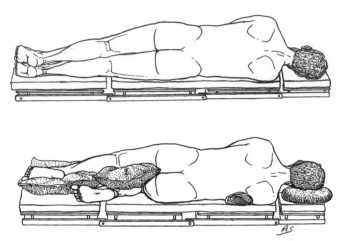

The standard lateral decubitus position. Improper padding/support is shown in the upper figure. Proper head support, axillary roll, and leg pillow arrangement are shown on lower figure. Down-side leg is flexed at hip and knee to stabilize torso. Retaining straps and pad for down-side peroneal nerve are not shown. *(From Martin JT, editor: Positioning in anesthesia and surgery, ed 2, Philadelphia, 1987, WB Saunders.)*

12. What is the principal hazard in the sitting position, and how should the patient be monitored to avoid this complication?

A *venous air embolism* (VAE) is the principal hazard in the sitting position (see the figure on page 71). Air can enter the venous system by a negative pressure gradient created when the operative site is above the level of the heart. Most cases of VAE occur during intracranial surgery, but VAE also may occur with head and neck surgery, open cardiac procedures, and laparoscopy with insufflation. Two factors that affect symptom severity are the volume of air entrained and the rate of entrainment. The incidence of VAE in the sitting position may be 30%, although it does not always contribute to increased morbidity or mortality. A precordial Doppler ultrasound placed over the second or third intercostal space to the right of the sternum is a sensitive noninvasive indicator of the presence of intracardiac air. If the classic "mill-wheel" murmur is audible, the size of the VAE is large and requires immediate intervention. Transesophageal echocardiography is slightly more sensitive but is more invasive. Continuous end-tidal carbon dioxide monitoring detects decreases in end-tidal carbon dioxide and increases in end-tidal nitrogen. Placement of a right atrial catheter allows access for aspiration of entrained air.

If a VAE is suspected, nitrous oxide should be discontinued, and 100% oxygen should be administered. The surgical field should be flooded with saline to limit air entrainment, while the anesthetist attempts to aspirate the air through the central venous catheter. Intravenous volume infusion and inotropic support may be necessary if cardiorespiratory instability occurs.

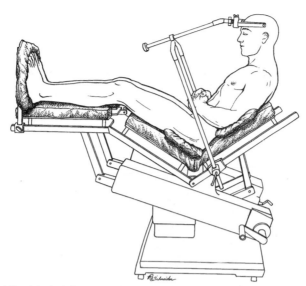

Elevation of the head shifts abdominal viscera away from the diaphragm and improves ventilation of the lung bases. According to the gradient above the heart, pressure in arteries of the head and neck decreases; pressure in the accompanying veins may become subatmospheric.

13. Name potentially detrimental cardiac effects of the sitting position.

In the sitting position, pooling of blood in the lower body decreases the central blood volume, leading to a decrease in cardiac output and blood pressure.

14. Why must both legs be moved simultaneously in the lithotomy position?

Both legs must be moved at the same time in the lithotomy position because raising or lowering them separately may cause peroneal nerve injury, hip dislocation, or torsion stress on the lumbar spine and pelvis (see the figure on page 72). Bringing the legs together in midline and lowering them slowly allows the circulatory system to adjust to changes in vascular capacitance.

15. Explain the thoracic outlet syndrome and how it is related to positioning.

The thoracic outlet syndrome is associated with a person's inability to raise the arms above the head without experiencing tingling, numbness, or pain in one or both arms. The syndrome occurs due to compression of the brachial plexus and subclavian vessels near the first rib. These patients are at an increased risk of brachial plexus injury.

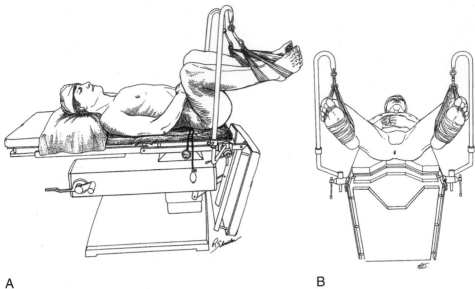

A

B

A, Standard lithotomy position with "candy cane" extremity support. Thighs are flexed approximately 90 degrees on abdomen; knees are flexed enough to bridge lower legs grossly parallel to the torso section of the tabletop. Arms are retained on boards, crossed on the abdomen, or snugged at the sides of the patient. Padding of the ankles, feet, and lower legs should be implemented (not shown). *B,* Perineal view. *(From Martin JT, editor: Positioning in anesthesia and surgery, ed 2, Philadelphia, 1987, WB Saunders.)*

Key Points

- Safe patient positioning is a team effort shared by the anesthetist, surgeon, and operating room nurses.
- Risk factors that increase probability of injury include extremes of age, obesity, concurrent cardiac or respiratory disease, and prolonged surgery.
- The most common physiological outcome of positioning is postural hypotension.
- The four peripheral nerves commonly injured by improper positioning are ulnar, brachial plexus, radial, and common peroneal nerve.
- The supine position produces minimal effects on circulation and ventilation.
- In the Trendelenburg position, special attention must be paid to the cephalad movement of the abdominal viscera, pushing the diaphragm up, diminishing pulmonary compliance and functional residual capacity. Myocardial workload may increase, and cardiac output may decrease.
- In the prone position, special attention must be paid to position of head and neck, eyes, compression of abdomen, venous pooling, pressure on breasts and genitalia, and most importantly the airway.

Key Points   *continued*

- In the lateral position, special attention must be paid to compression of the neurovascular bundle in the axilla; the stretching of the brachial plexus; the compression of nerves in lower extremities; and the dependent eye, ear, and breast.
- VAE is the principal hazard in the sitting position.
- In the lithotomy position, both legs should be moved simultaneously to avoid nerve injury and changes in vascular capacitance.

Internet Resources

Virtual Anaesthesia Textbook:
http://www.virtual-anaesthesia-textbook.com/

Surgical-tutor.org (UK): Prevention of injuries in the anaesthetised patient:
http://www.surgical-tutor.org.uk/default-home.htm?core/preop1/
perioperative_injuries.htm~right

GasNet Search: Patient Positioning:
http://www.gasnet.org/about/search.php?p1=patient+positioning

ASA Practice Advisory: Prevention of Perioperative Peripheral Neuropathy:
http://anesthesiologyinfo.com/articles/02062002.php

Bibliography

Alexander C, Vandam L: Positioning of patients for operation. In Longnecker DB, Tinker JH, Morgan GE, editors: *Principles and practice of anesthesiology*, ed 2, St Louis, 1998, Mosby, pp 680-699.

Beeson M: Positioning. In McIntosh LW, editor: *Essentials of nurse anesthesia*, New York, 1997, McGraw-Hill, pp 171-189.

Britt B, Joy N, Mackay MB: Anesthesia-related trauma caused by patient malpositioning. In Gravenstein N, Kirby R, editors: *Complications in anesthesiology*, ed 2, Philadelphia, 1996, Lippincott-Raven, pp 365-389.

Martin JT: The physiology of patient posture. In Collins V, editor: *Principles of anesthesiology: general and regional anesthesia*, ed 3, Philadelphia, 1993, Lea & Febiger, pp 163-173.

Martin JT, Warner MA: Patient positioning. In Barash PG, Cullen BF, Stoelting RK, editors: *Clinical anesthesia*, ed 3, Philadelphia, 1997, Lippincott Williams & Wilkins, pp 595-620.

Monti EJ: Positioning for anesthesia and surgery. In Nagelhout JJ, Zaglaniczny KL, editors: *Nurse anesthesia*, ed 2, Philadelphia, 2001, WB Saunders, pp 365-381.

Morgan GE, Mikhail MS, Murray MJ: *Clinical anesthesiology*, ed 3, Stamford, 2002, Appleton & Lange, pp 757-759.

Stoelting RK, Miller RD: *Basics of anesthesia*, ed 4, NewYork, 2000, Churchill Livingstone, pp 196-208.

Wilson AT, et al: Anaesthesia and the obese patient, *Int J Obes* 17:427-435, 1993.

Section II

Clinical Pharmacology

Chapter 9

Inhalational Anesthetics

Timothy L. Murry

1. What are the molecular structures of halothane, enflurane, isoflurane, desflurane, and sevoflurane?

The molecular structures are shown in the following figure.

Chemical structures of common inhaled anesthetics.

2. What gas laws describe the behavior of inhalational agents?

- *Boyle's law:* At a constant temperature, the volume of a given mass of gas varies inversely with the absolute pressure.
- *Charles' law:* At a constant pressure, the volume of a gas varies directly with the temperature.
- *Gay-Lussac's law:* At a constant volume, the absolute pressure of a gas varies directly with the absolute temperature.
- *Dalton's law of partial pressures:* The total pressure exerted by a mixture of gases is equal to the sum of the partial pressures exerted by the individual gases.
- *Henry's law:* At a constant temperature, the amount of a gas dissolved in a liquid is directly proportional to the partial pressure of the gas in equilibrium with the liquid.

3. What is the Ostwald solubility coefficient, and how does it relate to inhalational agents?

The Ostwald solubility coefficient is the measure of the volume of gas that dissolves in a unit volume of liquid at ambient temperature; this is closely related to partition coefficients. The partition coefficient is the ratio of the volume of gas that can dissolve in the same volume of a liquid phase, such as blood or tissue. These concepts can be applied to the uptake of inhaled anesthetic agents and aid in predicting the speed at which the agents will work. The higher the blood:gas partition coefficient, the longer it takes to induce anesthesia and the longer it takes to emerge from anesthesia. The agent follows a series of partial pressure gradients to reach its target, the brain: delivered > inspired > alveolar > arterial > brain and tissue.

4. Define minimal alveolar concentration (MAC).

MAC is the amount of inhaled anesthetic, or concentration, needed to provide immobility in 50% of patients exposed to surgical stimulation. An agent's MAC may be considered to be that agent's effective dose. MAC is measured as the inhaled anesthetic's alveolar partial pressure, which reflects the partial pressure at the site of action, the brain. MAC values provide a means of discussing different agents at equal potent doses. In addition, MAC values are additive: 0.5 MAC of one agent + 0.5 MAC of another agent = 1 MAC of the first agent alone.

5. Explain what determines an inhaled agent's alveolar partial pressure.

Major determinants of the inhaled agent's alveolar partial pressure include the following:
- *Delivered partial pressure:* The delivered concentration (selected vaporizer setting) influences the alveolar partial pressure by making more or less inhaled agent available for uptake.
- *Inhaled partial pressure:* Initially a high inspired concentration is needed to offset the uptake of an inhaled agent by blood and tissue. The effect the inhaled partial pressure has on the alveolar partial pressure is called the *concentration effect*. The higher the inhaled partial pressure, the more rapidly the alveolar partial pressure approaches the inhaled partial pressure.
- *Alveolar ventilation:* The greater the rate and volume of the ventilation (minute volume), the faster the rate of rise of alveolar partial pressure to inhaled partial pressure. High fresh gas flows reduce the dilution of inspired gas by expired gas and facilitate a more rapid rise in alveolar partial pressure with anesthetic induction.
- *Characteristics of the breathing system:* The solubility of the agent in the breathing system can affect the rate of rise of the alveolar concentration. Today's breathing systems are made of materials that absorb very little agent.

6. What is the second gas effect?

The second gas effect is the ability of the high-volume uptake of one gas to increase the alveolar partial pressure of a second gas. A high inhaled partial pressure of the first gas results in a higher alveolar partial pressure of the first and second gases. Nitrous oxide (N_2O) is the classic example of the first gas in this phenomenon. In clinical practice, even at high concentrations, the effect on the second gas is minimal.

7. Anesthetic uptake depends on which variables?

SOLUBILITY OF THE ANESTHETIC IN THE BLOOD

Volatile anesthetic solubility is expressed as the blood:gas partition coefficient (see the following table), which is the degree that an agent can partition itself between a liquid and a gaseous phase at equilibrium. The blood acts as an inactive reservoir for inhaled agents. The more insoluble an agent (e.g., N_2O, desflurane, sevoflurane), the less it is taken up by the blood, and the sooner equilibrium with the alveolar partial pressure is achieved. An insoluble agent produces a more rapid anesthetic induction. A more soluble agent (e.g., halothane, isoflurane, enflurane) takes longer to reach equilibrium with the alveolar partial pressure, which results in a prolonged induction of anesthesia.

Physical Properties of Anesthetic Gases

	Halothane	Enflurane	Isoflurane	Desflurane	Sevoflurane	Nitrous Oxide
Vapor pressure (20°C)	243	175	250	670	157	39,000
Partition coefficient (37°C)						
Blood:gas	2.4	1.9	1.4	0.42	0.65	0.47
Oil:gas	224	98.5	97.8	18.7	53.4	1.4
Fat:blood	60	36	52	29	50	2.3
Minimal alveolar concentration (%)	0.75	1.7	1.3	6	2	110
Metabolism	15–20%	2.4–6%	0.2%	0.02–0.2%	2–5%	0.005%

CARDIAC OUTPUT

In general, with a high cardiac output, more blood is exposed to the alveoli, and more agent is removed from the alveoli. This situation results in a longer time to reach equilibrium of alveolar and blood partial pressures and prolongs the induction of anesthesia. Conversely, if the cardiac output is low, less agent is taken away from the lungs, equilibrium is reached more quickly, and the anesthetic induction is faster. Alterations in cardiac output influence the rate of anesthetic uptake of soluble agents to a greater degree than insoluble agents.

ANESTHETIC UPTAKE BY TISSUE

The amount of agent taken up by the tissues affects the concentration of agent in the venous blood and its capacity for taking more agent from the alveoli (alveolar-to-venous anesthetic partial pressure difference). Tissue uptake depends on the solubility of the agent in tissue, tissue blood flow, and the partial pressure difference of the arterial blood and the tissue. The induction of anesthesia may not be affected by tissue uptake, depending to a greater degree on the agent's blood gas solubility coefficient. Emergence can be prolonged for agents that have high tissue:blood partition coefficients because large amounts of agent can be sequestered in tissues during the anesthetic, then reenter the circulation during emergence.

8. N$_2$O is 34 times more soluble than nitrogen. In what circumstances should N$_2$O be avoided?

N$_2$O leaves the blood and enters an air-filled cavity 34 times faster than nitrogen can leave. This results in either the volume or the pressure of the cavity increasing depending on if the cavity's walls are compliant (intestine, pleural space, pulmonary blebs) or noncompliant (middle ear, cerebral ventricles, supratentorial space). The increase in pressure or volume depends on the concentration of N$_2$O delivered, blood flow to the cavity, and duration of delivery. N$_2$O delivered as a 75% mixture doubled the size of a pneumothorax in 10 minutes in animal studies. For this reason, patients with any of the following conditions should not receive N$_2$O:
- Acute intestinal obstruction
- Pneumothorax
- Air emboli
- Pneumocephalus
- Air cysts
- Intraocular air bubbles (avoid for 5 days postoperatively)
- Intraocular gas bubbles (avoid for 10 days postoperatively with sulfur hexafluoride and for 15 to 30 days postoperatively with perfluoropropane)

For procedures involving tympanic grafts, N$_2$O should be discontinued at least 30 minutes before graft application.

9. Do volatile anesthetics affect the cerebral circulation?

At greater than 0.5 MAC and with normocapnia, volatile anesthetics cause decreased cerebral vascular resistance, cerebral vasodilation, and a dose-dependent increase in cerebral blood flow (CBF). Halothane starts to show a significant increase in CBF at 0.5 MAC. Isoflurane does not show a significant increase in CBF until the MAC is greater than 1.

10. Explain why isoflurane may offer cerebral protection.

Volatile anesthetics, especially isoflurane, decrease cerebral metabolic requirements. During isoflurane-induced hypotension, minimal changes in CBF, in concert with decreased cerebral metabolic oxygen requirements, provide a favorable cerebral oxygen supply-to-demand ratio.

11. Volatile agents produce dose-dependent decreases in mean arterial pressure (MAP) by what mechanism?

Volatile agents decrease MAP primarily by decreasing systemic vascular resistance. The exception is halothane, which reduces MAP, at least in part, by decreasing myocardial contractility and cardiac output.

12. What is the coronary steal syndrome?

Coronary steal may be observed when normal coronary vessels dilate and divert or "steal" blood away from already maximally dilated and underperfused vessels. It has been suggested that isoflurane may contribute to coronary steal, but the clinical significance of this is controversial.

13. How are volatile agents metabolized?

Volatile anesthetics undergo oxidative metabolism by the liver cytochrome P-450 enzyme system and to a lesser extent by metabolism in the kidneys and lungs. Halothane also is capable of reductive metabolism. All volatile agents (except sevoflurane) can produce acetylated proteins capable of evoking antibody formation and hepatotoxicity, as described with halothane. The incidence of hepatotoxicity seems to be related to the degree of agent metabolism: halothane > enflurane > isoflurane > desflurane. There have been rare reports of hepatic injury after sevoflurane with no causal relationship established.

Nephrotoxicity from free fluoride metabolites first was described with methoxyflurane. Enflurane and sevoflurane produce a free fluoride metabolite, but they undergo less metabolism than methoxyflurane and produce much less fluoride ion. Sevoflurane also has less intrarenal production of fluoride than enflurane. Intrarenal fluoride production may play a greater role in the development of nephrotoxicity than increased fluoride from hepatic metabolism.

14. What degradation process is unique to sevoflurane?

Sevoflurane interacts with carbon dioxide absorbents (soda lime and barium hydroxide lime) to form compound A. Compound A is a dose-dependent nephrotoxin in rats. When using sevoflurane, it is recommended that a fresh gas flow rate of at least 1 L be used for the first 2 MAC hours, followed by at least 2 L of fresh gas flow for any additional administration. Higher gas flows are beneficial because they dilute the concentration of compound A in the breathing circuit.

15. Which agent may interfere with DNA synthesis?

Bone marrow changes have been found in patients who have been exposed to N_2O for 24 hours. N_2O interferes with methionine synthetase, which is necessary for the synthesis of DNA. Despite this, studies have failed to show consistent findings that N_2O causes teratogenic, carcinogenic, or mutagenic effects.

16. What effects do inhalational anesthetics have on the major organ systems?

Organ system effects of inhalational anesthetics are listed in the following table.

Organ System Effects of Anesthetic Gases

	Halothane	Enflurane	Isoflurane	Desflurane	Sevoflurane	Nitrous Oxide
Cardiovascular						
Blood pressure	↓↓	↓↓	↓↓	↓↓	↓	N/C
Heart Rate	↓	↑	↑	↑ or N/C	N/C	N/C
SVR	N/C	↓	↓↓	↓↓	↓	N/C
Respiratory						
Tidal volume	↓↓	↓↓	↓↓	↓	↓	↓
Respiratory rate	↑↑	↑↑	↑	↑	↑	↑
Renal						
RBF	↓↓	↓↓	↓↓	↓	↓	↓↓
Urinary output	↓↓	↓↓	↓↓	?	?	↓↓
Hepatic						
Blood flow	↓↓	↓↓	↓	↓	↓	↓

N/C, no change; RBF, renal blood flow; SVR, systemic vascular resistance.
Adapted from Morgan GE, Mikhail MS, Murray MJ: Clinical anesthesiology, inhalational anesthetics, ed 3, New York, 2002, Lange Medical Books/McGraw-Hill.

 Key Points

- Five gas laws describe the behavior of inhalational anesthetics:
  - Boyle's law
  - Charles' law
  - Gay-Lussac's law
  - Dalton's law of partial pressure
  - Henry's law

Key Points   *continued*

- The Ostwald solubility coefficient is the measure of the volume of gas that dissolves in a unit volume of liquid at ambient temperature.
- An inhalational agent follows a series of partial pressure gradients to reach its target, the brain: delivered > inspired > alveolar > arterial > brain and tissue.
- MAC is the amount of inhaled anesthetic, or concentration, needed to provide immobility in 50% of patients exposed to surgical stimulation. MAC values provide a means of discussing different agents at equal potent doses.
- The second gas effect is the ability of the high-volume uptake of one gas to increase the alveolar partial pressure of a second gas.
- Anesthetic uptake depends on:
  - Blood gas partition coefficient
  - Cardiac output
  - Anesthetic uptake by tissue
- N_2O is 34 times more soluble than nitrogen.
- Patients with any of the following conditions should not receive N_2O: acute intestinal obstruction, pneumothorax, air emboli, pneumocephalus, air cysts, intraocular air bubbles, intraocular gas bubbles with sulfur hexafluoride, and perfluoropropane. For procedures involving tympanic grafts, N_2O should be discontinued at least 30 minutes before graft application.
- At greater than 0.5 MAC and with normocapnia, volatile anesthetics cause decreased cerebral vascular resistance, cerebral vasodilation, and a dose-dependent increase in CBF.
- Isoflurane offers cerebral protection by decreasing cerebral metabolic requirements.
- Volatile agents decrease MAP, primarily by decreasing systemic vascular resistance.
- The incidence of hepatotoxicity seems to be related to the degree of agent metabolism: halothane > enflurane > isoflurane > desflurane.
- Sevoflurane interacts with carbon dioxide absorbents (soda lime and barium hydroxide lime) to form compound A. Compound A is a dose-dependent nephrotoxin in rats.

Internet Resources

Search GASNet: Inhalational Anesthetics:
http://www.gasnet.org/about/search.php?p1=inhalational+anesthetics

Virtual Anaesthesia Textbook:
http://www.virtual-anaesthesia-textbook.com/

Nurse-Anesthesia.com:
http://www.nurse-anesthesia.com/

Continued

Internet Resources *continued*

Anaesthetist.com:
Volatile Anaesthetics: http://www.anaesthetist.com/anaes/drugs/volatile.htm

Anesthesia Pharmacology:
http://www.anesthesia2001.com/

Pharmacology of General Anesthesia:
http://www.neuro.nwu.edu/meded/m2/anesthesia.htm

Bibliography

Davis PD, Parbrook GD, Kenny GNC: *Basic physics and measurement in anesthesia*, ed 4, Oxford, 1999, Butterworth-Heinemann.

Gold ME, Finander LS: Inhaled anesthetics. In Waugaman WR, Foster SD, Rigor BM Sr, editors: *Principles and practice of nurse anesthesia*, ed 3, Stamford, 1999, Appleton & Lange, pp 363-380.

Morgan GE, Mikhail MS, Murray MJ: *Clinical anesthesiology, inhalational anesthetics*, ed 3, New York, 2002, Lange Medical Books/McGraw-Hill.

Stevens WC, Kingston HGG: Inhalation anesthesia. In Barash PG, Cullen BF, Stoelting RK, editors: *Clinical anesthesia*, ed 3, Philadelphia, 1997, Lippincott-Raven, pp 359-383.

Stoelting RK: *Pharmacology and pathophysiology in anesthetic practice*, ed 3, Philadelphia, 1999, Lippincott-Raven.

Induction Drugs

Sass Elisha

1. Are there differences between the mechanisms of action of propofol, thiopental, etomidate, and ketamine?

Propofol, thiopental, and *etomidate* produce their sedative-hypnotic effects through stimulation of gamma-aminobutyric acid (GABA) receptors. Activation of GABA receptors produces an inhibitory effect that is associated with a decreased level of consciousness. GABA receptor stimulation increases the influx of chloride ion, which hyperpolarizes the membrane potential in presynaptic and postsynaptic neurons in the central nervous system (CNS).

Ketamine stimulates N-methyl-D-aspartate (NMDA) receptors within the CNS, which is the proposed mechanism for its dissociative anesthetic effects. Various areas of the brain are depressed (cerebral cortex and thalamus), whereas other areas are stimulated (limbic system). Ketamine also may produce opioid receptor stimulation.

2. How do common anesthetic agents affect cerebral blood flow (CBF) and cerebral metabolic rate of oxygen consumption (CMRO$_2$)?

Ketamine increases CBF by approximately 60% to 80%. As a result of the excitatory effects produced within the CNS and the stimulation of sympathetic tone, ketamine increases CMRO$_2$. For this reason, ketamine is not recommended for patients with increased intracranial pressure. Another CNS effect associated with ketamine is emergence delirium. The incidence of emergence delirium can be decreased with the concurrent administration of benzodiazepines.

Thiopental, propofol, and etomidate produce CNS depression, a decrease in CMRO$_2$, and cerebral vascular vasoconstriction. Etomidate has been associated with epileptiform activity and should be used with caution in patients with a history of epilepsy.

3. Describe the pharmacokinetic profile of common induction agents after rapid intravenous injection.

When anesthetic induction agents are administered as an intravenous bolus, the blood concentration peaks rapidly. Because these drugs are highly lipid soluble,

CNS depression and loss of consciousness are achieved quickly due to the rapid uptake into the brain (vessel-rich group). Redistribution occurs rapidly as the drug begins to concentrate in lean tissue (primarily muscle), then in adipose tissue (see the following figure). During this period, the cerebral concentration of the induction agent decreases, and awakening occurs. Elimination begins to occur as the drug, which is sequestered in tissues, reenters the central circulation and is metabolized in the liver.

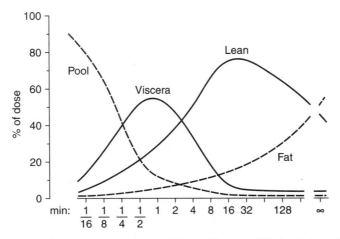

Time and percent dose differences concerning redistribution of thiopental from central blood pool, viscera (brain), lean tissue, and fat after bolus intravenous administration. *(From Price HL, Kovnat PJ, Safer JN, et al: The uptake of thiopental by body tissues and its relation to the duration of narcosis, Clin Pharmacol Ther 1(16), 1960.)*

4. Why is etomidate contraindicated in a patient with adrenocortical suppression?

A single bolus dose of etomidate (0.3 mg/kg intravenously) can cause adrenocortical suppression for 12 hours. This phenomenon is caused by the inhibition of 11β-hydroxylase, which is the enzyme necessary to complete the conversion of cholesterol intermediaries to cortisol and aldosterone. The degree of adrenocortical suppression is dose dependent and temporary.

5. Discuss the effects the induction agents have on the respiratory system.

Thiopental and *propofol* are potent respiratory depressants and cause dose-dependent decreases in minute ventilation. The respiratory depressant effects are caused by central inhibition of the pontine and medullary centers in the brain. In addition, the ventilatory response to carbon dioxide is decreased.

Etomidate has minimal effects on the central ventilatory centers. The respiratory depressant effects are less compared with thiopental or propofol. Respiratory arrest occurs, however, when a full bolus induction dose is administered.

Ketamine generally does not produce respiratory depression, and the ventilatory response to carbon dioxide is preserved. Respiratory depression can occur, however, when large bolus doses are administered. Ketamine produces broncho-dilation, as evidenced by a decrease in total airway resistance. Muscarinic receptor stimulation by ketamine can cause an increase in upper airway secretions.

Each of these induction agents can cause apnea when clinical dosages are administered as a bolus injection. The frequency of respiratory depression is increased with the concomitant use of narcotics or benzodiazepines.

6. Which induction agent is contraindicated in a patient with acute intermittent porphyria?

Acute intermittent porphyria is an inborn error in the metabolism of porphyrins. The production of the heme portion of hemoglobin and cytochromes depends on porphyrin synthesis. The enzyme, aminolevulinic acid synthetase, accelerates the production of porphobilinogen, which is toxic to the CNS and peripheral nervous system. Barbiturates, such as *thiopental,* can induce increased activity of aminolevulinic acid synthetase and provoke an acute exacerbation of the disease.

7. Compare the hemodynamic effects of the common induction agents, propofol, thiopental, etomidate, and ketamine.

Of the four induction agents, *propofol* has the greatest negative inotropic effect and causes the largest decrease in systemic vascular resistance (SVR). The decreased SVR is accentuated by blunting of the baroreceptor reflex.

The decreased blood pressure observed after administration of *thiopental* is due to peripheral vasodilation (depression of the medullary vasomotor center) and a moderate direct myocardial depressant effect. After the administration of a bolus dose of sodium thiopental, mild-to-moderate increases in heart rate occur.

Etomidate has minimal myocardial depressant effects and may be administered to patients with decreased cardiac reserve. With normal induction doses, etomidate produces a mild decrease in SVR and may decrease the blood pressure by approximately 15%. Clinically significant myocardial depression and decreases in SVR can occur with large induction doses.

Ketamine increases sympathetic nervous system tone by inhibiting reuptake of catecholamines. As a result, ketamine is associated with increases in heart rate, blood pressure, and cardiac output. Myocardial oxygen consumption also is increased. Patients who are catecholamine depleted (e.g., critically ill) may not exhibit these cardiovascular responses with ketamine administration (see the table on page 88).

With each of these induction agents, severe hypotension can occur in hypovolemic patients.

Cardiovascular, Respiratory, and Cerebral Effects of Commonly Used Anesthetic Induction Agents						
	Cardiovascular		Respiratory		Cerebral	
Agent	**HR**	**MAP**	**VENT**	**BRON DIL**	**CBF**	**CMRO₂**
Thiopental	↑↑	↓↓	↓↓↓	0	↓↓↓	↓↓↓
Propofol	0	↓↓↓	↓↓↓	0	↓↓↓	↓↓↓
Etomidate	0	↓	↓	0	↓↓↓	↓↓↓
Ketamine	↑↑	↑↑	↓	↑↑↑	↑↑↑	↑

0 = no effect.
↑ = increase (mild, moderate, severe).
↓= decrease (mild, moderate, severe).
BRON DIL, bronchodilation; CBF, cerebral blood flow; CMRO₂, cerebral metabolic rate of oxygen consumption; HR, heart rate; MAP, mean arterial pressure; VENT, ventilation rate.

8. Which induction agent is the drug of choice for a patient with asthma?

Ketamine is the induction agent of choice. It produces bronchodilation as a result of beta$_2$-receptor agonism caused by the central release of catecholamines.

9. Which induction agent may cause burning after rapid intravenous administration?

Burning immediately after intravenous injection can occur with *propofol* and *etomidate*. This effect can be decreased with the administration of lidocaine before rapid intravenous administration.

10. Why is it recommended that propofol be administered within 6 hours after it is drawn up into a syringe?

Propofol is formulated as a 1% aqueous solution, in a fat emulsion consisting of soybean oil, glycerol, and egg lecithin. As a result of the presence of fat in the preparation, microbial growth can occur, despite the presence of preservative agents. Propofol should be drawn into a syringe using aseptic technique, and the drug should not be used if it has been drawn up for greater than 6 hours. The prepackaged propofol (Diprivan) filled syringe system may decrease the possibility of microbial growth.

11. Discuss the differences and potential physiological effects of trade versus generic preparations of propofol.

The preservative used to formulate the Diprivan (AstraZeneca) form of propofol is ethylenediaminetretraacetic acid (EDTA). The preservative used to formulate the generic preparation of propofol (Baxter, Liberty Corners) is sodium met-abisulfite. Propofol with metabisulfite has been implicated in causing broncho-constriction as a result of histamine release. Controversy exists, however, as to whether propofol with metabisulfite increases airway resistance to a greater degree than propofol (Diprivan) with EDTA. There is conflicting evidence as to whether the concentration of metabisulfite in propofol is sufficient to cause increased airway resistance. Because of this concern, it may be prudent to administer the Diprivan formula to patients who are predisposed to increased airway resistance and have a potential for airway hyperactivity.

12. Which induction agent would be most appropriate under the following conditions?

- A 27-year-old woman with no significant medical history, scheduled for a laparoscopic tubal ligation as an outpatient.
  - The induction agent of choice for outpatient anesthesia is *propofol*. The half-life of propofol is considerably shorter compared with the other induction agents (0.5 to 1.5 hours). Awakening occurs more quickly due to the short distribution half-life (2 to 8 minutes). In addition, this patient is at higher risk for nausea and vomiting due to predisposing factors, which include female gender and laparoscopic surgery. Propofol has antiemetic properties.
- An 84-year-old man with a history of coronary artery disease scheduled for a bowel resection.
  - The only anesthetic induction agent that is *contraindicated* for a patient with known coronary artery disease is *ketamine*. The sympathomimetic effects of this drug may increase myocardial oxygen consumption. Clinically, propofol, etomidate, or thiopental could be administered to this patient. Because of the patient's increased age, history of coronary artery disease, and hypovolemic state after a bowel preparation, hypotension is likely to occur. *Etomidate* may be the best choice for an induction agent due to its minimal effects on the cardiovascular system.
- An 18-year-old man who has sustained a gunshot wound to the chest; signs and symptoms include shortness of breath and hypotension; he is awake and alert.
  - The induction agent of choice is *ketamine* due to this drug's ability to increase cardiac contractility and blood pressure.

The decision to use a specific induction agent or anesthetic technique must always be based on the immediate and specific patient circumstances.

13. Why are larger initial doses of thiopental and propofol recommended for pediatric patients?

Total body water content of a pediatric patient is approximately 10% to 30% greater than that of an adult. For this reason, thiopental and propofol have a larger volume of distribution in the pediatric patient, and a greater initial dose of these agents is required for the induction of anesthesia.

14. **A patient has experienced an anaphylactic reaction after eating eggs. Is propofol administration contraindicated for this patient?**

In most cases when patients have egg allergies, it is the egg white (egg albumin) that is likely the cause of the response. Egg lecithin, which is a component of the egg yolk, is used to formulate propofol. Despite this, the prudent approach is to avoid the use of propofol in all patients with egg allergies because alternative induction agents exist.

Key Points

- Propofol, thiopental, and etomidate produce their sedative-hypnotic effects by stimulation of GABA receptors.
- Ketamine stimulates NMDA receptors to produce its dissociative anesthetic effects and opioid receptors to produce analgesia.
- Ketamine increases CBF and $CMRO_2$.
- Thiopental, propofol, and etomidate produce CNS depression, decreased $CMRO_2$ and cerebral vascular vasoconstriction.
- Etomidate has been associated with epileptiform activity and should be used with caution in patients with a history of epilepsy.
- A single bolus dose of etomidate (0.3 mg/kg intravenously) can cause adrenocortical suppression for 12 hours.
- In ranked order, propofol has the greatest cardiovascular effects followed by thiopental and etomidate; ketamine has minimal cardiovascular effects.
- Ketamine is the induction agent of choice in asthmatics.
- Propofol can contain metabisulfite and could result in bronchoconstriction in susceptible patients.
- Propofol and thiopental have a larger volume of distribution in pediatric patients.

Internet Resources

Anesthesia Pharmacology Units:
http://www.anesthesia2001.com/learning2.htm

International Society for Anaesthetic Pharmacology:
http://www.isaponline.org/isap/default.asp.

Anesthesia & Analgesia Search: Pharmacology:
http://www.anesthesia-analgesia.org/cgi/collection/pharmacology?page=28.

Pharmacology of General Anesthesia:
http://www.neuro.nwu.edu/meded/m2/anesthesia.htm

Bibliography

Brown RH, Greenberg RS, Wagner EM: Efficacy of propofol to prevent bronchoconstriction: effects of preservative, *Anesthesiology* 94:851-855, 2001.

Desnick RJ: The porphyrias. In Fauci AS, Braunwald E, et al, editors: *Harrison's principles of internal medicine,* ed 14, New York, 1998, McGraw-Hill, pp 2152-2158.

Fallacaro NA, Fallacaro MD: Intravenous induction agents. In Nagelhout JJ, Zaglaniczny KL, editors: *Nurse anesthesia,* ed 2, Philadelphia, 2001, WB Saunders, pp 115-135.

Morgan GE Jr, Mikhail MS, Murray MJ: *Clinical anesthesiology,* ed 3, New York, 2002, McGraw-Hill, pp 151-177.

Price HL, Kovnat PJ, Safer JN, et al: The uptake of thiopental by body tissues and its relation to the duration of narcosis, *Clin Pharmacol Ther* 1(16), 1960.

Reeves GJ, Glass PSA, Lubarsky DA: Nonbarbiturate intravenous agents. In Miller RD, editor: *Anesthesia,* ed 5, Philadelphia, 2000, Churchill Livingstone, pp 229-272.

Sarton E, Teppema LJ, Oliever C, et al: The involvement of the mu-opioid receptor in ketamine induced respiratory depression and antinociception, *Anesth Analg* 93:1495-1500, 2001.

Schenarts CL, Burton JH, Riker RR: Adrenocortical dysfunction following etomidate induction in emergency department patients, *Acad Emerg Med* 8:1-7, 2001.

Sprung J, Ogletree-Hughes ML, McConnell BK, et al: The effect of propofol on the contractility of failing and nonfailing human heart muscle, *Anesth Analg* 93:550-559, 2001.

Sprung J, Ogeltree-Hughes ML, Moravec CS: The effects of etomidate on contractility of failing and nonfailing human heart muscle, *Anesth Analg* 91:68-75, 2000.

Stoelting RK: *Pharmacology and physiology in anesthetic practice,* ed 3, Philadelphia, 1999, Lipincott-Raven, pp 140-157.

Wagner LE, Gingrich KJ, Kulli JC, et al: Ketamine blockade of voltage-gated sodium channels: evidence for a shared receptor site with local anesthetics, *Anesthesiology* 95:1406-1413, 2001.

Xinli S, Hong L, White PF, et al: Bisulfite-containing propofol: is it a cost-effective alternative to Diprivan for induction of anesthesia? *Anesth Analg* 91:871-875, 2000.

Narcotics and Benzodiazepines

Sass Elisha

1. What is the definition of an opiate?

The term *opiate* refers to all drugs that are derived from poppy. Opiate compounds stimulate opiate receptors within the body and cause a variety of physiological responses, including analgesia. Endogenous opiate receptor agonists include endorphins, enkephalins, and dynorphins. Exogenous opiate receptor agonists are divided into several chemical classes, two of which are used in anesthetic practice: phenanthrenes and benzylisoquinolines.

2. Describe the relative potency and elimination half-life of commonly used intravenous narcotics.

The *potency* of an opiate agonist depends on the specific drug's affinity for an opiate receptor. Factors that determine the *elimination* half-life include degree of ionization, protein binding, lipid solubility, and hepatic and renal clearance (see the following table).

Potency and Elimination of Common Narcotics		
Drug	**Potency**	**Elimination Half-Life (Approximate Time in Minutes)**
Morphine	1	160
Meperidine	0.1	240
Alfentanil	20	90
Fentanyl	100	180
Sufentanil	1000	150
Remifentanil	100	10

3. Classify the various opiate receptor subtypes and their physiological effects.

There are three types of opiate receptors: *mu, kappa,* and *delta*. Stimulation of different receptors produces different physiological responses (see the table on page 94).

Classification of Opiate Receptors

	Mu$_1$	Mu$_2$	Kappa	Delta
Clinical Effect	Supraspinal analgesia, euphoria, bradycardia, sedation	Spinal analgesia, euphoria, respiratory depression, pruritus	Spinal and supraspinal analgesia, dysphoria, sedation, delirium	Spinal and supraspinal analgesia, respiratory depression, dysphoria
Agonists	Morphine, synthetic opiates, endorphins	Morphine, synthetic opiates, endorphins	Morphine, nalbuphine, dynorphin, butorphanol	Enkephalin, endorphin
Antagonists	Naloxone, naltrexone, nalmefene	Naloxone, naltrexone, nalmefene	Naloxone, naltrexone, nalmefene	Naloxone, naltrexone, nalmefene

4. **Summarize effects of opiates on the cardiovascular system, respiratory system, and central nervous system (CNS).**

   Cardiovascular, respiratory, and CNS effects are summarized in the table below.

Physiological Effects of Commonly Used Narcotic Agents

	Cardiovascular		Respiratory		Cerebral	
Agent	**HR**	**MAP**	**VENT**	**BRON DIL**	**CBF**	**CMRO$_2$**
Morphine	↓	↓	↓↓↓	0*	↓	↓
Meperidine	↑	↓↓	↓↓↓	0	↓	↓
Alfentanil	↓↓	↓↓	↓↓↓	0	↓	↓
Fentanyl	↓↓	↓↓	↓↓↓	0	↓	↓
Sufentanil	↓↓	↓↓	↓↓↓	0	↓	↓
Remifentanil	↓↓	↓↓	↓↓↓	0	↓	↓

0 = no effect.
↑ = increase (mild, moderate, severe).
↓ = decrease (mild, moderate, severe).
* Bronchoconstriction may occur due to histamine release.
BRON DIL, bronchodilation; CBF, cerebral blood flow; CMRO$_2$, cerebral metabolic rate of oxygen consumption; HR, heart rate; MAP, mean arterial pressure; VENT, ventilation rate.

5. Which of the commonly used intravenously administered narcotics induce histamine release?

Morphine is associated with histamine release. It should be administered with caution to patients with hyperreactive airway disease, including asthma. The phenylpiperidine analogues (e.g., meperidine) do not produce significant histamine release.

6. Which narcotics cause the greatest degree of sphincter of Oddi spasm?

All narcotics can increase smooth muscle contractility of the biliary tree. The degree of increased biliary tree pressure depends on the dose and type of narcotic administered (see the following figure). Narcotics that increase biliary pressure and create sphincter of Oddi spasm in order from the greatest degree to least degree are as follows: fentanyl > morphine > demerol. Due to the rapid metabolism of remifentanil, smooth muscle spasm of the biliary tree is alleviated rapidly by drug discontinuation.

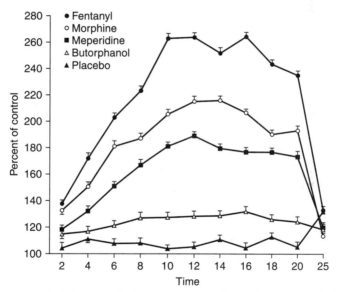

Varied increases in common bile duct pressure after intravenous administration of opiate agonists and opiate agonist-antagonist. *(From Radnay PA, Duncalf D, Nakaovic M, et al: Common bile duct pressure changes after fentanyl, morphine, meperidine, butorphanol and naloxone, Anesth Analg 63:441-444, 1984.)*

Increased biliary pressure and spasm of the sphincter of Oddi can increase the difficulty of performing an intraoperative cholangiogram. This situation occurs in approximately 3% of patients who receive narcotics and undergo an intraoperative cholangiogram. Treatment for narcotic-induced sphincter of Oddi spasm includes the administration of an opiate antagonist (naloxone), agonist/antagonist (nalbuphine, butorphanol), glucagon, anticholinergic agents, or nitrates.

7. Discuss the differences between opiate antagonists and opiate agonist-antagonists.

Opiate antagonists (e.g., naloxone, naltrexone, nalmefene) have a high affinity for all groups of opiate receptors. These drugs displace opiate agonists, competitively bind to opiate receptors, and reverse the physiological effects of narcotics. Clinically the most widely used opiate antagonist is naloxone (Narcan). Because of its relatively short half life (30 to 45 minutes), repeat doses may be required to prevent renarcosis and respiratory depression.

Opiate agonist-antagonists (e.g., pentazocine, butorphanol, nalbuphine, buprenorphine, nalorphine, dezocine, meptazinol) exert their antagonist effects by binding with mu receptors. In addition, these drugs produce an agonist effect at kappa and delta opiate receptor subtypes. Opiate agonist-antagonists may reverse the sedative and respiratory depressant effects of narcotics, while partially maintaining the analgesic properties.

8. Discuss the advantages and disadvantages of remifentanil.

Remifentanil is an ultrashort-acting opiate receptor agonist. This drug's chemical structure is similar to the phenylpiperidine derivatives (e.g., meperidine, fentanyl). It is unique because of its ester linkage. Metabolism of remifentanil is rapid due to hydrolysis by nonspecific blood and tissue esterases at the ester linkage site. An advantage of remifentanil is the rapid dissipation of respiratory and CNS depression after discontinuation of an infusion. Alternative strategies for postoperative pain relief may be required, owing to the absence of an analgesic effect on termination of the drug.

9. What are the effects of administering narcotics into the subarachnoid space?

Opiate administration into the subarachnoid space produces analgesia by inhibiting substance P and other pain neurotransmitters and by decreasing the neuroendocrine response to noxious stimuli. Opiate binding to receptors (mu, kappa, and delta) within the substantia gelatinosa interrupts afferent pain impulses *in the dorsal horn of the spinal cord*. When combined with local anesthetic agents, intrathecal narcotics may increase the intensity and duration of spinal anesthesia.

10. What effect does lipid solubility have on the degree of the cephalad spread of narcotics within the subarachnoid space?

After injection into the subarachnoid space, narcotics diffuse into the spinal cord and spinal nerve roots. The degree of binding to these structures depends on the lipid solubility of the narcotic. Narcotics that are lipophilic (e.g., fentanyl, sufentanil) diffuse readily into lipid-rich tissues, leaving a smaller percentage of free drug available within the cerebrospinal fluid. More hydrophilic narcotics (e.g., morphine) are less lipid soluble. These drugs do not diffuse as readily into lipid-rich tissues, leaving a higher fraction of free drug within the cerebrospinal fluid. The higher the concentration of narcotic within the cerebrospinal fluid, the greater the likelihood of cephalad spread and centrally mediated respiratory depression. Although respiratory depression is more common with hydrophilic opioids, such as morphine, respiratory depression also can occur with lipophilic drugs.

11. Describe the side effects associated with neuraxial opiate administration.

Side effects that can occur with neuraxial opiate administration include the following:
• Respiratory depression
• Urinary retention
• Nausea and vomiting
• Pruritus
• Sedation

Naloxone is the definitive treatment for patients who experience respiratory depression due to neuraxial opiate administration. Administration of naloxone also inhibits analgesia caused by narcotics. Alternative treatments are available for pruritus (e.g., diphenhydramine) and nausea and vomiting (e.g., serotonin receptor antagonists).

12. Which narcotic should not be administered to patients who have a history of seizures?

Meperidine should not be administered to patients with seizure disorders. Normeperidine, a metabolite of meperidine, has twice the CNS excitatory effects as the parent compound and has been associated with seizure activity. Normeperidine is excreted principally by the kidney. Decreased renal clearance and prolonged dosing regimens increase the seizure potential associated with meperidine administration in susceptible patients.

13. Why is meperidine administration contraindicated in patients taking monoamine oxidase (MAO) inhibitors?

MAO is a naturally occurring enzyme that is present in autonomic nerve endings, liver, gastrointestinal tract, kidneys, and lungs. MAO inactivates bioactive amines, such as epinephrine. MAO inhibitors are antidepressant drugs that inhibit the breakdown of epinephrine, norepinephrine, and serotonin at nerve endings. Patients taking MAO inhibitors have increased amounts of these neurotransmitters within the synaptic junction. Meperidine decreases the reuptake of serotonin. The combination of meperidine and MAO inhibitors can result in large amounts of free serotonin within the synaptic cleft. Side effects that may be associated with this drug combination include the following:
• Headache
• Muscle rigidity
• Hyperpyrexia
• Hypertension

- Convulsions
- Coma
- Death

14. Which narcotic is associated with persistent or recurrent respiratory depression during the postoperative period?

Fentanyl is associated with secondary peaks in plasma concentration that potentially can cause respiratory depression in the postoperative period. There are three proposed mechanisms for the delayed respiratory depression, which can occur 4 hours after the last dose:

- Sequestration of fentanyl in gastric fluid can be reabsorbed into the central circulation.
- Increased fentanyl uptake from the lungs can occur when normal physiological ventilation and perfusion is reestablished in the postoperative period.
- Large amounts of fentanyl that have distributed to muscle tissue reenter the circulation after patients become active in the recovery room.

15. Discuss the mechanism of action of benzodiazepines.

Benzodiazepines produce their sedative-hypnotic effects through stimulation of gamma-aminobutyric acid (GABA) receptors. GABA receptor stimulation increases the influx of chloride ion, causing hyperpolarization of postsynaptic neurons in the CNS. Activation of GABA receptors produces an inhibitory effect that is associated with anxiolysis and sedation.

16. Describe the distribution, metabolism, and excretion of benzodiazepines.

Benzodiazepines are lipid-soluble drugs and rapidly produce CNS depressant effects. After an intravenous dose of midazolam, high concentrations of the drug are present within the brain. Benzodiazepines are metabolized in the liver by oxidation and conjugation reactions. Patients with liver disease or renal insufficiency may have decreased metabolism and clearance and exhibit prolonged sedation (see the following table).

Comparison of Commonly Used Benzodiazepines

	Volume Distribution (L/kg)	Clearance (mL/kg/min)	Elimination Half- Life (hr)
Midazolam	1–1.5	6–8	1.5–2.5
Lorazepam	1–1.5	0.2–0.5	12–22
Diazepam	0.8-1.3	0.7–1	20–50

17. Summarize the clinical effects of benzodiazepines on the CNS, cardiovascular system, and respiratory system.

CENTRAL NERVOUS SYSTEM

Benzodiazepines produce anxiolysis, sedation, and anterograde (moving forward) amnesia. As a result of CNS depressant effects, they decrease cerebral metabolic rate of oxygen consumption and cerebral blood flow. Midazolam and diazepam have anticonvulsant properties, making them particularly useful agents for patients with seizure histories.

CARDIOVASCULAR SYSTEM

Benzodiazepines have minimal to no effect on myocardial contractility. They have a modest effect, however, in decreasing systemic vascular resistance, which is responsible for a slight decrease in blood pressure after rapid intravenous administration. The combined use of benzodiazepines and narcotics produces a synergistic effect, resulting in a greater decrease in mean arterial pressure than if either drug was administered independently. A proposed mechanism of action for this phenomenon includes a greater decrease in sympathetic tone with this combination of drugs.

RESPIRATORY SYSTEM

Respiratory depression can occur after the administration of benzodiazepines due to their ability to decrease the ventilatory response to carbon dioxide. Apnea can occur when benzodiazepines are administered with narcotics because of the additive ventilatory depressant effects in the central respiratory center. In addition, older patients may have increased sensitivity even after administration of small intravenous doses of benzodiazepines. For this reason, all patients who receive intravenous benzodiazepines must be monitored closely for respiratory depression.

18. Relate the pharmacological properties of flumazenil.

Flumazenil is a benzodiazepine receptor antagonist that reverses all of the pharmacological effects of benzodiazepines in a dose-dependent manner. Because of flumazenil's short half-life (approximately 45 to 90 minutes), benzodiazepine-induced sedation and respiratory depression can recur. Flumazenil itself does not exert significant cardiovascular effects, but the increased sympathetic nervous system activity associated with benzodiazepine reversal may increase

Diazepam   Lorazepam   Midazolam   Flumazenil

Chemical structures of benzodiazepines and antagonist.

plasma catecholamine levels and increase myocardial oxygen consumption. Reversal of benzodiazepines in patients with epilepsy may increase the risk of withdrawal seizures. The chemical structure of flumazenil is similar to drugs in the benzodiazepine class (see the figure on page 99).

Key Points

- Opiate compounds stimulate opiate receptors within the body and cause a variety of physiological responses, including analgesia.
- Endogenous opiate receptor agonists include endorphins, enkephalins and dynorphins.
- Exogenous opiate receptor agonists are divided into several chemical classes, two of which are used in anesthetic practice: phenanthrenes and benzylisoquinolines.
- The potency of an opiate agonist depends on the specific drug's affinity for an opiate receptor.
- There are three types of opiate receptors: mu, kappa, and delta. Stimulation of different receptors produces different physiological responses.
- All narcotics can increase smooth muscle contractility of the biliary tree; in order from the greatest degree to least degree are fentanyl > morphine > meperidine.
- Opiate antagonists (e.g., naloxone, naltrexone, nalmefene) displace opiate agonists, competitively bind to opiate receptors, and reverse the physiological effects of narcotics.
- Opiate agonist-antagonists (e.g., pentazocine, butorphanol, nalbuphine, buprenorphine, nalorphine, dezocine, meptazinol) exert their antagonist effects by binding with mu receptors.
- The degree of binding of narcotics to the spinal nerve roots depends on the lipid solubility of the narcotic.
- Meperidine should not be administered to patients with seizure disorders.
- Fentanyl is associated with secondary peaks in plasma concentration that potentially can cause respiratory depression in the postoperative period.
- Benzodiazepines produce their sedative-hypnotic effects through stimulation of GABA receptors.
- Benzodiazepines produce anxiolysis, sedation, and anterograde (moving forward) amnesia.
- Flumazenil is a benzodiazepine receptor antagonist that reverses all of the pharmacologic effects of benzodiazepines in a dose-dependent manner.

Internet Resources

Internet Resources   *continued*

GasNet Search: Opioid:
http://www.gasnet.org/about/search.php?p1=opioid

Anesthesiology INFO: Intravenous Anesthetics:
http://anesthesiologyinfo.com/articles/01072002.php

Virtual Anaesthesia Textbook:
http://www.virtual-anaesthesia-textbook.com/

Bibliography

Bailey PL, Talmage DE, Theodore SH: Intravenous opioid anesthetics. In Miller RD, editor: *Anesthesia*, ed 5, Philadelphia, 2000, Churchill Livingstone, pp 273-376.

Carr DB, Cousins MJ: Spinal route of analgesia: opioids and future options. In Cousins MJ, Bridenbaugh PO, editors: *Clinical anesthesia and management of pain*, ed 3, Philadelphia, 1998, Lippincott-Raven, pp 915-983.

Fragen RJ, Vilich F, Spies SM, et al: The effect of remifentanil on biliary tract drainage into the duodenum, *Anesth Analg* 89:1561-1567, 1999.

Kamijo Y, Masuda T, Nishikawa T, et al: Cardiovascular response to stress reaction to flumazenil injection in patients under infusion with midazolam, *Crit Care Med* 28:318-323, 2000.

Morgan GE Jr, Mikhail MS, Murray MJ: *Clinical anesthesiology,* ed 3, New York, 2002, McGraw-Hill, pp 160-169.

Radnay PA, Duncalf D, Navakovic M, et al: Common bile duct pressure changes after fentanyl, morphine, meperidine, butorphanol and naloxone, *Anesth Analg* 63:441-444, 1984.

Reeves GJ, Glass PSA, Lubarsky DA: Nonbarbiturate intravenous agents. In Miller RD, editor: *Anesthesia*, ed 5, Philadelphia, 2000, Churchill Livingstone, pp 229-272.

Stoelting RK: *Pharmacology and physiology in anesthetic practice,* ed 3, Philadelphia, 1999, Lippincott-Raven, pp 77-112, 126-139.

Wilson WO: Opioid agonists and antagonists In Nagelhout JJ, Zaglaniczny KL, editors: *Nurse anesthesia,* ed 2, Philadelphia, 2001, WB Saunders, pp 157-170.

Neuromuscular Blocking Drugs

Le-Lan Le

1. How did neuromuscular blocking agents become part of the anesthesia practitioner's arsenal?

Flaccid muscle paralysis was first described in 1516, when Amazon tribesmen instilled a vine derivative, curare, in their arrows to poison their enemies. In 1856, studies first confirmed that the site of pharmacodynamic action of curare was at the neuromuscular junction. In 1942, curare was introduced into anesthesia practice for the purpose of muscle relaxation.

2. Briefly describe the functional anatomy of the neuromuscular junction.

The point at which a motor nerve fiber meets a skeletal muscle fiber is termed the *neuromuscular junction* (NMJ) (see the following figure). The end of the nerve fiber, called the *terminal button,* houses packets of the neurotransmitter acetylcholine (ACh), which are released into the synaptic cleft in response to depolarization of the nerve fiber. ACh crosses the 20- to 30-nm-wide cleft and activates ACh receptors on the motor end plate, the specific site on the muscle fiber membrane with receptors.

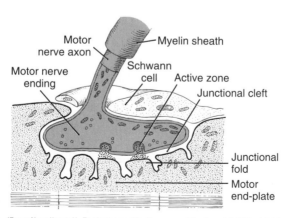

Neuromuscular junction. *(From Nagelhout JJ, Zaglaniczny. KL: Nurse anesthesia. ed 2, Philadelphia, 2001, WB Saunders, p. 717.)*

3. Discuss the synthesis and metabolism of the neurotransmitter, ACh.

SYNTHESIS
ACh is the principal neurotransmitter involved in muscle fiber activation. It is synthesized in the nerve endings of cholinergic nerve fibers from acetyl coenzyme A and choline. Choline acetyltransferase catalyzes the reaction.

$$acetyl\text{-}CoA + choline \Rightarrow ACh$$

When synthesized, about 10,000 molecules of ACh are stored in vesicles in the terminal button, awaiting release.

METABOLISM
After release from cholinergic nerve endings, ACh is rapidly hydrolyzed by the enzyme acetylcholinesterase into choline and acetate. Choline returns to the nerve terminal to be recycled for future ACh synthesis.

4. List the sequence of events leading to muscle fiber contraction.
- An impulse travels down the nerve axon and opens voltage-gated calcium channels at the terminal button.
- Calcium influx from the synaptic cleft enhances fusion of ACh vesicles to the nerve membrane, and ACh is released into the cleft.
- ACh binds to ACh receptors on the motor end plate.
- Binding causes ACh-gated channels to open and allows influx of primarily Na^+ and Ca^{2+}.
- Influx of cations causes an end plate potential that spreads along the muscle fiber to initiate muscle contraction.

5. Does neuromuscular blockade alter consciousness?
No. Neuromuscular blocking drugs have their pharmacodynamic effect only at the NMJ. Muscle relaxants may enhance hearing by affecting muscles of the middle ear. Consciousness and sensorium are intact, even in the presence of total neuromuscular blockade.

6. Discuss the two classes of neuromuscular blocking agents currently in use.
The two classes of neuromuscular blocking agents are the *nondepolarizing agents* and the *depolarizing agents*. These classes differ primarily in their mechanism of action at the NMJ. They also vary in their onset of action, duration of action, metabolism, and side effects. Both classes of drugs resemble ACh in their structure but act at the receptor in different ways.
- Nondepolarizing agents are quaternary compounds that are classified further into aminosteroids or benzylisoquoliniums.
- Depolarizing agents are quaternary compounds and include the drug succinylcholine.

7. How are neuromuscular blocking agents compared pharmacologically?

The ED_{95} is the effective dose at which 95% suppression of the single twitch response is achieved. In practice, approximately twice the ED_{95} dose is recommended for tracheal intubation (see the following table).

Neuromuscular Blocking Agents

Drug	Intubating Dose (mg/kg)	Maintenance Dose (mg/kg)	Onset (min)	Duration (min)
Short-Acting Agents				
Succinylcholine	1–2	NA	30–60 sec	3–10
Mivacurium	0.15–0.2	0.1	1.5–3	12–20
Intermediate-Acting Agents				
Atracurium	0.4–0.5	0.1–0.2	2–3	20–35
Cisatracurium	0.1–0.15	0.03	2–3	20–35
Rocuronium	0.6–1.2	0.1–0.2	1–2	20–35
Vecuronium	0.08–0.1	0.01–0.04	2–3	20–35
Long-Acting agents				
Pancuronium	0.08–0.12	0.01	2–3	60–90
Pipecuronium	0.06–0.1	0.01–0.015	3–5	60–120

8. Which muscles are most sensitive to neuromuscular blocking drugs?

Muscles of the eyes, digits, upper airway, and larynx are more sensitive to neuromuscular blocking drugs than larger muscles, such as the abdominal muscles, muscles of the arms and legs, and diaphragm. The diaphragm is the least sensitive and most resistant muscle to neuromuscular blocking drugs. This is significant because reversal of muscle paralysis in the surgical patient may result in adequate return of diaphragmatic function, but incomplete reversal of the more profoundly blocked laryngeal and upper airway muscles. Extubation under these conditions can result in a compromised respiratory status.

9. Discuss the mechanism of the depolarizing neuromuscular blocking agent, succinylcholine.

Succinylcholine is actually two molecules of ACh. It binds and activates ACh receptors on the motor end plate to generate an action potential. In contrast to ACh, succinylcholine is not metabolized by acetylcholinesterase in the synaptic cleft; the cleft concentration does not decrease as rapidly. This results in a prolonged motor end plate depolarization, manifesting clinically as fasciculations followed by paralysis.

10. How is succinylcholine metabolized?

Plasma cholinesterase is an enzyme that hydrolyzes succinylcholine. It is produced by the liver.

11. List factors that decrease plasma cholinesterase levels and prolong neuromuscular blockade.

- *Inherited*—atypical plasma cholinesterase
- *Physiologic*—pregnancy, infancy, advanced age
- *Acquired*—liver dysfunction, renal dysfunction, malnutrition, burn injury, malignancy
- *Iatrogenic*—echothiophate, neostigmine, pyridostigmine, trimethaphan, cyclophosphamide, propanolol, birth control pills, plasmapheresis, cardiopulmonary bypass, estrogen

12. What is atypical plasma cholinesterase?

Atypical plasma cholinesterase is abnormal cholinesterase that results in impaired metabolism of succinylcholine. The incidence of heterozygous atypical plasma cholinesterase is 1 in 50 patients. These patients may have prolonged muscle blockade lasting 20 to 30 minutes. The incidence of homozygous atypical plasma cholinesterase has been reported as 1 in 3000 patients. These patients can have prolonged blockade of 6 to 8 hours.

13. Can individuals be tested for atypical plasma cholinesterase?

Yes. The dibucaine number was first described in 1957. Dibucaine is an amide local anesthetic that inhibits normal plasma cholinesterase and atypical plasma cholinesterase by 80% and 20%.

Dibucaine Number	
80	Indicates normal plasma cholinesterase
40–60	Indicates heterozygous atypical plasma cholinesterase
20	Indicates homozygous atypical plasma cholinesterase

14. Define phase II block.

Phase II block is a protracted succinylcholine-induced muscle paralysis that resembles a nondepolarizing blockade. The exact mechanism continues to be debated, but among the proposed theories are desensitization of the ACh receptor to succinylcholine, ion channel blockade at the NMJ, and succinylcholine accumulation inside the muscle fiber membrane. Phase II block can occur after an initial large dose of succinylcholine (>2 mg/kg), repeated doses, or a continuous infusion of succinylcholine. Phase II block is accentuated by nondepolarizing agents and is reversible by anticholinesterases.

15. Describe some of the side effects of succinylcholine.

- *Bradycardia:* Caused by stimulation of cholinergic sinoatrial node receptors by succinylmonocholine. Atropine may be administered prophylactically (20 mcg/kg) in a pediatric patient and before a second dose of succinylcholine in adults (0.4 mg).
- *Postoperative myalgia:* Fasciculations from succinylcholine may cause postoperative muscle aches. Some practitioners administer a "defasciculation

dose" of a nondepolarizer (usually {1/10} an intubating dose) to minimize fasciculations. Some studies have shown no correlation between fasciculations and postoperative myalgia.

- *Hyperkalemia:* Under normal conditions, succinylcholine-induced depolarization of the muscle fiber membrane causes enough potassium efflux to raise serum levels by 0.5 mEq/L. Patients with normal serum potassium levels can tolerate this increase in serum potassium. Conditions that lead to the development of extrajunctional receptors, such as immobility, stroke, and spinal cord injury, are associated with exaggerated potassium efflux after succinylcholine administration. In these patients, serum potassium levels of 11 mEq/L have been reported preceding cardiac arrest. Similar increases may be observed in cases of burn and trauma.
- *Increased gastric pressure:* Abdominal fasciculations from succinylcholine can cause increased intragastric pressure to 40 cm H_2O. Pressures exceeding 20 cm H_2O can compromise cardioesophageal sphincter tone and lead to aspiration of stomach contents.
- *Increased intraocular pressure:* Fasciculations of the extraocular muscles can cause increased pressure in the globe. The injured eye may not tolerate increases in pressure. After succinylcholine administration, intraocular pressure increases within 60 seconds, peaks at 2 to 3 minutes, and decreases to baseline at 5 to 7 minutes.
- *Malignant hyperthermia:* Succinylcholine is a known trigger agent for malignant hyperthermia and should be avoided in all patients with a known or suspected familial malignant hyperthermia history.
- *Increased intracranial pressure:* Succinylcholine increases intracranial pressure, electroencephalogram activity, and cerebral blood flow. The increase in intracranial pressure secondary to laryngoscopy is greater than that seen with succinylcholine administration.

16. If there are so many undesired side effects, why is succinylcholine still used?

Despite unpleasant side effects, succinylcholine has remained a steadfast member of the airway management arsenal for more than 50 years. An appreciation for the historical discovery of complications may shed light on the apparent "comfort" of so many practitioners with succinylcholine. Complications from succinylcholine were noted gradually, allowing anesthesia providers to become familiar with the causes and treatment of each complication. Succinylcholine comes closest to meeting the criteria of the ideal muscle relaxant (i.e., it has a specific route of action, has a rapid onset of action, is easily titrated, exhibits a wide margin of safety between muscle relaxation and respiratory arrest, and allows a rapid rate of recovery). Despite the cited side effects, it remains cost-effective.

The longevity of succinylcholine is probably due to its favorable pharmacokinetics, gradual appreciation of known complications, and cost considerations. Succinylcholine can cost as little as 19¢ compared with rocuronium, which can cost more than $3 per vial.

17. State the primary indications for succinylcholine.

Succinylcholine is indicated in circumstances in which rapid airway control is needed. Patients with a full stomach, parturients, obese patients, patients presenting with nausea, patients with a hiatal hernia or uncontrolled reflux, and patients with impaired airway reflexes may be candidates for succinylcholine.

18. List the absolute contraindications to succinylcholine.

- Known or suspected history of malignant hyperthermia
- Prolonged bed rest
- Crush injuries
- Burn injury
- Spinal cord injury
- Stroke
- Hyperkalemia

19. Is succinylcholine indicated for pediatric general anesthesia?

Most anesthetists avoid succinylcholine in pediatric patients. Reports of cardiac arrest after administration of succinylcholine in some pediatric patients led to recommendations to avoid succinylcholine as an elective muscle relaxant in this patient group. Succinylcholine may be used under emergent conditions, such as laryngospasm. One tenth of an intubating dose intravenously or 4 to 5 mg/kg intramuscularly is usually effective. If intravenous succinylcholine is indicated in a pediatric patient, atropine, 20 mcg/kg intravenously, should be given before succinylcholine administration to prevent bradycardia. Intramuscular atropine also should be given with intramuscular succinylcholine when this route is the only one available.

20. Explain the pharmacodynamic action of nondepolarizing agents.

Nondepolarizing drugs also bind to ACh receptors on the motor end plate. In contrast to succinylcholine, however, they are unable to activate the receptors and do not facilitate depolarization of muscle fiber membrane. This mechanism of action classifies them as competitive antagonists at the NMJ.

21. How are nondepolarizing muscle blockers metabolized?

Metabolism of nondepolarizing muscle blocking agents depends primarily on redistribution, metabolism, and excretion (see the table on page 109).

22. Name common side effects of the nondepolarizing benzylisoquiniliniums.

Atracurium and mivacurium can cause histamine release, which can precipitate bronchospasm and hypotension. D-tubocurarine and metocurine cause even greater histamine release, but they are seldom used in current practice.

Metabolism of Nondepolarizing Muscle Blockers Agents

Drug	Metabolism	Excretion
Pancuronim, doxacurium, pipecuronium	Negligible	Renal
Vecuronium	Liver	Renal, bile
Atracurium	Hoffman elimination, non-specific esterases	Bile, renal (laudanosine)
Cisatracurium	Hoffman elimination	Bile, renal (laudanosine)
Rocuronium	Liver	Bile, renal
Mivacurium	Plasma cholinesterase	Renal (minor)

23. **Name common side effects of the nondepolarizing aminosteroids.**

    Pancuronium shows vagolytic effects at an intubating dose, resulting in significant tachycardia. Rocuronium also may transiently increase the heart rate after higher (1 to 1.2 mg/kg intravenously) doses. Vecuronium has no significant vagolytic properties.

24. **List some medications administered in the perioperative period that potentiate nondepolarizing blockade.**

    - Aminoglycosides (amikacin, gentamicin, kanamycin, streptomycin, tobramycin)
    - Antiarrhythmics (lidocaine, calcium channel blockers, procainamide)
    - Polypeptides (polymyxin B, polymyxin E)
    - Tetracyclines
    - Volatile agents
    - Local anesthetics
    - Magnesium sulfate
    - Diuretics
    - Lithium
    - Cyclosporine

25. **What are some other perioperative conditions that may affect the pharmacodynamics of neuromuscular blockade?**

    - Hypothermia prolongs muscle blockade by decreasing hepatic, biliary, and renal blood flow. Hypothermia also prolongs the duration of atracurium by impairing temperature-dependent Hoffman elimination. Hypokalemia, hypocalcemia, and hypermagnesemia can prolong muscle blockade.
    - Differentiation between a priming dose and a defasciculating dose of a nondepolarizing muscle blocker needs to be done.

- A priming dose is used to accelerate the onset of a nondepolarizing muscle relaxant. Generally, one tenth of the intubating dose of a nondepolarizer is administered 3 to 4 minutes before the remaining intubation dose. Some patients may become weak, dysphagic, or apneic after the priming dose, and immediate airway control should be available.
- A defasciculating dose is one tenth of an intubating dose of a nondepolarizer, administered 1 to 3 minutes before succinylcholine is given. The occupation of some ACh receptors by the nondepolaring relaxant may prevent succinylcholine-induced fasciculations.

26. What is laudanosine?

Laudanosine is the metabolite of atracurium and cisatracurium degradation from Hoffman elimination. Laudanosine peaks at 2 minutes after intravenous administration, and it is cleared by the liver. Animal studies revealed central nervous system stimulant effects of laudanosine, which caused epileptic activity and seizures. However, human peak plasma levels are 20 times less than the levels tested in animals.

27. With the availability of rocuronium for rapid-sequence induction, why do some surveys show that succinylcholine is still used three times as frequently?

Anesthesia delivery is a diverse and controversial practice. Whether rocuronium or succinylcholine is chosen for rapid-sequence induction is based partly on preference, past training, and experience. Some studies have shown no significant difference in onset and laryngeal relaxation between rocuronium and succinylcholine. Electromyography studies at the adductor laryngeal muscles have shown, however, a faster onset of laryngeal muscle relaxation (and quicker ideal intubating conditions) with succinylcholine (1.5 mg/kg intravenously) than with rocuronium (0.6 to 0.9 mg/kg intravenously). Additionally, the duration of action with rocuronium may be unacceptable in the event of a difficult airway.

 Key Points

- In 1942, curare was introduced into anesthesia practice for muscle relaxation.
- The point at which a motor nerve fiber meets a skeletal muscle fiber is termed the *neuromuscular junction.*
- ACh is synthesized in the nerve endings of cholinergic nerve fibers from acetyl coenzyme A and choline.
- ACh is rapidly hydrolyzed by the enzyme acetylcholinesterase into choline and acetate.
- The two classes of neuromuscular blocking agents are the nondepolarizing agents and the depolarizing agents.

Key Points   *continued*

- Nondepolarizing agents are quaternary compounds that are classified further into aminosteroids or benzylisoquinoliniums.
- Depolarizing agents are quaternary compounds and include the drug succinylcholine.
- Plasma cholinesterase is an enzyme that hydrolyzes succinylcholine.
- The dibucaine number is a test for atypical plasma cholinesterase.
- Phase II block is a protracted succinylcholine-induced muscle paralysis that resembles a nondepolarizing blockade.
- Side effects of succinylcholine include bradycardia, myalgia, hyperkalemia, increased gastric pressure, increased intraocular pressure, increased intracranial pressure, and malignant hyperthermia.
- Succinylcholine is indicated in circumstances in which rapid airway control is needed.
- Absolute contraindications to succinylcholine are known malignant hyperthermia, crush injuries, burn injury, spinal cord injury, stroke, and hyperkalemia.
- Nondepolarizing drugs are competitive antagonists at the NMJ.
- The benzylisoquinoliniums, atracurium, mivacurium, D-tubocurarine, and metocurine, cause histamine release.
- Nondepolarizing muscle relaxants are potentiated by aminoglycosides, antiarrhythmics, polypeptides, tetracyclines, volatile agents, local anesthetics, magnesium sulfate, diuretics, lithium, and cyclosporine.
- A priming dose is used to accelerate the onset of a nondepolarizing muscle relaxant.
- A defasciculating dose is one tenth of an intubating dose of a nondepolarizer.

Internet Resources

Anesthesia Pharmacology:
http://www.anesthesia2001.com/

Virtual Anaesthesia Textbook:
http://www.virtual-anaesthesia-textbook.com/

Anesthesiology INFO: Intravenous Anesthetics: Muscle Relaxants:
http://anesthesiologyinfo.com/articles/01072002d.php

GasNet Search: Anesthesia and Muscle Relaxants:
http://gasnet.med.yale.edu/about/search.php?p1=anesthesia+and+muscle+relaxants

Bibliography

Cook DR: Can succinylcholine be abandoned? *Anesth Analg* 90:S24-S28, 2000.

Dexter F, et al: Cost identification analysis for succinylcholine, *Anesth Analg* 92:693-699, 2001.

Donnelly AJ, et al: *Anesthesiology and critical care handbook,* ed 3, Cleveland, 2001, Lexi-comp, pp 1120-1124.

Guyton AC: Excitation of skeletal muscle: neuromuscular transmission and excitation-contraction coupling. In: *Medical physiology,* ed 10, Philadelphia, 2000, WB Saunders, pp 80-82.

Katz RL: Succinylcholine: its past, present, and future. In *Muscle relaxants: basic and clinical aspects,* Orlando, 1985, Grune & Stratton, pp 69-85.

Laurin EG, et al: A comparison of succinylcholine and rocuronium for rapid-sequence intubation of emergency department patients, *Acad Emerg Med* 7:1362-1369, 2000.

Maged S, Morgan GE, Mikhail MS: Muscle relaxants. In *Clinical anesthesiology,* ed 3, Stamford, 2001, Appleton & Lange, pp 149-164.

O'Flynn RP, et al: Masseter muscle rigidity and malignant hyperthermia susceptibility in pediatric patients: an update on management and diagnosis, *Anesthesiology* 80:1228-1233, 1994.

Stoelting RK: Neuromuscular-blocking drugs. In *Pharmacology and physiology in anesthetic practice,* ed 3, Philadelphia, 1998, Lippincott Williams & Wilkins, pp 182-223.

Wimberly JS: Neuromuscular blockade. In Hurford WE, et al, editors: *Clinical anesthesia procedures of the Massachusetts General Hospital,* ed 6, Philadelphia, 2002, Lippincott Williams & Wilkins, pp 181-203.

Cholinesterase Inhibitors and Anticholinergic Drugs

James B. Hicks

1. Cholinesterase inhibitors act on which type of receptors?

Primarily, cholinesterase inhibitors act on *nicotinic receptors.* Secondarily, they act on *muscarinic receptors.*

2. How do cholinesterase inhibitors reverse the effects of nondepolarizing muscle relaxants?

Cholinesterase inhibitors block the activity of acetylcholinesterase, leading to an increased level of acetylcholine at the neuromuscular junction (NMJ). The overabundance of acetylcholine at the NMJ competes with the nondepolarizing muscle relaxant and displaces it from the receptor site, allowing the receptor to respond to acetylcholine.

3. Can the practitioner effectively reverse a neuromuscular blockade at any time with cholinesterase inhibitors?

No. A peripheral nerve stimulator should always be used when administering muscle relaxants. If there is no detectable twitch, reversal of neuromuscular blockade should not be attempted.

4. Outline features of the cholinesterase inhibitors and anticholinergic drugs that are used for reversal of neuromuscular blockade.

Common reversal agents are outlined in the following table.

Common Reversal Agents for Neuromuscular Blockade			
	Edrophonium	**Neostigmine**	**Pyridostigmine**
Reversal dose (mg/kg)	0.5–1	0.06	0.25
Maximum dose (mg)	40	5	30
Speed of onset (min)	<1	<3	2–5
Duration (min)	5–20	40–60	90
Dose of atropine (mcg/kg)	15	15	15
Dose of glycopyrrolate (mcg/kg)	Not recommended	7	7

5. Why is the administration of glycopyrrolate with edrophonium not recommended?

Edrophonium has a more rapid onset of action than glycopyrrolate. The muscarinic effects of edrophonium occur before glycopyrrolate can block them. *Atropine* has an onset time more similar to edrophonium. It is a better choice to offset the muscarinic effects of edrophonium.

6. Why are cholinesterase inhibitors useful in the treatment of myasthenia gravis?

Myasthenia gravis is a disorder of skeletal muscle weakness that results from a decreased number of acetylcholine receptors at the NMJ. Cholinesterase inhibitors stop the activity of acetylcholinesterase, leading to an increase of acetylcholine at the NMJ. Neostigmine and pyridostigmine are the most common cholinesterase inhibitors used in the treatment of myasthenia gravis.

7. Anticholinergic drugs act on which type of receptors?

Anticholinergic drugs act on *muscarinic receptors.*

8. Why should the anesthetist administer cholinesterase inhibitors and anticholinergics together?

Cholinesterase inhibitors produce an effect on muscarinic and nicotinic receptors. The muscarinic effects include excessive salivation, bradycardia, and bronchial constriction. Concurrent use of anticholinergic drugs with cholinesterase inhibitors decreases or prevents the undesirable muscarinic effects that occur when cholinesterase inhibitors are administered alone.

9. Describe central anticholinergic syndrome.

- *Red as a beet* refers to atropine flush, which is due to dilation of cutaneous blood vessels.
- *Wild as a hare* refers to central nervous system stimulation. Stimulation may present as agitation, excitation, restlessness, or hallucinations.
- *Dry as a bone* refers to the antisialagogue effect associated with anticholinergic drugs, drying respiratory tract secretions from the nose to the mucosa.

Other signs and symptoms include atropine fever (inhibition of sweat glands leading to a rise in body temperature) and impaired vision (inhibition of near vision and promotion of pupillary dilation).

10. Discuss anticholinesterase medications that can cause central anticholinergic syndrome.

Scopolamine is the most likely anticholinergic drug to cause central anticholinergic syndrome. *Atropine* produces the syndrome but to a lesser extent than scopolamine. Both drugs are tertiary amines and are able to cross the blood-brain barrier. Scopolamine is approximately eight times more potent than atropine in regard to its effects on the central nervous system. Glycopyrrolate does not cause central anticholinergic syndrome because it is a synthetic quaternary ammonium compound and is unable to cross the blood-brain barrier.

11. Which drug effectively treats central anticholinergic syndrome?

Physostigmine is a tertiary amine cholinesterase inhibitor and crosses the blood-brain barrier. Intravenous physostigmine may be administered at a dose of 10 to 30 mcg/kg and given 1 mg/min.

12. Which anticholinergic drug would be the best choice as a preoperative medication to dry oral secretions?

Scopolamine has the best antisialagogue effect compared with atropine and glycopyrrolate. Scopolamine also produces the most sedation. Glycopyrrolate is the best choice when the practitioner desires the antisialagogue effect without sedation.

Key Points

- Cholinesterase inhibitors act on nicotinic and muscarinic receptors.
- Cholinesterase inhibitors block the activity of acetylcholinesterase, leading to an increased level of acetylcholine at the NMJ.
- If there is no detectable twitch, reversal of neuromuscular blockade should not be attempted.
- Atropine, not glycopyrrolate, should be used with edrophonium to reverse neuromuscular block.
- Cholinesterase inhibitors are useful in the treatment of myasthenia gravis.
- Anticholinergic drugs act on muscarinic receptors.
- Use of anticholinergic drugs with cholinesterase inhibitors decreases or prevents the undesirable muscarinic effects that occur when cholinesterase inhibitors are administered alone.
- Central anticholinergic syndrome is characterized by flushing, central nervous system stimulation, severe dryness in the respiratory tract, increased body temperature, and impaired vision.
- Scopolamine is the most likely anticholinergic drug to cause central anticholinergic syndrome.
- Physostigmine is a tertiary amine cholinesterase inhibitor and is the treatment for central anticholinergic syndrome
- Scopolamine has the best antisialagogue effect compared with atropine and glycopyrrolate. Scopolamine also produces the most sedation. Glycopyrrolate is the best choice when the practitioner desires the antisialagogue effect without sedation.

Internet Resources

Anesthesia Pharmacology:
http://www.anesthesia2001.com/

Virtual Anaesthesia Textbook:
http://www.virtual-anaesthesia-textbook.com/

GasNet:
http://www.gasnet.org/

Update in Anaesthesia Issue Index:
http://www.nda.ox.ac.uk/wfsa/html/pages/up_issu.htm#1

Bibliography

Morgan GE Jr, Mikhail MS, Murray MJ: *Clinical anesthesiology*, ed 3, New York, 2002, Lange Medical Books/McGraw-Hill, pp 199-211.

Omoigui S: *Anesthesia drugs handbook,* ed 3, Massachusetts, 1999, Blackwell Science, Malden, MA.

Stoelting RK, Dierdorf SF: *Anesthesia and co-existing disease,* ed 4, New York, 2002, Churchill Livingstone, pp 505-550.

Stoelting RK, Miller RD: *Basics of anesthesia,* ed 4, Philadelphia, 2000, Churchill Livingstone, pp 104-105.

Inotropic and Vasoactive Drugs

Tim Palmer

1. How are adrenergic receptors classified, and what are their physiologic functions?

The major adrenergic receptor types are *alpha, beta,* and *dopaminergic.* Two types of *alpha receptors* have clinical importance—alpha$_1$ and alpha$_2$. Alpha$_1$-receptor stimulation results in mydriasis, relaxation of gastrointestinal smooth muscle, increased gastrointestinal and bladder sphincter tone, increased sweating and salivation, and vasoconstriction. Alpha$_2$ receptors reside presynaptically and postsynaptically. Presynaptic alpha$_2$-receptor stimulation promotes platelet aggregation and suppression of insulin and renin release. Alpha$_2$-receptor stimulation hyperpolarizes neurons, reducing anesthetic requirements.

Beta receptors are postsynaptic. Beta$_1$ stimulation affects primarily the heart and results in increased heart rate, contractility, automaticity, and conduction velocity. Beta$_2$-receptor stimulation produces increased renin and insulin secretion, lipolysis, glycogenolysis, and smooth muscle relaxation (bronchodilation, uterine relaxation, peripheral vasodilation, gastrointestinal and bladder relaxation). Beta$_2$-receptor stimulation also promotes intracellular movement of potassium.

Dopamine, a precursor of norepinephrine, is a central nervous system and peripheral nervous system neurotransmitter. Two major *dopaminergic* subtypes have been defined—D$_1$ and D$_2$. D$_1$ receptors are postsynaptic and found in the smooth muscle of the renal, mesenteric, cerebral, and coronary vasculature. D$_2$ receptors are presynaptic and when stimulated suppress norepinephrine release. Stimulation of D$_1$ and D$_2$ receptors results in vasodilation. The table on page 118 outlines the use of common sympathomimetics for acute cardiac failure.

2. Define inotropicity, chronotropicity, dromotropicity, and lusitropicity.

- *Inotropicity* refers to the intrinsic myocardial strength of contraction.
- *Chronotropicity* is the rate of cardiac contraction.
- *Dromotropicity* refers to the rate of electrical impulse conduction to the contractile elements.
- *Lusitropicity* describes the degree or effectiveness of diastolic function.

Sympathomimetic Inotropes for Acute Cardiac Failure Therapy

Drugs and Mediating Receptors	Dobutamine ($\beta_1 > \beta_2 > \alpha$)	Dopamine (Dopaminergic > β; High Dose α)	Norepinephrine ($\beta_1 > \alpha > \beta_2$)	Epinephrine ($\beta_1 = \beta_2 > \alpha$)	Isoproterenol ($\beta_2 > \beta_1$)	Amrinone (PDE Inhibitor)	Milrinone (PDE Inhibitor)	Phenylephrine (α-Agonist)
Dose infusion (mcg/kg/min)	2–15	2–5 renal effect 5–10 inotropic 10–20 SVR ↑	0.01–0.03; maximum 0.1	0.01–0.03; maximum 0.1–0.3	0.01–0.1	Bolus 750 (3 min) Drip 2–10	Bolus 50–75 (10 min) Drip 0.375–0.75	0.2–0.3
Elimination half-life (min)	2.4	2.0	3.0	2.0	2.0	240*	150*	20
Inotropic effect	↑↑	↑↑	↑	↑↑	↑↑↑	↑	↑	0
Arteriolar vasodilation	↑	↑↑	0	↑	↑	↑↑	↑↑	→
Vasoconstriction	HD↑	HD↑↑	↑↑	HD↑	0	0	0	↑↑↑
Chronotropic effect	↑	0, ↑	↑	↑↑	↑↑↑	0	0	0
Blood pressure effect	↑	DH↑	↑	0, ↑	↑	↑	→	↑↑↑
Diuretic effect (direct)	0	↑↑	↑	0	0	0	0	0
Arrhythmia risk	↑↑	HD↑	↑	↑↑↑	↑↑↑	↑↑	↑	0

* Note duration of action of milrinone is 3–5 hours versus amrinone; 30–120 minutes.
↑, Increase; 0, ro change, ↓, decrease.
HD, high dose; PDE, phosphodiesterase; SVR, systemic vascular resistance.
From Opie L: Drugs for the heart, ed 5, Philadelphia, 2001, WB Saunders.

3. What is the second messenger system associated with beta-adrenergic stimulation?

Adrenergic receptor occupation stimulates regulatory proteins, called *G proteins*, which activate the enzyme adenyl cyclase. Adenyl cyclase catalyzes the conversion of adenosine triphospate (ATP) to cyclic adenosine monophosphate (cAMP), the second messenger. Phosphodiesterase (PDE) III catalyzes the breakdown of cAMP.

4. Define sympathomimetic and sympatholytic. What is meant by indirect sympathomimetic activity?

A *sympathomimetic agent* is one that elicits an autonomic sympathetic response similar to stimulation of the receptor by a natural catecholamine. A *sympatholytic agent* is one that blocks a response that would normally result from receptor stimulation by a natural catecholamine.

An *indirect-acting sympathomimetic agent* evokes release of norepinephrine into the synaptic cleft. A direct-acting sympathomimetic activates the receptor directly. Indirect-acting sympathomimetic agents typically show alpha and beta activity. These agents include ephedrine, mephentermine, and metaraminol. Ephedrine, at titrated doses of 5 to 25 mg intravenously in adults, is used to treat hypotension from regional blockade and other anesthetic agents.

5. Explain the mechanism of action of angiotensin-converting enzyme (ACE) inhibitors.

ACE inhibitors interfere with the conversion of angiotensin I to angiotensin II. Angiotensin II causes vasoconstriction and sodium retention (by increasing aldosterone release). By inhibiting the formation of angiotensin II, ACE inhibitors produce vasodilation and effectively lower the blood pressure. Fibrosis and myocardial hypertrophy imposed on the ventricular architecture due to chronic increased afterload also are attenuated. ACE inhibitors are effective agents in the treatment of hypertension and acute and chronic heart failure. Enalapril (Vasotec) is an ACE inhibitor that is available parenterally. A typical dose of enalapril is 0.625 to 1.25 mg intravenously over 10 minutes. Response time usually is within 15 minutes, and the duration of action is 4 to 6 hours. Side effects of ACE inhibitors include hypotension, hyperkalemia, and cough. Oral preparations of ACE inhibitors include captopril (Capoten), fosinopril (Monopril), and lisinopril (Zestril, Prinivil).

6. What is the mechanism of action of epinephrine, and how is it used clinically?

Epinephrine is an endogenous catecholamine released from the adrenal medulla. It directly stimulates alpha and beta receptors. Effects of epinephrine include increased heart rate, enhanced myocardial contractility, vascular and smooth muscle constriction, glandular secretion, glycogenolysis, and lipolysis. Epinephrine

is 2 to 10 times more potent at the beta receptor than norepinephrine. As a clinical preparation, effects of epinephrine are dose dependent, as follows:
- 0.03 mcg/kg/min (pure beta)
- 0.15 mcg/kg/min (mixed alpha and beta)
- Greater than 0.15 mcg/kg/min (pure alpha)

The increased heart rate observed with epinephrine is due largely to increased phase IV depolarization, which may precipitate dysrhythmias. Systolic time is shortened more than diastolic time, enhancing coronary blood flow. In the intermediate dosing range, intense vasoconstriction (alpha effect) is offset by beta receptor–mediated vasodilation; systemic vascular resistance (SVR) remains stable or may be slightly decreased. At higher dosing schedules, mesenteric and renal arterial vasoconstriction may occur.

7. Describe the actions of norepinephrine.

Norepinephrine is a natural catecholamine and the primary postganglionic sympathetic neurotransmitter. It is a molecular precursor of epinephrine. Clinically, norepinephrine produces vasoconstriction, with marked increases in SVR and mean arterial pressure and compensatory bradycardia. Renal and mesenteric vessels are affected.

A standard preparation is 4 mg in 250 mL of intravenous solution. Infusion generally is initiated at 0.01 to 1.0 mcg/kg/min. Onset time is immediate, and duration of action is short (minutes). Norepinephrine is indicated for aggressive maintenance of SVR and systemic blood pressure in states of critical physiologic decompensation (e.g., shock, sepsis) (see the figure on page 121). It also is used during weaning from cardiopulmonary bypass.

Norepinephrine can precipitate congestive heart failure and angina in a patient with a susceptible myocardium. It should be administered only via a central line because extravasation from a peripheral vein causes localized tissue necrosis.

8. What is the action of phenylephrine, and how is it used clinically?

Phenylephrine is an alpha-receptor agonist and potent vasoconstrictor. Intravenous administration produces abrupt increases in mean arterial pressure and SVR. In the presence of an intact baroreceptor reflex, bradycardia may occur.

The usual concentration for infusion is 10 mg/250 mL (40 mcg/mL); it is initiated at 0.2 to 0.3 mcg/kg/min. Bolus doses of 20 to 40 mcg commonly are used to treat episodes of intraoperative hypotension. Onset is immediate, and the elimination half-life is 20 minutes. Phenylephrine is not indicated for treatment of hypotension in parturients (uterine vasoconstriction), in patients with congestive heart failure, in patients with renal insufficiency (renal artery vasoconstriction), and in patients with an internal mammary coronary artery bypass graft (vasoconstriction).

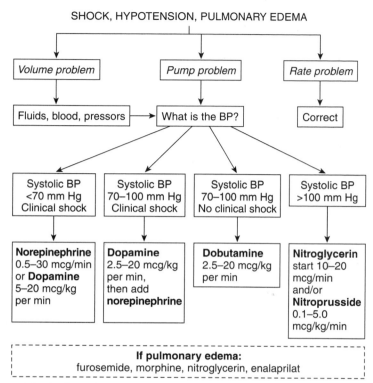

SHOCK, HYPOTENSION, PULMONARY EDEMA

| Volume problem | Pump problem | Rate problem |

| Fluids, blood, pressors | → | What is the BP? | | Correct |

| Systolic BP <70 mm Hg Clinical shock | Systolic BP 70–100 mm Hg Clinical shock | Systolic BP 70–100 mm Hg No clinical shock | Systolic BP >100 mm Hg |

| **Norepinephrine** 0.5–30 mcg/min or **Dopamine** 5–20 mcg/kg per min | **Dopamine** 2.5–20 mcg/kg per min, then add **norepinephrine** | **Dobutamine** 2.5–20 mcg/kg per min | **Nitroglycerin** start 10–20 mcg/min and/or **Nitroprusside** 0.1–5.0 mcg/kg/min |

If pulmonary edema:
furosemide, morphine, nitroglycerin, enalaprilat

Algorithm for shock, hypotension, and acute pulmonary edema. Note the important role of clinical judgment decision making in management. For details of this approach, see the statement of the American Heart Association Emergency Cardiac Care Committee, *Journal of the American Medical Association* 268:2199-2241, 1992. *(From Opie L: Drugs for the heart, ed 5, Philadelphia, 2001, WB Saunders.)*

9. Describe the clinical uses of intravenous dopamine.

Dopamine is used for its positive inotropic effects, to support systemic blood pressure, and to promote mesenteric and renal perfusion. Dopamine exhibits dose-dependent, receptor-mediated responses, as follows:
- 2 to 5 mcg/kg/min: primarily dopaminergic receptor stimulation with minor beta-receptor activity
- 5 to 10 mcg/kg/min: predominantly beta-receptor activity with some minor alpha-receptor stimulation
- Greater than 10 mcg/kg/min: predominantly alpha-receptor activity; effect similar to that seen with norepinephrine

Side effects of dopamine infusion include hypokalemia and supraventricular and ventricular arrhythmias. Low-dose, prophylactic infusion of dopamine ("renal dopamine") traditionally has been used in perioperative renal preservation strategies, particularly during aortic cross-clamping, during cardiopulmonary bypass, and in patients at high risk for sustaining an intraoperative renal insult. The efficacy of "renal dose" dopamine has been called into question. Current strategies for renal protection emphasize combination therapy and include optimizing renal oxygen delivery (cardiac output), suppressing reflex vasoconstriction (intravenous hydration), and use of osmotic diuretics, calcium channel blockers, ACE inhibitors, and dopaminergic agents.

10. Name and describe two dopaminergic agents currently available.

Fenoldopam is a selective D_1 agonist that produces dopaminergic receptor–mediated vasodilation. It is relatively devoid of alpha adrenergic–mediated vasoconstrictive or central nervous system effects. It has a rapid onset and offset when administered intravenously at 0.1 to 0.5 mcg/kg/min. It induces significant diuresis and natriuresis.

Dopexamine is a synthetic analogue of dopamine with potent D_2 and $beta_2$ receptor agonist activity. Dopexamine also inhibits presynaptic reuptake of norepinephrine. In general, dopexamine reduces cardiac afterload and promotes renal and splanchnic blood flow. In contrast to dopamine, there is minimal activity at the $beta_1$ receptor and no alpha agonist activity. Dopexamine has been shown to increase inotropicity and vasodilation with a modest increase in heart rate. Left and right ventricular afterload is reduced, and augmented renal blood flow is seen with doses of 1 to 5 mcg/kg/min. Infusion rates greater than 4 mcg/kg/min may result in tachycardia.

11. Describe the mechanisms of action of dobutamine.

Dobutamine is a synthetic sympathomimetic amine and potent beta-receptor agonist. It increases cardiac contractility and heart rate in a dose-dependent manner. Dobutamine may offer the same beneficial inotropic effects as dopamine without the tendency for peripheral vasoconstriction.

The recommended infusion range is 2 to 20 mcg/kg/min. Its half-life is short (2 minutes). Potential side effects include decreased mean arterial pressure due to excessive vasodilation, ventricular ectopy, and increased myocardial oxygen consumption secondary to tachycardia.

12. Discuss important perioperative considerations for the patient taking digoxin.

Digitalis preparations increase myocardial contractility; increase automaticity and excitability of the atria and ventricles; and decrease conduction velocity in the atria, ventricles, and atrioventricular node. These drugs have a narrow therapeutic index. An accepted normal plasma digoxin level (adult) is 1 to 2 ng/mL. Significant signs and symptoms of digitalis toxicity include nausea and vomiting, fatigue, confusion, malaise, arrhythmias, atrioventricular block, and sinus bradycardia. Hypokalemia, hypercalcemia, and hypomagnesemia sensitize the myocardium to side effects of digitalis. Elderly patients, patients with underlying cardiac disease, and patients with renal failure are at increased risk for digitalis toxicity.

13. What role do PDE III inhibitors play in the management of heart failure?

PDE III inhibitors produce inodilation, concurrent inotropicity, and vasodilation. The breakdown of cAMP in cardiac and smooth muscle is inhibited by PDE III inhibitors. Increased cAMP results in augmented myocardial contractility and arterial and venous dilation. These agents have become valuable adjuncts in the acute management of heart failure, particularly in the setting of receptor desensitivity, which may occur with chronic heart failure, with chronic beta-receptor blockade, and post cardiopulmonary bypass.

14. What PDE III inhibitors are currently available?

Amrinone and *milrinone* are PDE III inhibitors that are available for clinical use. In moderate doses, both drugs increase cardiac output, decrease peripheral vascular resistance, and decrease preload. Milrinone is more stable in solution and relatively devoid of the thrombocytopenia-inducing activity associated with amrinone. Milrinone has largely superseded its predecessor amrinone in clinical utility. Milrinone is administered intravenously initially as a bolus (50 mcg/kg over 10 minutes) followed by a titratable infusion (0.375 to 0.75 mcg/kg/min). Hypotension associated with milrinone infusion may require the concurrent infusion of a peripheral vasoconstrictor, such as norepinephrine, phenylephrine, or vasopressin.

15. Describe the vasodilatory effects of nitrates.

The formation of nitric oxide in the vessel wall accounts for the vasodilatory activity of nitrates. Nitrates produce vasodilation in the coronary and the peripheral circulation, which accounts for their use as antianginal and antihypertensive agents.

16. Differentiate between nitroglycerin and nitroprusside in terms of effect, dose, and utility.

At the lower dose range (0.5 to 2 mcg/kg/min), nitroglycerin dilates the capacitance (venous) circulation, decreasing preload and reducing myocardial wall stress. Coronary blood flow also is enhanced. At higher doses (5 to 10 mcg/kg/min), nitroglycerin exerts effects on the resistance (arterial) circulation, affecting afterload.

Within a normal dose range (<2 mcg/kg/min), nitroprusside affects resistance and capacitance vessels, but has a more profound effect on resistance vessels. Nitroprusside should be avoided in patients with ischemic heart disease because of a "steal" phenomenon it may induce.

17. List and describe precautions associated with the use of intravenous nitroglycerin and nitroprusside perioperatively.

Marked hypotension and baroreceptor-mediated tachycardia may be associated with nitroprusside and nitroglycerin. High-dose nitroglycerin may result in heparin resistance. Nitroprusside is associated with cyanide toxicity, particularly at higher doses over prolonged periods (>10 mcg/kg/min over 10 minutes). Manifestations of cyanide toxicity include tachycardia, convulsions, coma, cardiovascular instability, and metabolic acidosis. Because of the need for continuous monitoring, light sensitivity, and risk of cyanide toxicity, nitroprusside is being largely replaced in the management of acute heart failure by inodilators, such as milrinone, and in hypertensive crises by calcium channel blockers, ACE inhibitors, and dopaminergic agonists.

18. Describe the actions of calcium channel blockers.

Calcium channel blockers reduce the entry of calcium into cardiac and vascular smooth muscle. The result is a reduction in cardiac contractility and vascular tone. Intracardiac electrical conduction also is slowed due to the blockade of Ca^{2+} influx into sinoatrial and atrioventricular nodes during phase II of the cardiac action potential.

19. What other cardiovascular effects do calcium channel blockers possess?

Calcium channel blockers are antidysrhythmic and antianginal. Verapamil and diltiazem are examples of calcium channel blockers with antidysrhythmic properties through inhibition of atrioventricular nodal activity. Other calcium channel blockers exert significant vasodilatory activity (e.g., nicardipine, nifedipine, felodipine) and are used primarily in the management of hypertension or, in the case of nicardipine, cerebral artery vasospasm.

20. Identify contraindications to verapamil or diltiazem.

Verapamil and diltiazem are contraindicated in patients with sick sinus syndrome, ventricular tachycardia, and digitalis toxicity and patients with a history of Wolff-Parkinson-White syndrome. Caution also is advised in patients receiving beta-adrenergic blockers.

21. Describe the use of intravenous calcium as an inotropic agent.

Intravenous administration of calcium increases SVR and mean arterial pressure. Cardiac contractility may be transiently increased in some patients.

22. What is the mechanism of action of hydralazine?

Hydralazine is a direct-acting arterial smooth muscle relaxant. Onset after an intravenous dose is 15 minutes, and duration is 3 to 4 hours. Hydralazine may be used to treat intraoperative hypertension with titratable adult doses of 10 to 40 mg.

23. Describe the mechanism of action of labetalol. How is it administered?

Labetalol (Trandate, Normodyne) is a rapid-acting antihypertensive agent with alpha and beta adrenergic blocking capacity. The ratio of beta to alpha receptor blockade is 7:1. Labetalol should not be used in patients with bradydysrhythmias and heart block. The usual intravenous bolus dose in an adult is 2.5 to 10 mg titrated slowly.

24. What are indications for the use of esmolol, and how is it infused?

Esmolol is an ultrashort-acting intravenous beta adrenergic blocker with a half-life of 9 minutes. It is metabolized by nonspecific plasma esterases. Indications for its use are short-term management of sinus tachycardia, supraventricular tachycardia, and severe hypertension. This drug is attractive for its rapid on-off beta blockade capability. A typical infusion schedule is 500 mcg/kg bolus administered over 1 minute followed by an infusion of 50 mcg/kg/min.

 Key Points

- Adrenergic receptor types are alpha, beta, and dopaminergic.
- All three types of receptors are subdivided into two groups:
  - Alpha$_1$-receptor stimulation results in mydriasis, relaxation of gastrointestinal smooth muscle, increased gastrointestinal and bladder sphincter tone, increased sweating and salivation, and vasoconstriction.
  - Alpha$_2$ receptors reside presynaptically and postsynaptically. Presynaptic alpha$_2$-receptor stimulation promotes platelet aggregation and suppression of insulin and renin release and hyperpolarizing neurons, reducing anesthetic requirements.
  - Beta$_1$ stimulation affects primarily the heart and results in increased heart rate, contractility, automaticity, and conduction velocity.
  - Beta$_2$-receptor stimulation produces increased renin and insulin secretion, lipolysis, glycogenolysis, smooth muscle relaxation, and intracellular movement of potassium.
  - D$_2$-receptor stimulation suppresses norepinephrine release.
  - Stimulation of D$_1$ and D$_2$ receptors results in vasodilation.
- ACE inhibitors interfere with the conversion of angiotensin I to angiotensin II.
- ACE inhibitors produce vasodilation and effectively lower the blood pressure.
- Epinephrine is an endogenous catecholamine released from the adrenal medulla. It directly stimulates alpha and beta receptors.
- Norepinephrine is a molecular precursor of epinephrine and produces vasoconstriction, with marked increases in SVR and mean arterial pressure and compensatory bradycardia.
- Phenylephrine is an alpha receptor agonist and potent vasoconstrictor.
- Fenoldopam is a selective D$_1$ agonist that produces dopaminergic receptor–mediated vasodilation.

Continued

Key Points   *continued*

- Dopexamine is a synthetic analogue of dopamine that reduces cardiac afterload and promotes renal and splanchnic blood flow.
- Dobutamine is a synthetic sympathomimetic amine, and it increases cardiac contractility and heart rate in a dose-dependent manner.
- Digitalis preparations increase myocardial contractility, automaticity, and excitability of the atria and ventricles and decrease conduction velocity in the atria, ventricles, and atrioventricular node.
- PDE III inhibitors produce inodilation, concurrent inotropicity, and vasodilation.
- Amrinone and milrinone are PDE III inhibitors that are available for clinical use. Both drugs increase cardiac output, decrease peripheral vascular resistance, and decrease preload.
- The formation of nitric oxide in the vessel wall accounts for the vasodilatory activity of nitrates.
- Nitroglycerin dilates the capacitance (venous) circulation, decreasing preload and reducing myocardial wall stress. Coronary blood flow also is enhanced.
- Nitroprusside affects resistance and capacitance vessels, but has a more profound effect on resistance vessels.
- Calcium channel blockers reduce the entry of calcium into cardiac and vascular smooth muscle. The result is a reduction in cardiac contractility and vascular tone.
- Hydralazine is a direct-acting arterial smooth muscle relaxant.
- Labetalol is a rapid-acting antihypertensive agent with alpha and beta adrenergic blocking capacity.
- Esmolol is an ultrashort-acting intravenous beta adrenergic blocker.

Internet Resources

Anesthesia Pharmacology:
http://www.anesthesia2001.com/

Virtual Anaesthesia Textbook:
http://www.virtual-anaesthesia-textbook.com/

Nurse-Anesthesia.com:
http://www.nurse-anesthesia.com/

Anesthetist.com: Drugs and Volatiles:
http://www.anaesthetist.com/anaes/drugs/index.htm

Pharmacology 2000: Medical Pharmacology Chapters:
http://www.pharmacology2000.com/learning2.htm

Introduction to Autonomic Pharmacology:
http://www.harcourt-international.com/e-books/pdf/225.pdf

Adrenergic Pharmacology:
http://www.mc.uky.edu/pharmacology/instruction/pha824ar/PHA824ar.html

Bibliography

Bristow MR, Ginsburg R, Minobe W, et al: Decreased late catecholamine sensitivity and beta-adrenergic receptor density in failing human hearts, *N Engl J Med* 307:205-211, 1982.

Cummins RO, Hazinski MF, et al: Guidelines 2000 for cardiopulmonary resuscitation and emergency cardiovascular care, international consensus on science. *Circulation* 102(suppl): 1-11, 2000.

Hollenberg SM: Heart failure and cardiac pulmonary edema. In Albert RK, Dries DJ, Hall JB, et al, editors: *ACCP/SCCM combined critical care course,* Des Plaines, Ill., 2001, Society of Critical Care Medicine, pp 85-95.

Opie L: *Drugs for the heart,* ed 5, Philadelphia, 2001, WB Saunders.

Pagel PS, Grossman W, Hearing JM, et al: Left ventricular diastolic function in the normal and diseased heart (part one), *Anesthesiology* 79:836-854, 1993.

Pagel PS, Grossman W, Hearing JM, et al: Left ventricular diastolic function in the normal and diseased heart (part two), *Anesthesiology* 79:1104-1120, 1993.

Prielipp RC, McGregor DA, Butterworth JF IV, et al: Pharmacodynamics and pharmacokinetics of milrinone adminstration to increase oxygen delivery in critically ill patients, *Chest* 109:1291-1301, 1996.

Royster RL, Butterworth JF IV, Prough DS, et al: Preoperative and intraoperative predictors of inotropic support and long-term outcome in patients having coronary artery bypass grafting, *Anesth Analg* 72:729-736, 1991.

Wagoner LE, Walsh RA: Inotropic therapy for systolic heart failure, *Compr Ther* 21:367-377, 1995.

Local Anesthetics

John Nagelhout

1. How are the local anesthetics classified?

The local anesthetics are commonly classified two ways—by their *chemical structure* and by their *duration of action* (see the table below). These are both useful clinical categorizations because they convey important information about a particular drug's action.

Chemically the local anesthetics are divided into two groups based on the type of group present on the intermediate chain of the molecule: the esters and the amides. Membership in either of these two chemical groups yields significant clinical differences in pharmacologic action. The ester-type local anesthetics are metabolized more readily in the body by hydrolysis catalyzed by plasma cholinesterases. The amide-type drugs are broken down in the liver by cytochrome mixed-function oxidase enzymes. The ester-type drugs are safer in the sense that due to their rapid metabolism in plasma and tissue they are less likely to result in significant blood levels, which can lead to toxicity. The amides require hepatic extraction, however, and are more prone to high blood levels and toxicity. In addition, the esters tend to be shorter acting than the amides.

Local Anesthetic Classification

Drug Name	Chemical Class	Duration of Action
Cocaine	Ester	Short
Procaine (Novocaine)	Ester	Short
Chloroprocaine (Nesacaine)	Ester	Short
Tetracaine (Pontocaine, others)	Ester	Intermediate
Lidocaine (Xylocaine)	Amide	Intermediate
Articaine (Septocaine)	Amide	Intermediate
Mepivacaine (Carbocaine, Polocaine)	Amide	Intermediate
Levobupivacaine (Chirocaine)	Amide	Long
Etidocaine (Duranest)	Amide	Long
Ropivacaine (Naropin)	Amide	Long
Bupivacaine (Marcaine, Sensorcaine)	Amide	Long

The second classification according to the duration of action includes three subtypes:
• Short-acting drugs lasting approximately 30 to 60 minutes
• Intermediate-acting drugs lasting 60 to 120 minutes
• Long-acting drugs lasting 2 to 6 hours

The clinical duration can vary depending on the dose, site of injection, and addition of vasoconstrictors.

2. How do local anesthetics work?

Local anesthetics exert their action by blocking neuronal sodium channels. To reach their site of action, they require three characteristic properties. *First,* they must have a lipid-soluble or lipophilic portion of their chemical structure. *Second,* they must have a water-soluble or hydrophilic portion. These two portions of the molecule are separated by the *third* structural requirement, an intermediate ester or amide chain. When injected, the local anesthetic molecule, depending on its pK_a, proportions itself into ionized and nonionized fractions. The nonionized fraction is lipid soluble and passes through the neuronal cell membrane. When inside the nerve cell, the drug reequilibrates, and the ionized fraction is able to access the inside of the sodium channel and bind to the local anesthetic receptor. Blockade of the sodium channel inhibits the ability of the nerve to reach an action potential, rendering it reversibly blocked.

3. Discuss the properties of local anesthetic drugs that affect their clinical action.

Three drug properties influence a local anesthetic's effect:
• Lipid solubility
• Protein binding
• pK_a

Potency of a local anesthetic drug is directly related to its *lipid solubility*: the more lipid soluble, the more potent.

There is a relationship between a local anesthetic's ability to bind to plasma, nerve, and tissue proteins and clinical duration of action. The higher the degree of *protein binding* a local anesthetic exhibits, the longer the duration of action. Local anesthetics bind to a large extent to the plasma protein alpha$_1$-acid glycoprotein. Agents such as bupivacaine, etidocaine, ropivacaine, and levobupivacaine all are 95% to 99% protein bound and are long-acting drugs.

The *pK_a* relates to onset of action because it influences the amount of nonionized lipid-soluble fraction available to cross the nerve cell membrane and reach the local anesthetic receptor. The local anesthetics are basic compounds with pK_a values ranging from 7.5 to 9.3. The closer the individual drug's pK_a is to the physiologic pH 7.4, the higher the fraction of nonionized, lipid-soluble molecules, and the faster the onset of action. The exception to this pattern is chloroprocaine. Chloroprocaine has a high pK_a but the most rapid onset of action. This exception is likely due to the higher concentrations used clinically (see the following table).

Protein Binding and pK_a Values

Drug Name	Protein Binding (%)	pK_a (25° C)
Procaine (Novocaine)	6	9.05
Chloroprocaine (Nesacaine)	N/A	9.3
Tetracaine (Pontocaine, others)	75	8.46
Lidocaine (Xylocaine)	64	7.91
Mepivacaine (Carbocaine, Polocaine, others)	77	7.76
Levobupivacaine (Chirocaine)	97	8.09
Etidocaine (Duranest)	95	7.7
Ropivacaine (Naropin)	95	8.2
Bupivacaine (Marcaine, Sensorcaine)	96	8.16
Articaine (Septocaine)	60	7.8

4. Describe the effect of the addition of epinephrine to local anesthetic solutions.

Epinephrine is added to local anesthetics for several reasons. The addition of epinephrine and the attendant vasoconstriction reduce the speed of local anesthetic absorption away from the injection site area, reducing blood levels and toxicity. Reducing absorption from the injection site also results in a longer duration of action. Other epinephrine effects include a more rapid onset time (with the exception of spinal anesthesia) and increased degrees of sensory and motor blockade. Absorption of epinephrine can cause minor transient hypertension and tachycardia; concentrations should be monitored carefully.

5. Explain the factors surrounding allergic reactions to local anesthetic drugs.

The incidence of true allergy to local anesthetics is small. There is, however, a difference in the incidence of allergy between the two chemical types of local anesthetics. The ester-type drugs and their metabolites are implicated in true allergic reactions much more frequently than the amide-type drugs. Local anesthetic molecules are not antigenic; however, they can form haptens. Repeated exposure to a local anesthetic drug or similar compound may elicit an allergic reaction. There does not seem to be any cross-allergy between chemical classes. A patient who is allergic to an ester-type drug may receive an amide and vice versa. Another common issue regards the history of what commonly is referred to as "dentist allergy." This reaction occurs when a patient receives a local anesthetic containing epinephrine for a dental office procedure. Epinephrine absorption from the highly vascular oral mucosa produces transient restlessness, anxiety, and an overall jittery feeling; flushing; tachycardia; palpitations; and an increase in blood pressure. Patients may mistake this reaction for a local anesthetic allergy.

Skin testing, although not definitive, can be helpful when the diagnosis of a true local anesthetic allergy is clinically essential. Additives such as methylparaben and sodium metabisulfite also have been implicated in local anesthetic anaphylaxis.

6. How does cocaine differ from the other local anesthetics?

Cocaine was the first local anesthetic drug used clinically. Because of toxicities associated with its injection, its use is reserved for topical application. Cocaine differs from the other local anesthetics in that it is naturally occurring and promotes the blockade of the reuptake of norepinephrine. This blockade results in prolonged sympathomimetic responses, such as vasoconstriction, hypertension, tachycardia, arrhythmias, and euphoria.

7. What is the maximal safe dose for the local anesthetics in common use?

Limiting the total dose of local anesthetic injected is one of the hallmarks of safe practice. Adhering to an "upper safe dose," regardless of the type of block performed, lowers the risk that the rate of absorption from the injection area will result in systemic toxic blood levels. The rate of absorption is affected by the lipid solubility, protein binding, vascularity of the injection area, injection rate, and total dose. An exception occurs during tumescent anesthesia for liposuction, when large doses of dilute local anesthetics are used in the wetting solution. Techniques to minimize the possibility of inadvertent intravascular injection, such as frequent aspiration, intermittent slow injection, use of test doses, and addition of vasoconstrictors, are part of routine clinical practice. Exact maximal safe doses in humans are estimates; upper safe doses are given in the following table.

Maximal Safe Doses

Drug Name	Maximal Safe Dose (mg/kg)
Cocaine	3 (topical)
Procaine (Novocaine)	12
Chloroprocaine (Nesacaine)	14
Tetracaine (Pontocaine, others)	1
Lidocaine (Xylocaine)	7
Mepivacaine (Carbocaine, Polocaine)	7
Levobupivacaine (Chirocaine)	3
Etidocaine (Duranest)	4
Ropivacaine (Naropin)	3
Bupivacaine (Marcaine, Sensorcaine)	3
Articaine (Septocaine)	7

8. Describe the signs, symptoms, and treatment for a local anesthetic overdose.

Preparation for treatment of an accidental overdose of a local anesthetic drug must be part of any regional anesthetic. A properly functioning intravenous line and basic airway management equipment and resuscitative drugs must be immediately available when injecting significant quantities of local anesthetic agents. The extent to which toxicity manifests depends on the blood (brain) level produced. The higher the blood level, the greater the severity of toxic manifestations. Recognition of premonitory signs is essential when injecting the drugs. Except for bupivacaine (which is discussed later), local anesthetic toxicity is characterized by initial central nervous system (CNS) disinhibition resulting in excitatory CNS signs. Symptoms include fear, anxiety, restlessness, confusion, tinnitus, numbness of the mouth or tongue (circumoral), lightheadedness, visual disturbances, and muscular twitching. As the blood level continues to rise, symptoms include seizures followed by profound CNS, respiratory, and cardiac depression and coma.

Treatment should be initiated as soon as possible and includes discontinuation of the injection and administration of anticonvulsants, such as a benzodiazepine or barbiturate. Proper airway management must be maintained to ensure oxygenation. Symptomatic treatment of hypotension and heart rate changes is accomplished with common resuscitative agents. As long as a patent airway and oxygenation are maintained, the effects of the overdose are generally short lived, and full patient recovery may be expected. Hypoxia, hypercarbia, and acidosis increase toxicity.

Special populations are more prone to toxicity. Pregnant patients are at increased risk secondary to progesterone-induced changes in cardiac sensitivity and reduced hepatic blood flow from the gravid uterus. Pediatric and geriatric patients are at increased risk due to lower alpha$_1$-acid glycoprotein levels. A reduction in the usual dose in these patients is prudent.

9. Explain why bupivacaine toxicity is different.

Early case reports of patients who had overdosed with bupivacaine indicated a different pattern of symptoms as the toxicity progressed. Patients exhibited cardiac arrest before the usual CNS symptoms. Subsequent animal and human investigations showed that bupivacaine elicits a unique pattern of toxicity. The drug strongly binds to cardiac muscle and interrupts conduction. Several hours of resuscitative efforts may be required when attempting to counteract this toxicity. Avoiding high concentrations, such as 0.75%, and slow injection with frequent aspiration have greatly minimized the occurrence of this problem. Newer long-acting agents have been developed in an attempt to minimize this unique cardiac toxicity.

10. How do the newer local anesthetics compare with existing agents?

Levobupivacaine and ropivacaine have been introduced more recently as long-acting agents. These two drugs were developed specifically to retain the desirable properties of bupivacaine while reducing cardiac toxicity. Ropivacaine is a derivative of and levobupivacaine is the purified isomer of racemic bupivacaine. Both agents are similar to bupivacaine in potency, efficacy, and duration of action; however, they are less cardiac toxic. The order of cardiac toxicity seems to be bupivacaine > levobupivacaine > ropivacaine.

11. Describe the two clinical situations in which "ion trapping" is an issue.

Ion trapping of local anesthetics refers to a pharmacokinetic phenomenon that occurs when a difference in pH exists in two body compartments. The more acidotic the pH, the greater the fraction of local anesthetic, which is a basic compound, that ionizes. Ionized compounds are water soluble and cannot easily pass biologic membranes. When the local anesthetic becomes more ionized and water soluble, it becomes less able to leave the body compartment. If a patient who has CNS toxicity due to a local anesthetic overdose, is improperly managed, and becomes hypoxic with accompanying acidosis, the local anesthetic becomes trapped in the CNS, retarding its redistribution out of the brain and further enhancing toxicity. Another situation in which ion trapping may occur is in pregnant patients because fetal pH is lower than maternal pH. The local anesthetic molecules tend to accumulate in the fetus due to a greater degree of ionization.

Key Points

- Local anesthetics commonly are classified by chemical structure and duration of action.
- Chemically the local anesthetics are divided into two groups: esters and amides.
- Classification according to the duration of action includes three subtypes: (1) short-acting drugs lasting approximately 30 to 60 minutes, (2) intermediate-acting drugs lasting 60 to 120 minutes, and (3) long-acting drugs lasting 2 to 6 hours.
- Local anesthetics exert their action by blocking neuronal sodium channels. Blockade of the sodium channel inhibits the ability of the nerve to reach an action potential, rendering it reversibly blocked.
- To reach their site of action, local anesthetics must have a lipid-soluble or lipophilic portion of their chemical structure, a water-soluble or hydrophilic portion, and an intermediate ester or amide chain.
- A local anesthetic's effect is influenced by (1) lipid solubility, (2) protein binding, and (3) pK_a.
- The addition of epinephrine and the attendant vasoconstriction reduces the speed of local anesthetic absorption away from the injection site area, reducing blood levels and toxicity and prolonging duration of action.
- True allergy to local anesthetics is rare. The ester-type drugs and their metabolites are implicated in true allergic reactions much more frequently than the amide-type drugs.
- The rate of absorption is affected by the lipid solubility, protein binding, and vascularity of the injection area; injection rate; and total dose.

Key Points   *continued*

- Local anesthetic toxicity is characterized by initial CNS disinhibition resulting in excitatory CNS signs. Symptoms include fear, anxiety, restlessness, confusion, tinnitus, numbness of the mouth or tongue (circumoral), lightheadedness, visual disturbances, and muscular twitching.
- Treatment includes discontinuation of the injection and administration of anticonvulsants, such as a benzodiazepine or barbiturate. Proper airway management must be maintained to ensure oxygenation.
- Bupivacaine elicits a unique pattern of toxicity. The drug strongly binds to cardiac muscle and interrupts conduction, resulting in cardiac arrest.
- Levobupivacaine and ropivacaine were developed specifically to retain the desirable properties of bupivacaine, while reducing cardiac toxicity.
- Ion trapping of local anesthetics results in the local anesthetic becoming trapped in the body compartment, retarding its redistribution and further enhancing toxicity.

Internet Resources

Anesthesia Pharmacology: Local Anesthesics:
http://www.anesthesia2001.com/Central/Local_Anes/LAobj1.htm

Update in Anesthesia. Bukbirwa H, Conn DA: Toxicity from Local Anesthetic Drugs. Issue 10 (1999), Article 8:
http://www.nda.ox.ac.uk/wfsa/html/u10/u1008_01.htm

Virtual Anaesthesia Textbook:
http://www.virtual-anaesthesia-textbook.com/

Bibliography

Burm AJL, van Kleef JW: Local anesthetics. In Bovill JG, Howie MB, editors: *Clinical pharmacology for anaesthetists,* London, 1999, WB Saunders, pp 157-172.

Howe JP: Local anaesthetics. In McCaughey W, Clark RSJ, Fee JPH, et al, editors: *Anaesthetic physiology and pharmacology,* New York, 1997, Churchill Livingstone, pp 83-100.

Liu SS, Hodgson PS: Local anesthetics. In Barash PG, Cullen BF, Stoelting RK, editors: *Clinical anesthesia,* ed 4, Philadelphia, 2001, Lippincott Williams & Wilkins, pp 449-472.

Mosby Drug Consult: Available online: http://www.mosbysdrugconsult.com. St. Louis, 2002, Mosby.

Mulroy M: Local anesthesia toxicity: have we solved the problems? *Audio-Digest Anesthesiology* 44(4), 2002.

Tetzlaff JE: *Clinical pharmacology of local anesthetics,* Boston, 2000, Butterworth Heinemann.

Tetzlaff JE: Local anesthesia: are the new agents any better? *Audio-Digest Anesthesiology* 44(4), 2002.

Williams JR: Local Anesthetics. In Nagelhout JJ, Zaglaniczny K, editors: *Nurse anesthesia,* ed 2, Philadelphia, 2001, WB Saunders, pp 136-156.

Diuretics and Antiemetics

Colleen M. Beauchamp and Anne Marie Hranchook

DIURETICS

1. **Identify the various pharmacological classes of diuretics, their site of action, and their mechanism of action.**

   The following table summarizes the pharmacological classes, site of action, and mechanism of action of diuretics.

Pharmacological Classes, Site of Action, and Mechanism of Action of Diuretics			
Type of Diuretic	**Prototype**	**Site of Action**	**Mechanism of Action**
Thiazide diuretics	Hydrochlorothiazide	Distal convoluted tubule	Inhibits luminal cotransport (Na^+, Cl^-)
Loop diuretics	Furosemide	Cortical and medullary thick ascending loop of Henle	Inhibits luminal cotransport (Na^+, K^+, Cl^-)
Potassium-sparing diuretics	Spironolactone	Cortical collecting tubule	Competes for aldosterone receptor
Carbonic anhydrase inhibitors	Acetazolamide	Proximal tubule	Inhibits carbonic anhydrase and increases HCO_3^- excretion
Osmotic diuretics	Mannitol	Proximal tubule Descending loop of Henle	↓ Na^+ resorption by osmotic action ↑ In medullary blood flow and medullary hypertonicity

2. **Do all patients receiving diuretics require potassium supplementation?**

   In general, ambulatory hypertensive patients who have been on long-term diuretic therapy do not require potassium supplementation to maintain serum potassium levels within a safe range. The serum potassium usually does decrease in these patients, but the hypokalemia is not progressive and is rarely pronounced.

The overall decrease in total body potassium rarely exceeds 10% and is generally well tolerated. The current opinion is that corrective measures for ambulatory patients are necessary only if the patient is symptomatically hypokalemic or if the serum level declines to less than 3 mEq/L.

The following circumstances may warrant potassium supplementation:
- Hypokalemia predisposes digitalized patients to digitalis intoxication. Modest decreases in serum potassium can precipitate serious cardiac toxicity.
- Cirrhotic patients commonly have secondary hyperaldosteronism resulting in low serum potassium levels, which may precipitate hepatic coma.
- Hypokalemic diabetic patients are at risk for accelerated glucose intolerance. During periods of excessive diuresis, a rapid decrease in serum potassium produces symptoms more frequently than a reduction that occurs over a longer time.

3. What role do diuretics play in the treatment of hypertension?

Diuretics have been used as monotherapy or in combination with other classes of antihypertensive agents, such as beta-adrenergic blockers, in a stepped-care approach to the treatment of hypertension. Thiazide diuretics in particular are often used for the initial management of hypertension. Thiazide diuretics have long been known for possessing diuretic and mild vasodilator properties.

In 1997, the Joint National Committee on Prevention, Detection, Evaluation, and Treatment of High Blood Pressure reemphasized its previous recommendation that a thiazide diuretic or beta-blocker be used initially for patients with uncomplicated hypertension because only these classes of antihypertensive agents have been shown clearly to reduce associated cardiovascular morbidity and mortality. Diuretics enhance the efficacy of many agents, particularly angiotensin-converting enzyme inhibitors. Patients being treated with powerful vasodilators, such as hydralazine or minoxidil, may require simultaneous administration of diuretics because vasodilators may cause significant volume retention and sometimes edema.

4. Which class of diuretics is associated with the development of ototoxicity?

The loop diuretics can cause dose-related hearing loss. Tinnitus, reversible or permanent hearing impairment, and reversible deafness have occurred as a result of rapid intravenous administration of furosemide in doses exceeding the usual therapeutic range of 20 to 40 mg. This rare complication is most likely to occur with prolonged elevations of the plasma concentration of these drugs. Drug-induced changes in the electrolyte composition of the endolymph is a possible mechanism. Ototoxicity is more common in patients with diminished renal function and patients who also are receiving other ototoxic agents, such as aminoglycoside antibiotics.

It is suggested that administering furosemide by slow intravenous infusion rather than as a bolus injection may reduce the likelihood of otic effects by preventing high peak plasma concentrations. The rate of administration for adults should not exceed 4 mg/min.

5. Describe the effect diuretics have on neuromuscular blockade.

Diuretic-induced hypokalemia has been associated with enhancement of the effects of nondepolarizing neuromuscular blocking drugs. Low extracellular concentrations of potassium potentiate nondepolarizing muscle relaxants and diminish the ability of anticholinergic drugs to antagonize the block. This may occur due to an increase in end plate transmembrane potential, which results from a higher ratio of intracellular to extracellular potassium. In addition, furosemide may act on presynaptic nerve terminals, decreasing the release of acetylcholine and potentiating nondepolarizing blocking drugs. Mannitol seems to have no direct effect on nondepolarizing neuromuscular blockade.

6. Summarize common therapeutic uses for the various classes of diuretics.

Therapeutic uses are summarized in the following table.

Therapeutic Uses of Diuretics

Type of Diuretic	Use
Thiazide diuretics	Hypertension Congestive heart failure (mild) Renal calculi Nephrotic diabetes insipidus Chronic renal failure
Loop diuretics	Hypertension with impaired renal function Congestive heart failure (moderate to severe) Acute pulmonary edema Chronic or acute renal failure Nephrotic syndrome Hyperkalemia
Potassium-sparing diuretics	Chronic liver failure Congestive heart failure with hypokalemia
Carbonic anhydrase inhibitors	Alkalinize tubular urine Counteract respiratory alkalosis Glaucoma
Osmotic diuretics	Acute renal failure ↓ Intraocular or intracranial pressure

7. **What cardiovascular considerations are important when administering osmotic diuretics to patients?**

Osmotic diuretics, such as mannitol, are distributed rapidly to the extracellular compartment causing extraction of water from the intracellular compartment. Before diuresis, expansion of the extracellular fluid volume and hyponatremia occur. Rapid expansion of the extracellular compartment increases the workload of the heart. Patients with poor left ventricular function are especially vulnerable, and pulmonary edema may develop. Underlying heart disease in the absence of frank congestive heart failure is not an absolute contraindication to osmotic diuretic administration, but it is a serious risk factor.

Osmotic diuretics should not be administered until the adequacy of the patient's renal function and urine flow has been established. A test dose may be used for this purpose. The cardiovascular status of the patient should be evaluated before administration. Renal function, urine output, fluid balance, serum sodium and potassium concentrations, and, when appropriate, central venous pressure should be monitored during administration of osmotic diuretics. The osmotic diuretic should be slowed or discontinued if decreased urine output, elevated blood pressure, elevated central venous pressure, or other evidence of circulatory overload is present.

ANTIEMETICS

8. **What are the risk factors for a prolonged Q-T interval with antiemetics and other drugs?**

Droperidol should not be considered a first-line antiemetic agent for patients with risk factors for a prolonged Q-T interval. Droperidol is contraindicated in men with a baseline Q-T interval greater then 440 msec and in women with a Q-T interval greater than 450 msec to minimize the risk of torsades de pointes. Preexisting hypokalemia and hypomagnesemia are risk factors and should always be corrected before droperidol administration. Other serious risk factors include bradycardia, diuretic use, congestive heart failure, cardiac hypertrophy, and concomitant use of other medications that prolong the Q-T interval. Major classes of drugs that prolong the Q-T interval include antiarrhythmics (e.g., amiodarone [Cordarone], sotalol [Betapace], procainamide [Procanbid]), antidepressants (e.g., desipramine [Norpramin], doxepin [Sinequan], fluoxetine [Prozac], paroxetine [Paxil], and sertraline [Zoloft]), some quinolone antibiotics (e.g., sparfloxacin [Zagam]), and erythromycin. Antipsychotics (e.g., chlorpromazine [Thorazine], haloperidol [Haldol], pimozide [Orap], ziprasidone [Geodon], mesoridazine [Serentil]), antimigraines (e.g., sumatriptan [Imitrex], naratriptan [Amerge], zolmitriptan [Zomig]), and antiemetics (e.g., dolasetron [Anzemet], ondansetron [Zofran]) also have been shown to prolong the Q-T interval. The website www.torsades.org maintains a list of other agents affecting the Q-T interval. Age greater than 65 years, alcohol abuse, use of benzodiazepines, volatile anesthetics, and intravenous opiates also increase risk. The electrocardiogram should be monitored for at least 2 to 3 hours after droperidol administration.

9. **Discuss the proper application, common adverse effects, and contraindications of transdermal scopolamine (Transderm Scōp) when used for prevention of postoperative nausea and vomiting (PONV).**

The patch should be *applied* to the hairless area behind the ear at least 4 hours before needed and removed after 24 hours. Patients and health care providers handling the patch should wash their hands after application or removal and avoid eye contact to prevent mydriasis, photophobia, and blurred vision.

The most common *adverse effects* are dry mouth (66%) and drowsiness (17%).

Transderm Scōp is *not* recommended for children younger than 12 years old, and patches should not be cut in half. Other *contraindications* include narrow-angle glaucoma, myasthenia gravis, obstructive gastrointestinal disease, obstructive uropathy, paralytic ileus/intestinal atony, ulcerative colitis/toxic megacolon, and reflux esophagitis.

10. **Compare and contrast the available serotonin antagonist antiemetics.**

Dolasetron has the lowest acquisition cost and longest duration of action (see the following table).

Serotonin Antagonist Antiemetics

Generic/Trade Name	Intravenous Dose	Onset/Peak (min)	Half-Life (hr)
Dolasetron/Anzemet	12.5 mg	10–15/20–35	8–9
Granisetron/Kytril	20–40 mcg/kg	4–10/20	4–5
Ondansetron/Zofran	4 mg	3–5/5–10	3–5
Tropisetron/Novoban	Only available orally		

11. **How should surgical patients at high risk for PONV be managed?**

Combination therapy, including a serotonin antagonist and a corticosteroid, droperidol, scopolamine, or metoclopramide, should be considered for high-risk patients. Combined therapy has a reported efficacy of greater than 70%. If patients experience breakthrough PONV, a drug from a group other than the one used for prophylaxis should be considered for rescue.

12. **List risk factors for PONV.**
   - Young age—a 10-year increase in age decreases PONV risk by 13%
   - Female gender—PONV risk of men is one third that of women
   - General anesthesia—risk 11 times greater than with regional or local
   - Duration of general anesthesia
   - History of motion sickness or PONV

- Opioid analgesics
- Type of surgery—strabismus; plastic; laparoscopy; orthopedic shoulder; dental; ear, nose, and throat; and thyroid

13. Is PONV prophylaxis for all surgical patients justifiable?

Routine prophylaxis for low-risk patients is difficult to justify. Early symptomatic treatment of PONV for low-risk patients results in outcomes (e.g., time to discharge, patient satisfaction, time to return to normal daily activities) that are similar to outcomes achieved with prophylaxis. Adverse effects of antiemetic agents are not innocuous. Serotonin antagonists have the most favorable adverse-effect profile. Surgical procedures that pose a low risk for PONV include cataract and cornea surgery; knee, ankle, wrist, or hand procedures; and minor gynecologic or urologic procedures.

14. Discuss the mechanism of action of metoclopramide (Reglan) in the prevention of PONV.

Metoclopramide is a dopamine antagonist that acts centrally at the chemoreceptor trigger zone and peripherally in the gastrointestinal tract. It is contraindicated in patients in whom stimulation of gastrointestinal motility might be dangerous (e.g., in the presence of mechanical gastrointestinal obstruction or perforation). Extrapyramidal reactions may occur in patients receiving metoclopramide and apparently are mediated via blockade of central dopaminergic receptors involved in motor function. They most frequently consist of feelings of motor restlessness, but also can be accompanied by dysphoria and anxiety and usually subside within 24 hours after discontinuance of the drug. Metoclopramide is contraindicated in patients receiving medications likely to cause extrapyramidal reactions (e.g., phenothiazines, butyrophenones). It also should be used with caution in children and young adults because extrapyramidal reactions occur most frequently in these age groups. Metoclopramide may exacerbate symptoms in patients with Parkinson's disease.

 Key Points

- The five pharmacological classes of diuretics are:
  - Thiazide diuretics
  - Loop diuretics
  - Osmotic diuretics
  - Potassium-sparing diuretics
  - Carbonic anhydrase inhibitors
- The role of diuretics in treating hypertension is vasodilation and intravascular fluid volume reduction.

Key Points   *continued*

- Diuretic-induced hypokalemia has been associated with enhancement of the effects of nondepolarizing neuromuscular blocking drugs.
- Osmotic diuretics, such as mannitol, can cause expansion of the extracellular fluid volume and hyponatremia. Rapid expansion of the extracellular compartment increases the workload of the heart.
- Droperidol is contraindicated in men with a baseline Q-T interval greater than 440 msec and in women with a Q-T interval greater than 450 msec to minimize the risk of torsades de pointes.
- Transderm-Scōp can be used effectively for prevention of PONV.
- Risk factors for PONV include:
  - Age
  - Gender
  - History of PONV
  - Type and duration of anesthesia
  - Use of opioid analgesics
  - Type of surgical procedure
- Metoclopramide is a dopamine antagonist that acts centrally at the chemoreceptor trigger zone and peripherally in the gastrointestinal tract.

Internet Resources

Anesthesia Pharmacology:
http://www.anesthesia2001.com/

Dr. Joseph F. Smith Medical Library: Diuretics:
http://www.chclibrary.org/micromed/00045620.html

NetPharmacology: Diuretics:
http://lysine.pharm.utah.edu/netpharm/netpharm_00/notes/diuretics.html

American Academy of Family Physicians: Practical Selection of Antiemetics:
http://www.aafp.org/afp/20040301/1169.html

Center for Pharmacy: 5-HT3 Antagonists for the Treatment of Chemotherapy-Induced Nausea and Vomiting in Adults: An Inpatient and Outpatient Management Tool:
http://www.centerforpharmacy.com/resources/newsletter/5HT3.htm

Bibliography

Ives HE: Diuretic agents. In Katzung BG, editor: *Basic and clinical pharmacology,* New York, 2001, McGraw-Hill, pp 245-264.

McEvoy GK, Litvak K, Welsh OH, Snow EK, editors: American Hospital Formulary Service Drug Information 2000, Bethesda, MD, pp 2386-2437.

MedWatch: www.torsades.org. Accessed April 01, 2002.

Micromedex HealthCare Series, Vol 113, Greenwood Village, CO, 2002, Micromedex.

Okusa MD: Diuretics: drugs that increase the excretion of water and electrolytes. In Brody TM, Larner J, Minneman K, editors. *Human pharmacology: molecular to clinical,* St. Louis, 1998, Mosby-Year Book, pp 259-278.

Scuderi PE, James RL, Harris L, Mims GR: Antiemetic prophylaxis does not improve outcomes after outpatient surgery when compared to symptomatic treatment, *Anesthesiology* 90:360-371,1999.

U.S. Food and Drug Administration: www.fda.gov/medwatch/SAFETY/2001/inapsine.htm. Accessed April 01, 2002.

White PF, Watcha MF: Postoperative nausea and vomiting: prophylaxis versus treatment, *Anesth Analg* 89:1337-1339, 1999.

Herbal Products

Karen Zaglaniczny

1. Why do patients take herbal medications?

It is estimated that one in three adults uses herbal products to treat or prevent a variety of diseases. Reports of use in surgical patients range from 17% to 63%. Explanations for the increased popularity of herbal therapy include consumer interest in health, disease prevention, and fitness; consumer dissatisfaction with traditional medicine; media promotion; and consumer self-treatment and control of chronic or acute illnesses. A popular myth is that there are greater amounts of toxins in the environment due to the destruction of the ozone layer, and consumers need to take "antioxidants" to help ward off any long-term systemic effects. Another common belief is that "natural is better" and that herbal remedies, being natural, are good and safe to use.

2. Name the common herbal medications used by surgical patients.

The most commonly used herbal medications in the United States are echinacea, ephedra, gingko, garlic, ginseng, kava kava, St. John's wort, and valerian. There are more 2000 herbal products identified and in use.

3. Describe the potential risks for surgical patients taking herbal medications.

Multiple adverse effects are associated with herbal products. The risks of herbal medications during the perioperative period can include cardiovascular instability, increased bleeding, synergism with sedative drugs, altered fluid and electrolyte status, and altered drug metabolism.

4. Because herbal medications are sold over the counter, aren't they safe to use?

The safety and therapeutic effectiveness of herbal medications used in the United States are controversial, owing to the lack of rigorous scientific studies. Although these products have been widely used in Europe and Asia for centuries, the documented evidence for safety and efficacy is limited. In the United States, herbal medications are not regulated by the Food and Drug Administration (FDA) and are considered dietary supplements. The 1994 Dietary Supplement Health and Education Act provides regulations for herbal products. These regulations include requirements for labeling that the product is not intended to diagnose, treat, cure, or prevent any disease. The label must include all ingredients, directions for use, warnings, and a statement indicating that the FDA has not evaluated the product.

5. Discuss dangers associated with herbal medications.

Dangers associated with the manufacturing and distribution of herbal medications include the lack of regulations, contamination with other products, and drug interactions. Because these products are not regulated for content, some preparations do not contain the listed ingredients, and others have toxic ingredients. Adulteration of herbal medications with unlisted substances can create health hazards. Some ingredients found in herbal preparations include antiinflammatory agents, steroids, diuretics, antihistamines, tranquilizers, and hormones. Heavy metals, such as lead, arsenic, mercury, aluminum, and zinc, have been added to some of these products. Lead and arsenic poisoning have been reported in patients using products imported from Asian countries.

6. Which herbal medications are dangerous?

Dangerous herbs may include comfrey, ephedra, chaparral, pennyroyal, lobelia, sassafras, coltsfoot, yohimbe, licorice, and pau d'arco. Some herbal products contain constituents that may be carcinogenic or hepatotoxic. Herbs considered to be carcinogenic include borage, calamus, coltsfoot, comfrey, life root, and sassafras. These herbs, except for calamus and sassafras, contain pyrrolizidine alkaloids that have been found to produce hepatic carcinomas in animals. In July 2001, the FDA issued a warning regarding the use of comfrey and asked manufacturers to remove the product from the market. Carcinogenic potential has been documented for safrole in sassafras and cis-isoasarone in calamus in animal studies. Hepatotoxicity has been associated with the use of germander, chaparral, and life root.

7. Explain the pharmacological basis for herbal medications.

The pharmacological basis for herbal medicines is related to the active ingredients extracted from the herbal plant. The major plant constituents from herbs that provide the proposed active medicinal substance are acids, alkaloids, anthraquinone, bitters, coumarins, flavones, glycosides, lignans, phenols, saponins, and tannins. Herbal medicines are marketed in a variety of forms, including extracts, teas, powdered solutions, topical ointments, tablets, and capsules. Potency varies tremendously among the types of preparations. Teas can be brewed to provide a strong or weak mixture. Tablets can contain various concentrations of the active herbal ingredient. Therapeutic effectiveness associated with herbal medicines is related to many factors involving purity of substances, concentration, dose, and length of treatment.

8. What preoperative questions should be asked regarding herbal products?

During the preoperative assessment, it is essential to ask specific questions about the use of herbal products. Patients frequently are hesitant or embarrassed to

inform health care providers about herbal use. Specific questions should elicit information about the following:
* Length of ingestion
* Dose taken
* Side effects
* Type of preparation
* Source of herbal product

Identifying the source of the herbal product is important because of the lack of regulation in manufacturing and production. Patients often purchase their products from a health food store or the Internet, and ingredients and directions may be listed in a foreign language.

9. **Describe the guidelines for preoperative laboratory screening in elective cases.**

Routine laboratory screening is not recommended for all patients taking herbal products. If a patient is taking herbal medications that affect clotting, coagulation parameters should be assessed. Likewise, a patient taking herbal medications that could affect electrolyte balance should have electrolyte determinations made.

10. **Should an elective case be delayed if a patient is taking herbal medications?**

Patients should be assessed individually regarding their herbal medication history. If the patient is taking a product that affects clotting, hemodynamic parameters, or sympathetic nervous system function, a thorough assessment, including appropriate laboratory and diagnostic studies, must be completed.

11. **Name herbal medications that can cause problems with bleeding during surgical care.**

Herbal products that may affect clotting include the following:
* Alfalfa
* Capsicum
* Garlic
* Ginkgo biloba
* Chamomile
* Ginseng
* Feverfew
* Echinacea
* Dong quai
* Willow bark
* Ginger
* Goldenseal
* Guarana
* Fish oil

- Kava kava
- Horse chestnut

Preoperatively, coagulation studies should be evaluated to identify if a clotting abnormality exists. Elective surgical procedures should be delayed (typically 2 weeks) after product use or until normal hematological function returns.

12. List herbal medications that can affect blood glucose.

MAY LOWER BLOOD GLUCOSE
- Alfalfa
- Aloe
- Argimony
- Artichokes
- Chromium
- Coriander
- Dandelion root
- Devil's claw
- Eucalyptus
- Fenugreek
- Fo-ti
- Garlic
- Ginseng
- Grape seed
- Juniper
- Onions
- Periwinkle
- Yellow root

MAY INCREASE BLOOD GLUCOSE
- Ephedra

13. Describe the herbal medications that can affect the nervous system during anesthesia care.

Central nervous system stimulation effects may be observed with feverfew, St. John's wort, guarana, gotu kola, goldenseal, ma huang, milk thistle, and yohimbe. Consideration for potential vasoactive agent interactions with these products is essential. Sedative-hypnotic effects can be observed with celery, chamomile, goldenseal, kava kava, hawthorn, valerian, lemon verbena, mugwort, lavender, lemon balm, passion flower, and rauwolfia. These drugs may potentiate the central nervous system depressant effects associated with administration of anesthetic agents such as barbiturates, benzodiazepines, and opioids.

Herbal products that may have antidepressant actions include St. John's wort, passion flower, ma huang, mugwort, lemon balm, ginseng, and yohimbe. Caution is advised with the coadministration of tricyclic antidepressants, selective seratonin reuptake inhibitors, and monoamine oxidase inhibitors.

14. Summarize the guidelines for discontinuation of herbal medications?

Patients should be advised to discontinue herbal therapies before the scheduled surgical procedure. The American Society of Anesthesiologists recommends that herbal products be discontinued 2 weeks before surgery. More recently, a more targeted approach has been recommended (see the following table). Some of the active constituents found in herbal products are eliminated quickly and can be discontinued closer to the time of surgery. Abrupt discontinuation of some herbal products such as kava, when used for long-term therapy, may precipitate acute withdrawal.

Recommendations for Discontinuing Herbal Preparations Preoperatively

Herbs	Recommendation
Echinacea	Pharmacokinetics not fully studied. Discontinue as far in advance as possible before surgery when compromises in hepatic function or blood flow are anticipated
Ephedra	Elimination half-life: 5.2 hr, with 70–80% excreted unchanged in urine. Discontinue at least 24 hours before surgery
Garlic	Data insufficient. Potential for irreversible inhibition of platelet function warrants discontinuation 7 days before surgery, especially if postoperative bleeding is a concern or if other platelet inhibitors are given
Ginkgo	Contains terpenoids and flavonoids. Elimination half-life of terpenoids after oral administration is 3–10 hr. Based on the risk of bleeding, discontinue at least 36 hr before surgery
Ginseng	Elimination half-life 0.8–7.4 hr. Due to platelet inhibition, discontinue at least 7 days before surgery
Kava Kava	Peak plasma levels occur at 1.8 hr, elimination half-life of kavakactones is 9 hr. Possibility for potentiation of sedative effects of anesthetics. Discontinue at least 24 hr before surgery
St. John's wort	Peak plasma levels of hypercin and hyperforin 6 & 3.5 hr; elimination half-lives 43.1 and 9 hr. Discontinue at least 5 days before surgery
Valerian	Effects short-lived. Abrupt discontinuation may precipitate benzodiazepine-like withdrawal in dependent patients; taper dose. Discontinue at least 24 hr before surgery

15. Summarize the anesthetic implications and potential drug interactions found with commonly used herbal medications.

Drug interactions and anesthetic implications are summarized in the table on pages 150–152.

Drug Interactions and Anesthetic Implications

Herb	Uses	Drug Interactions and Anesthetic Implications	Side Effects
Black cohosh	Dysmenorrhea, premenopausal and menopausal symptoms	May potentiate antihypertensive agents and hypotension; avoid during pregnancy, may increase spontaneous abortion	May affect the hypothalamic-pituitary system, GI disturbances, hypotension, not to be used for > 6 mon
Horse chestnut	Varicose veins and other venous insufficiencies, soft tissue swelling, diarrhea, fever, hemorrhoids	Increased risk of bleeding with anticoagulants, aspirin; check coagulation profile	Pruritus, nausea, muscle spasm, nephropathy, urticaria, severe bleeding and bruising, shock, hepatotoxicity
Echinacea	Immunostimulant (colds, fever, bronchitis); antimicrobial; topical wound healing	Antagonistic interaction with immunosuppressant agents; increased bleeding time for patients on long-term warfarin; possible enhancement of hepatotoxicity with anabolic steroids, amiodarone, methotrexate; assess coagulation parameters	Severe allergic reactions in patients with a history of asthma, atopy, allergic rhinitis, and known allergy to members of the daisy family; hepatotoxicity; used for a maximum of 8 wk; potential immunosuppression with long-term use; avoid use with autoimmune diseases, multiple sclerosis, HIV
Ephedra	Asthma, colds, cough, bronchitis; flu; weight loss	Avoid use with MAOIs, antihypertensives, theophylline, cardiac glycosides (digoxin), oxytocin, decongestants, stimulants, beta blockers, phenothiazines; assess fluid and electrolyte status if used as dietary supplement; may need higher doses of anesthetic agents if recent ingestion; long-term use depletes endogenous catecholamines and may cause intraoperative CV instability	Dose-related; headache, irritability, motor restlessness, nausea, insomnia, tachycardia, urinary difficulties, kidney stones, headache, dizziness; high doses: HTN, myocardial infarction, stroke, dependence, arrhythmias, tachyphylaxis; use for short-term therapy, < 7 days; maximal dose: 24 mg/day
Feverfew	Migraines, arthritis, rheumatic diseases, dermatitis, menstrual problems, fever, asthma, allergies	May enhance effects of anticoagulants, antiplatelet drugs (aspirin), NSAIDs; assess coagulation parameters; discontinue before elective surgery	Gastric discomfort, minor oral mucosal ulceration, loss of taste; discontinuation may produce muscle and joint stiffness, rebound migraine symptoms, anxiety, sleeplessness; advised not to take for >4 mon without medical consultation

Drug Interactions and Anesthetic Implications *continued*

Herb	Uses	Drug Interactions and Anesthetic Implications	Side Effects
Garlic	Hyperlipidemia; prevention of atherosclerosis	May interact with hypoglycemic therapy; may enhance antithrombotic effects of antiinflammatory drug; assess coagulation parameters	Diaphoresis, dizziness, GI disturbances, allergic reactions, chronic or excessive use may lead to decreased hemoglobin production and lysis of red blood cells
Ginger	Motion sickness; nausea and vomiting; loss of appetite; antiinflammatory; CV stimulant; antioxidant	Risk of prolonged bleeding time, especially when used with antiplatelet drugs; discontinue before elective surgery; check coagulation parameters	Possible CNS depression or arrhythmias with overdose
Gingko	Cerebral and peripheral vascular disease, dementia; antioxidant	May enhance antiplatelet effects of aspirin, warfarin, NSAIDs; avoid concurrent use with MAOIs; assess coagulation parameters; discontinue before elective surgery	Hypersensitivity reactions, gastric disturbances, headache, vertigo, dizziness, spontaneous bleeding
Ginseng	Fatigue, debility, declining capacity to work and concentrate; aphrodisiac; antidepressant	Caution with warfarin, potential to increase risk of bleeding; red ginseng may potentiate the effect of caffeine and other stimulants; may reduce effects of certain antihypertensive agents; potential for hypoglycemia, avoid with hypoglycemic agents; avoid concomitant use with MAOIs	Contraindicated with HTN, chest pain, diarrhea, epistaxis, headache, impotence, insomnia, nausea, nervousness, palpitations; avoid in patients with CV disease; overdose can bring about ginseng abuse syndrome, characterized by sleeplessness, hypertonia, and edema; limit treatment to 3 mon
Kava kava	Anxiety, nervousness, stress and insomnia; contraindicated in patients with endogenous depression because it increases risk of suicide	Potentiates benzodiazepines, barbiturates, antipsychotics, and alcohol, sedation, oral and lingual dyskinesia, torticollis, ocular crisis, exacerbation of Parkinson's disease, painful twisting movements of trunk, rash; potential to increase sedative effects of anesthetics, potential for addiction, tolerance, and withdrawal	Changes in motor reflexes and judgment, visual disturbances; chronic use: decreased platelet count, dopamine antagonism, pulmonary HTN, vitamin B deficiency, reversible skin discoloration, eye disturbances; limited use for 1–3 mon in Australia and Germany; Canadian regulations prohibit use

Continued

Drug Interactions and Anesthetic Implications   *continued*

Herb	Uses	Drug Interactions and Anesthetic Implications	Side Effects
St. John's wort	Mild-to-moderate depression, anxiety; topical treatment wounds and burns; bronchial inflammation, insomnia, kidney	Potential interactions with MAOIs, SSRIs, vasopressors; induction of cytochrome P-450 enzymes may increase metabolism of cyclosporins, warfarin, steroids, calcium channel blockers, benzodiazepines	Photosensitivity; GI complaints, dry mouth, nausea and vomiting, headache, dizziness, allergic reaction, sedation, restlessness, increased heart rate, convulsions, shortness of breath, disorientation; avoid use with other antidepressants, alcohol, OTC cold and flu medications
Valerian	Anxiety, sleep disorders, mental strain, stress	Potentiates other CNS depressants; potential to increase sedative effect of anesthetics and increase anesthetic requirements with long-term use; may negate therapeutic effect to phenytoin and warfarin	Headaches, excitability, insomnia, mydriasis, cardiac disorders; dystonic reactions; hepatotoxicity with other herbs (skullcap, mistletoe); long-term use not advised; benzodiazepine-like acute withdrawal
Yohimbe	Sexual and erectile dysfunction; hallucinogenic	Potentiated by tricyclic antidepressants, central alpha$_2$-adrenergic blockers, centrally acting sympathomimetics, MAOIs, and antimuscarinic agents: avoid with OTC stimulants (additive); avoid with tyramine-containing foods (wine, cheese): high BP	High risk to benefit ratio; CNS stimulation, nervousness, palpitations, restlessness, hallucinations, anxiety, HTN, tachycardia, nausea/vomiting, cardiac failure; contraindicated in liver and kidney disease; avoid long-term use

BP, bloood pressure; CNS, central nervous system; CV, cardiovascular; GI, gastrointestinal; HIV, human immunodeficiency virus; HTN, hypertension; MAOIs, monoamine oxidase inhibitors; NSAIDs, nonsteroidal antiinflammatory drugs; OTC, over-the-counter; SSRIs, selective serotonin reuptake inhibitors.

Key Points

- Herbal medications are reported to be taken by 17% to 63% of surgical patients.
- The most commonly used herbal medications in the United States are echinacea, ephedra, gingko, garlic, ginseng, kava kava, St. John's wort, and valerian.
- The risks of herbal medications during the perioperative period include cardiovascular instability, increased bleeding, synergism with sedative drugs, altered fluid and electrolyte status, and altered drug metabolism.
- In the United States, herbal medications are not regulated by the FDA and are considered dietary supplements.
- Dangers associated with the manufacturing and distribution of herbal medications include the lack of regulations, contamination with other products, and drug interactions.
- Dangerous or unsafe herbs may include comfrey, ephedra, chaparral, pennyroyal, lobelia, sassafras, coltsfoot, yohimbe, licorice, and pau d'arco.
- In the preoperative interview, information should be elicited about the length of ingestion, dose taken, side effects, type of preparation, and source of herbal product.
- Herbal products should be discontinued 2 weeks before surgery. Abrupt discontinuance of some herbs could cause withdrawal symptoms.

Internet Resources

University of Wisconsin Department of Anesthesiology: Preoperative Anesthesiology Assessment Clinic: Herbal Medication and Anesthesia:
http://www.anesthesia.wisc.edu/Clinic/providerinfo/herbals.html

American Society of Anesthesiologists: Herbal Medicine:
http://www.asahq.org/patientEducation/vnr3.htm

Herbs and Anesthesia, by Abdul N. Naushad, MD, Indiana University School of Medicine:
http://www.brandianestesia.it/File%20PDF/herbs.pdf

Healthyinfo.com: Preoperative Evaluation: Herbals Away:
http://www.healthyinfo.com/clinical/herbal/herbals.away.shtml

Critical Care Nurse: Preoperative Considerations: Which Herbal Products Should Be Discontinued Before Surgery?
http://www.aacn.org/AACN/jrnlccn.nsf/Files/PharmacologyApr03/$file/Pharmacology.pdf

Bibliography

Gruenwald J, et al: *PDR for herbal medicines*, ed 2, Montvale, NJ, 2000, Medical Economics Company.

Mosby's drug consult: herbal and supplement information, St. Louis, 2003, Mosby, pp 1-49.

Murray MT, et al: Pharmacology of natural medicine. In Pizzorno JE, Murray MT, editors: *Textbook of natural medicine*, ed 2, New York, 1999, Churchill Livingstone, pp 551-1030.

Norred CL, et al: Use of complementary and alternative medicines by surgical patients, *AANA J* 68:13-18, 2000.

Skidmore-Roth L: *Mosby's handbook of natural supplements*, Philadelphia, 2001, Mosby.

Physiology, Pathophysiology, and Anesthetic Management

Cardiovascular Disease

Linda Callahan

1. What functional systemic changes should the anesthetist consider in a patient with hypertension?

Although hypertension is the most common cardiovascular disorder encountered by the nurse anesthetist, the disease is generally asymptomatic and insidious in onset. Almost two thirds of patients older than age 65 have hypertension. If hypertension is inadequately treated over the long-term, hypertensive cardiomyopathy and systolic ventricular dysfunction result from the organ changes associated with hypertension. Increased afterload from chronic vasoconstriction is a significant cause of congestive heart failure (CHF) and cardiomyopathy. Other risks in poorly controlled hypertension include stroke and nephrosclerosis.

2. Describe the pathological changes associated with untreated or poorly controlled hypertension.

Long-standing hypertension produces left ventricular hypertrophy due to chronic elevation of myocardial wall tension. As a result, subendocardial ischemia may result at blood pressures that would be adequate for perfusion in a normotensive individual. In addition to increased risk of stroke, hypertension may lead to an elevation of the lower pressure threshold for cerebrovascular autoregulation. This elevation further increases the risk for cerebral ischemia at mean arterial pressures that would not be problematic in a normotensive individual. The presence of proteinuria indicates a gradual decline in renal function in poorly controlled patients.

3. How do the functional changes associated with hypertension affect anesthetic management?

The decision to anesthetize a patient with hypertension for elective surgery is predicated on assessment of the degree of end-organ involvement and the level of blood pressure control currently present. Every patient with hypertension should be considered to have some degree of coronary artery disease (CAD). Even with adequate treatment, intraoperative hypertension remains a potential problem. Antihypertensive medications often decrease the effectiveness of hemodynamic compensatory mechanisms normally present in response to vasodilation that may occur during anesthetic induction. Often hypertensive patients are hypovolemic, and responses such as tachycardia and vasoconstriction to additional blood or fluid loss may be attenuated or lost. These patients may show an exaggerated response to common vasopressors used to correct the resultant hypotension.

4. Should antihypertensive medications be discontinued before surgery?

Antihypertensive medications should be continued up to the time of surgery to avoid serious side effects associated with discontinuation (e.g., rebound hypertension after discontinuation of clonidine, angina and tachycardia after withdrawal of beta blockers.)

5. Discuss the common pathologies of valvular heart disease.

In the normal heart, the valves allow blood to flow between chambers and the great vessels. A normal-sized valve orifice produces only a small degree of obstruction to flow and a hemodynamically insignificant gradient. The valvular lesions most commonly seen by the anesthetist produce pressure overloads (mitral stenosis, aortic stenosis) or volume overloads (mitral regurgitation, aortic regurgitation) in the left atrium or the left ventricle. Overall left-sided lesions produce impedance to forward blood flow into the systemic circulation. Right-sided valvular lesions occur less frequently.

6. How does valvular disease change overall cardiac function?

In general, valvular lesions increase cardiac work. In *valvular stenosis,* the opening of the valve becomes constricted and impedes the forward flow of blood through the valve. Additional pressure must be generated to overcome the increased resistance to blood flow across the stenosed valve; this increases pressure work. In *valvular regurgitation* (valvular insufficiency or incompetence), the valves fail to close securely, allowing backward flow of blood across the valve. Valvular regurgitation requires the heart to pump the additional regurgitant volume of blood, producing an increase in volume work. The responses of the cardiac muscle to increased pressure work and increased volume work are chamber dilation and muscular hypertrophy.

7. Discuss the specific functional pathological changes associated with mitral regurgitation.

Regurgitation may be caused by rheumatic heart fever, ischemia, or mitral valve prolapse. Chronic regurgitation produces left ventricular and atrial volume overload with resultant dilation and hypertrophy. Loss of left ventricular pressure occurs due to backflow through the valve into the left atrium. This produces increased left atrial pressure, pulmonary hypertension, and eventual right heart failure. In acute mitral regurgitation, the right heart is subjected to sudden increases in volume and pressure without time for compensatory ventricular dilation to occur. These sudden changes may produce acute pulmonary hypertension, pulmonary edema, and severe right-sided failure.

8. **What are the anesthetic concerns for patients with mitral regurgitation?**

Left ventricular volume overload is the primary problem; management should be designed to improve forward flow. Maintenance of a slightly elevated heart rate and the use of vasodilating drugs to decrease systemic vascular resistance are useful measures in meeting this goal.

9. **Describe the functional pathological changes of mitral stenosis.**

Mitral stenosis occurs progressively over 10 to 20 years and is most often associated with rheumatic disease. Pressure-volume inequality develops, in which left atrial pressure rises with resultant hypertrophy and dilation, while the left ventricle is volume overloaded because of obstruction to forward flow. Increased left atrial pressure produces pulmonary congestion and pulmonary hypertension with resultant right ventricular hypertrophy. Atrial fibrillation often occurs leading to decreased cardiac output. Stasis of blood in the dilated atrium predisposes the patient to thrombus formation with resultant emboli.

10. **What are the anesthetic considerations for a patient with mitral stenosis?**

Anesthetic management should focus on enhancing flow across the stenotic valve. Adequate volume must be ensured. Increases in pulmonary vascular resistance must be avoided to prevent right heart failure; vasopressors should be used with caution. Preoperative digitalization may be beneficial in producing a slower heart rate, which allows greater ventricular filling. A low-dose premedication should be used to avoid respiratory depression. Respiratory depression can produce hypercarbia or hypoxemia or both, which can lead to increased pulmonary vascular resistance. Circulatory time may be prolonged.

11. **Describe the functional pathological changes of aortic stenosis.**

The causes of aortic stenosis include congenital bicuspid valve, calcification, and rheumatic disease. The resultant scarring produces an obstruction to left ventricular ejection with pressure overload. The left ventricular muscle hypertrophies as a result of the increased intraventricular pressure and wall tension required to maintain forward ejection of blood. Early changes include decreased left ventricular compliance, but an increased preload mechanism and an atrial kick allow contractility maintenance with normal stroke volume. Progressive late changes include fibrosis with decreased contractility, left ventricular dilation, and decreased stroke volume as the ventricle fails to generate the excessive pressure required to move blood past the stenotic lesion.

12. **How do the symptoms associated with aortic stenosis manifest?**

Because of the ability of the left ventricle to undergo significant hypertrophy, the latency period to the development of significant symptoms may be 30 years. Increasing stenosis predisposes the patient to the development of ischemia even without the presence of CAD. This predisposition occurs because left ventricular hypertrophy produces increased oxygen demand, whereas ventricular dilation and overfilling may result in subendocardial compression decreasing perfusion during diastole. Aortic stenosis becomes hemodynamically significant when a pressure gradient of 50 mm Hg or greater is present across the valve, or a valvular orifice size of 0.8 cm or less is present. When symptoms of angina, dyspnea, syncope, and congestive heart failure are present, there is a 50% chance of death in 4 to 5 years. Aortic stenosis is associated with sudden death. Cardiovascular arrest is often not amenable to resuscitative attempts because of the excessive pressure on the chest wall that must be generated to move blood past an extremely stenotic aortic valve.

13. What are the anesthetic considerations for a patient with aortic stenosis?

Maintenance of adequate intravascular volume and normal cardiac rate and rhythm are essential. Cardiac output is relatively fixed by the stenotic valve. Even mild hypotension may lead to reduced coronary perfusion. Tachycardia should be avoided to ensure adequate time for atrial filling because the atrial "kick" may account for 40% of the left ventricular filling. Bradycardia can lead to overdistention of the left ventricle with resultant impaired perfusion of the myocardium during diastole. These patients are at increased risk for the development of CHF.

14. Describe specific functional pathological changes associated with aortic regurgitation.

Functional changes are related to the rapidity of the development of the regurgitation. Acute insufficiency subjects the left ventricle to rapid volume overload due to backflow into the ventricle. This overload produces elevated end-diastolic pressure with decreased overall contractility. In chronic regurgitation situations, stroke volume increases are due to ventricular hypertrophy with increased compliance. As hypertrophic functional limits are reached, dilation results in failure of the left ventricle to maintain forward flow. This situation defeats the ability of the mitral valve to protect the pulmonary circulation with resultant increases in pulmonary vascular resistance. The peripheral circulation is hyperdynamic.

15. Define CHF, and discuss the causes.

Classically, *heart failure* is defined as the inability of the heart to deliver a supply of oxygenated blood sufficient to meet the metabolic needs of the peripheral tissues at rest and during exercise (see the table on page 161). Clinically, cardiac failure may be studied in terms of the valvular defects or shunts that contribute to overburdening the right or left ventricle to the point of dysfunction. The ventricles can be overloaded by increased blood volume that must be ejected forward or increased resistance against which ejection must occur. Cardiomyopathies, ischemia, restrictive and congenital cardiac disease, and conduction defects also may be causative. Noncardiac causes of failure include hypertension, pulmonary emboli, and thyrotoxicosis.

Classifications of Heart Failure

Stage	Definition
A	No structural heart disease or symptoms but at high risk for failure due to coexisting conditions (e.g. hypertension, diabetes, rheumatic disease)
B	Structural heart disease, such as myocardial infarct; right or left ventricular dysfunction, without signs or symptoms of heart failure
C	Structural heart disease with past or current symptoms of heart failure.
D	Advanced structural heart disease with symptoms of heart failure at rest, despite medication.

Adapted from ACC/AHA practice guidelines for evaluation and management of chronic heart failure in the adult, J Am Coll Cardiol 38:2101–2113, 2001, available online: http://www.acc.org/clinical/topic/topic.htm#guidelines.

16. What symptoms are associated with CHF?

Early symptoms most often are dyspnea on exertion and excessive fatigue during exercise. A dry, nocturnal cough may be reported. Later symptoms include increasing dyspnea, particularly in the supine position, as the left ventricular end-diastolic pressure becomes more elevated. Rales are present when transudation of fluid from capillaries into the interstitial vessels and interalveolar spaces exceeds the removal capacity of the lymphatic system. The chest x-ray reveals cardiomegaly and increased pulmonary vascular markings. An S_3 gallop may be heard. Peripheral edema develops due to increased venous capillary pressure and decreased cardiac output with consequent fluid retention. Hepatomegaly also may be present. Low cardiac output in severe CHF produces low flow through capillary beds with resultant increased oxygen extraction and cyanosis.

17. How are treatment decisions made for patients with CHF?

The goals of pharmacological treatment are to decrease heart size, decrease wall stress, decrease cardiac work, decrease afterload and preload, and increase contractility resulting in increased overall cardiac output (see the following table). Nonpharmacological therapies such as sodium restriction in combination with diuretics are aimed at decreasing ventricular size by decreasing volume.

Suggested Pharmacological Treatment of Heart Failure

Stage	Treatment
A	Control risk factors and coexisting diseases; ACEI in patients with a history of athcrosclerosis, diabetes, or hypertension

Continued

Suggested Pharmacological Treatment of Heart Failure *continued*	
Stage	**Treatment**
B	Same as stage A; ACEI and beta blocker in patients with a history of recent MI regardless of ejection fraction; ACEI and beta blocker in patients with decreased ejection fraction without history of MI
C	Same as stage A; combination of diuretic with beta blocker and ACEI; digoxin to treat symptoms and increase exercise tolerance; if ACEI not tolerated, angiotensin receptor blocker plus diuretic, beta blocker, and digoxin may be given; discontinue NSAIDs and myocardial depressants, such as antiarrhythmics and calcium channel blockers
D	As in stage C, but may be able to tolerate only small doses of drugs; specialized treatment, such as mechanical circulatory support, continuous intravenous inotropic therapy, referral for cardiac transplantation

ACEI, angiotensin-converting enzyme inhibitor; NSAIDs, nonsteroidal antiinflammatory drugs; MI, myocardial infarction.
Adapted from ACC/AHA practice guidelines for evaluation and management of chronic heart failure in the adult, J Am Coll Cardiol 38:2101-2113, 2001, available online: http://www.acc.org/clinical/topic/topic.htm#guidelines.

18. When planning anesthesia care for a patient with CHF, what should the anesthetist consider?

Most importantly, optimization of cardiac function should be attained if possible. Patients with uncompensated cardiac failure are not candidates for elective surgery. In emergency situations in which anesthesia must be administered, invasive monitoring is necessary to assess continuously overall cardiac function and to control fluid administration. Monitoring also allows the anesthetist to assess the response of the patient to pharmacological agents that are administered. Intraoperative care should include the provision of adequate preload, while slowly treating electrolyte imbalances. Anesthetic agents that, in small doses, produce the least cardiac depression should be chosen. Techniques may include coadministration of low doses of ketamine and benzodiazepine agents. Etomidate or opioids also may be used in normovolemic or hypervolemic patients. Propofol and barbiturates generally are contraindicated because both may produce significant cardiac depression when administered in doses required to produce anesthesia.

19. In assessing a digitalized patient, what clinical findings would indicate toxicity?

- Symptoms include nausea, vomiting, or anorexia; abdominal pain; confusion, double vision or "floaters" in the visual path; and paresthesias.

- Electrocardiogram (ECG) abnormalities may be due to increased automaticity (multiple premature ventricular contractions or ventricular tachycardia) or delayed atrioventricular node conduction (varying degrees of heart block).
- Predisposing factors in the development of digitalis toxicity are hypokalemia, hypothyroidism, decreased renal function, increased age, and hypercalcemia.

20. Is there an increased risk of perioperative myocardial infarction in patients with a history of previous myocardial infarction, angina, or CAD?

Overall, perioperative risk is definitely increased in patients with known CAD. In patients undergoing major peripheral vascular or aortic surgery, the combined risk of death from cardiac causes can be 29%. In stable cardiovascular patients undergoing major noncardiac surgery, the predictors of increased risk from major cardiac complications include high-risk surgery, the presence of ischemic heart disease, a history of congestive heart failure, a previous cerebrovascular accident, the presence of insulin-dependent diabetes mellitus, or a serum creatinine concentration greater than 2 mg/dL. When assessing risk preoperatively, previous coronary artery bypass graft surgery, the presence of ST-T wave changes, current treatment with beta blockers, significant aortic stenosis, advanced age, and the presence of cardiac arrhythmia are significant considerations.

21. How may risk of myocardial ischemia be assessed preoperatively?

Overall exercise tolerance as established by the ability to climb a flight of stairs or undertake strenuous walking without symptoms is most useful in estimating tolerance of stress-related increases in heart rate, such as are experienced during surgery. A thorough history and physical examination with ECG are essential; specialized invasive and noninvasive tests, such as stress testing with or without thallium, computed tomography or magnetic resonance imaging, echocardiography, or radionucleotide ventriculography, should be employed only when the information gained would assist in making therapeutic choices that would maximize cardiac function before or during anesthesia. If noninvasive tests reveal significant cardiac ischemia during or after minimal exertion, a coronary artery revascularization procedure may be indicated before any other surgery is planned.

22. How is intraoperative management of heart rate and blood pressure best achieved in patients at risk for myocardial ischemia?

Balancing myocardial oxygen requirement against myocardial oxygen delivery is probably more important than any specific anesthetic technique or pharmacological therapy. Special considerations should be given to control during especially stressful periods, such as induction, intubation, and emergence. The heart rate and blood pressure should be maintained within 20% of the normal awake value. Selective intraoperative control of the heart rate and blood pressure may include many therapies (see the table on page 164). Before pharmacologic intervention, the volume status, depth of anesthesia, overall contractile function,

Treatment and Prevention of Myocardial Ischemia

Hemodynamic Abnormality	Treatment (Intravenous)
Hypertension, tachycardia	Nitroglycerin, beta blockade, labetalol
Hypertension, normal heart rate	Nitroglycerin, nifedipine, beta blockade
Normotension, tachycardia	Beta blockade, nitroglycerin
Hypotension, tachycardia	Alpha agonist to increase coronary perfusion pressure; when normotensive, beta blockade, nitroglycerin
Hypotension, bradycardia	Ephedrine, atropine, epinephrine, nitroglycerin after normotensive
Hypotension, normal heart rate	Alpha agonist for reduced SVR; specific inotrope as required; nitroglycerin when normotensive

SVR, systemic vascular resistance.
Adapted from Miller RD, editor: Atlas of anesthesia, vol 8; Philadelphia, 1999 Churchill Livingstone; Estafanous FG, Barish PG, Reves JG, editors: Cardiac anesthesia: principles and clinical practice, Philadelphia, 2001; Lippincott Williams & Wilkins.

systemic vascular resistance, and presence of complicating arrhythmias should be assessed and treated.

23. Describe the signs and symptoms of intraoperative cardiac ischemia.

In addition to routine blood pressure and pulse monitoring, the ECG remains the simplest, most cost-effective, and most reliable way to diagnose ischemia. A 1-mm depression or elevation in the ST-T wave segments is deemed diagnostic for ischemia. T-wave inversion and R-wave changes may be associated with ischemia or with other factors, such as electrolyte imbalance. The depth of the ST-segment depression is thought to parallel the depth of myocardial ischemia. Lead II, which reflects the area supplied by the right coronary artery, and the V_5 lead, which reflects the area of the left ventricle supplied by the left anterior descending coronary artery, detect the most significant ST-segment changes. Increases in heart rate to greater than 110 beats/min are more likely than episodes of hypertension to produce signs of ischemia on the ECG. Increases in heart rate decrease coronary filling and result in lower oxygen delivery. End-tidal carbon dioxide monitoring is important because hyperventilation with resultant hypocarbia may result in coronary artery vasoconstriction with resultant ischemia.

Key Points

- Functional systemic changes associated with hypertension are:
  - Cardiomyopathy
  - Systolic ventricular dysfunction
  - Heart failure
  - Stroke
  - Nephrosclerosis
- Pathological changes associated with untreated or poorly controlled hypertension are:
  - Left ventricular hypertrophy
  - Stroke
  - Subendocardial ischemia
  - Elevation of threshold for cerebrovascular autoregulation
- Antihypertensive medication should be continued to the time of surgery to avoid serious side effects associated with discontinuation.
- Valvular lesions produce pressure overloads (mitral stenosis, aortic stenosis) or volume overloads (mitral regurgitation, aortic regurgitation) in the left atrium or the left ventricle.
- Valvular lesions increase cardiac work in pressure and volume.
- Chronic mitral valve regurgitation produces left ventricular and atrial volume overload with resultant dilation and hypertrophy.
- The anesthetic management goal of a patient with mitral regurgitation is improving forward flow of blood volume.
- With mitral stenosis, left atrial pressure increases resulting in hypertrophy and dilation, while the left ventricle is volume overloaded because of obstruction to forward flow.
- Aortic stenosis predisposes the patient to the development of ischemia even without the presence of CAD.
- Symptoms of aortic stenosis are angina, dyspnea, syncope, and CHF.
- Anesthetic considerations in aortic stenosis are maintenance of adequate intravascular volume and normal cardiac rate and rhythm.
- Heart failure is defined as the inability of the heart to deliver a supply of oxygenated blood sufficient to meet the metabolic needs of the peripheral tissues at rest and during exercise.
- CHF can be caused by cardiomyopathies, ischemia, restrictive and congenital cardiac disease, and conduction defects. Noncardiac causes of CHF include hypertension, pulmonary emboli, and thyrotoxicosis.
- Symptoms of CHF are dyspnea on exertion and excessive fatigue during exercise; dry, nocturnal cough; rales; cardiomegaly; peripheral edema; hepatomegaly; and low cardiac output.
- Optimization of cardiac function is important to anesthetic planning. Patients with uncompensated cardiac failure are not candidates for elective surgery.

Continued

Key Points   *continued*

- Symptoms of digitalis toxicity include nausea, vomiting, or anorexia; abdominal pain; confusion; double vision or "floaters" in the visual path; and paresthesias.
- Overall perioperative risk is definitely increased in patients with known CAD.
- If noninvasive tests reveal significant cardiac ischemia during or after minimal exertion, a coronary artery revascularization procedure may be indicated before any other surgery is planned.

Internet Resources

GASNet Search: Anesthesia and Cardiovascular Disease:
http://gasnet.med.yale.edu/about/search.php?p1=anesthesia+and+cardiovascular+disease

Virtual Anaesthesia Textbook:
http://www.virtual-anaesthesia-textbook.com/

Nurse-Anesthesia.com:
http://www.nurse-anesthesia.com/

Update in Anaesthesia: Cumulative Index Arranged by Issue:
http://www.nda.ox.ac.uk/wfsa/html/pages/up_issu.htm

University of Chicago: Anesthesia and Critical Care: Vascular Thoracic Anesthesia Manual:
http://daccx.bsd.uchicago.edu/manuals/vtmanual/vtmanual.html

Bibliography

ACC/AHA practice guidelines update for perioperative cardiovascular evaluation for noncardiac surgery, 2002; available online: http://www.acc.org/clinical/topic/topic.htm#guidelines.

ACC/AHA practice guidelines for evaluation and management of chronic heart failure in the adult, *J Am Coll Cardiol* 38:2101-2113, 2001; available online: http://www.acc.org/clinical/topic/topic.htm#guidelines.

Atwell D, Mossad EB: Preoperative anesthesia evaluation in cardiac anesthesia. In Estafanous FG, Barash PG, Reves JG, editors: *Cardiac anesthesia: principles and clinical practice,* Philadelphia, 2001, Lippincott Williams & Wilkins, pp 153-173.

Bondy RJ, Wynands JE, Dorman BH, Reves JG: Anesthesia for coronary artery by-pass surgery. In Estafanous FG, Barash PG, Reves JG, editors: *Cardiac anesthesia: principles and clinical practice,* Philadelphia, 2001, Lippincott Williams & Wilkins, pp 541-555.

Felisher LA: Preoperative assessment. In Youngberg JA, editor: *Cardiac, vascular, and thoracic anesthesia,* New York, 2000, Churchill Livingstone, pp 3-19.

Frasco PE, DeBruijn NP: Valvular heart disease. In Estafanous FG, Barash PG, Reves JG, editors: *Cardiac anesthesia: principles and clinical practice,* Philadelphia, 2001, Lippincott Williams & Wilkins, pp 557-584.

Martin DE, Shanks GE: Strategies for the preoperative evaluation of the hypertensive patient, *Anesthesiol Clin N Am* 17:529-548, 1999.

McNulty SE: Preoperative evaluation of hypertension: anesthetic implications in patients with coronary disease, *Anesthesiol Clin N Am* 17:549-565, 1999.

Shanewise JS, Hug CG: Anesthesia for adult cardiac surgery. In Miller R, editor: *Anesthesia,* ed 5, New York, 2000, Churchill Livingstone, pp 1753-1804.

Stoelting RK, Dierdorf SF: *Anesthesia and co-existing disease,* ed 4, New York, 2002, Churchill Livingstone.

Troianos JS: Anesthesia for the cardiac patient, St. Louis, 2002, Mosby-Year Book.

Respiratory Disease

Karen F. Ricker

1. What are pulmonary function tests (PFTs)?

PFTs are diagnostic tools to evaluate lung function. They also are frequently used to differentiate between restrictive, obstructive, or mixed disorders of the lungs and to evaluate the effectiveness of treatments for these disorders.

The most commonly performed PFTs measure *airway function, lung volumes and ventilation, and diffusing capacity*. Most PFTs are patient effort–dependent and should include a notation by the technician as to the reliability of results. PFTs typically are reported in absolute values and as a predicted percentage of normal. Normal values vary depending on gender, race, age, weight, and height. It is not possible to interpret spirometry accurately without this patient information.

2. Name and define lung volume subdivisions.

Lung volumes are subdivisions of the maximal lung capacity (see the following figure). Combinations of volumes are termed *capacities* (see the table on page 170).

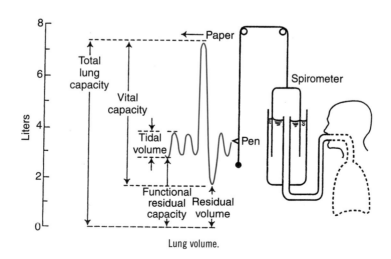

Lung volume.

Lung Volumes and Capacities*

Tidal volume (VT)	Volume of air that is inspired or exhaled with each normal breath (500 mL)
Inspiratory reserve volume (IRV)	Volume of air that can be inhaled above a normal tidal breath (3000 mL)
Inspiratory capacity (IC) = IRV + VT	Maximal amount of air a person can inspire (3500 mL)
Expiratory reserve volume (ERV)	Volume of air that can be exhaled by force at the end of a normal expiration (1100 mL)
Vital capacity (VC) = IC + ERV	Maximal amount of air that can be exhaled after a maximum inspiration (4600–5000 mL)
Functional residual capacity (FRC) = RV + ERV	Volume of air that remains in the lungs at the end of a normal expiration (2300 mL)
Residual volume (RV)	Volume of air remaining in the lung at the end of the most forceful expiration (1200 mL)
Closing volume (CV)	Portion of the VC that can be exhaled after the onset of airway closure
Closing capacity (CC) = CV + RV	Lung volume at which airways begin to close (1500 mL)
Total lung capacity (TLC) = VC + RV	Total lung volume after a maximal inspiration (5800 mL)

*Normal values are based on the age, height, and sex of the person being tested. Values in parentheses are typical approximate values for a healthy 70 kg adult.

3. How is FRC affected by anesthesia and surgery?

The FRC is affected by pharmacology, ventilation techniques, patient positioning, and patient preoperative health status. The supine position causes a 0.5 to 1 L (10% to 20%) decrease in FRC because of increased pulmonary vascular congestion and cephalad displacement of the diaphragm by the abdominal viscera. With the induction of general anesthesia, the FRC decreases an additional 15% to 20%, owing to the loss of respiratory and abdominal muscle tone.

4. Describe common pulmonary function tests.

Postbronchodilator challenges usually are performed during spirometry testing to determine if there is a reversible component to airway obstruction. A greater than 12% increase in the FEV_1 (an absolute improvement in FEV_1 of at least 200 mL) or the FVC after inhaling a beta agonist is generally considered a significant response (see the table on page 171).

Common Pulmonary Function Tests

Forced vital capacity (FVC)	Maximal amount of air that can be exhaled rapidly and forcefully after a full inspiration (60–70 mL/kg)
Forced expiratory volume in one second (FEV_1)	Volume of air expired during the first second of the FVC (4 L); often expressed as a percentage of the FVC (FEV_1/FVC%) (4 L/5 L = 80%); the FEV_1 is reduced in obstructive (increased airway resistance) and restrictive (low vital capacity) lung disease.
Peak expiratory flow rate (PEFR)	Maximal expiratory flow rate during a FVC maneuver (8–9 L/sec)
Forced midexpiratory flow rate (FEF25–75%) or maximal midexpiratory flow rate (MMF)	Average rate of airflow during the midportion of a FVC (4–5 L/sec). This is reduced in obstructive and restrictive disorders and is more effort independent.
Maximum voluntary ventilation (MVV)	Maximal amount of air exchanged during one min (125–170 L/min), reflects effort and overall pulmonary function.
Diffusing capacity of the lung for carbon monoxide (DLco)	Carbon monoxide can be used to measure the diffusing capacity across the alveolar-capillary membrane. DLco is decreased with COPD (especially emphysema). The normal value for a single-breath DLco is 25 mL/min/mm Hg

*Values in parentheses are typical approximate values for a healthy 70kg adult
COPD, chronic obstructive pulmonary disease.

5. Characterize and differentiate restrictive and obstructive disorders.

Restrictive disorders produce a decrease in lung volumes due to impaired expansion from lung or chest wall restriction. Patients with restrictive disorders have a reduced TLC and VC (<80% of the predicted values) and normal or decreased FRC. The reduction in TLC and VC are primarily caused by a reduction in IC. The PEFR, FEV_1, and FVC may be decreased with restrictive disease, but the FEV_1/FVC% is usually normal (see the following figure).

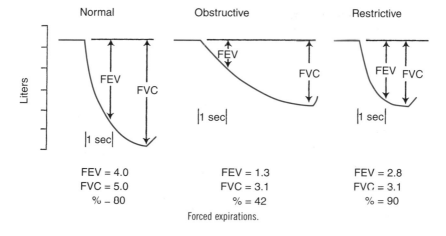

Forced expirations.

Patients with restrictive disease typically exhibit an increased work of breathing due to their abnormally low, minimally effective lung volumes. Reversible restrictive changes resulting from anesthesia and surgery include pain and residual muscle relaxant effects.

Patients with obstructive disorders have impeded airflow out of the lungs from causes such as bronchoconstriction, excess mucus production, and collapsible airways. Obstructive disease is characterized by increased TLC, FRC, and RV and decreased expiratory airflow rates (decreased PEFR and MMF). Principal diagnostic measurements for a patient with obstructive disease are FEV_1 less than 80% of the predicted value and $FEV_1/FVC\%$ less than 70% (see the following table).

Common Restrictive and Obstructive Disorders

Restrictive	Obstructive
Thickness or stiffening of lung parenchyma (pulmonary fibrosis, sarcoidosis)	COPD (Emphysema, Chronic Bronchitis)
Surgical removal of lung tissue (pneumonectomy or lobe resection)	Asthma
Pleural effusion	Cystic Fibrosis
Scoliosis, kyphoscoliosis	
Elevated diaphragm from morbid obesity, pregnancy, or ascites	
Intrathoracic and upper abdominal surgery	

COPD, chronic obstructive pulmonary disease.

6. **What is a flow volume loop, and what is its value in respiratory disease identification and management?**

During spirometry testing, the technician asks the patient to inhale fully, then exhale fully, then inhale fully again. With this maneuver, a flow volume loop tracing can be produced and displayed (see the figure on page 173). The shape of this curve from approximately 75% of FVC to maximal expiration is predominantly independent of patient effort. Flow during this time is determined by lung elastic recoil and resistance to flow. Small airways provide the primary resistance factor. In healthy subjects, the pattern of airflow limitation gives the curve a linear or slightly concave shape.

7. **Why is an emphysematous patient called a "pink puffer," and why is a patient with chronic bronchitis called a "blue bloater"?**

Chronic obstructive pulmonary disease (COPD) is one of the most common pulmonary disorders and is a major cause of disability and death in the United States. Clinical features of emphysema and chronic bronchitis are present in patients with COPD, although in many patients features of one predominate.

Emphysema is characterized by destruction of lung parenchyma and loss of radial traction within the alveolar walls, resulting in a loss of surface area for effective

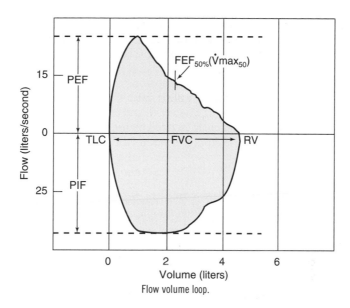

Flow volume loop.

gas exchange and reduced lung elastic recoil. The emphysematous alveoli become "baggy" similar to a balloon that has been repeatedly inflated; ultimately, this results in a decreased ability to exhale completely ("gas trapping") and overinflated lungs. Emphysematous patients tend to exhale against pursed lips in an attempt to keep their alveoli open longer (a self-generated positive end-expiratory pressure) for more complete exhalation. Despite the obstructive process, these patients usually preserve their ability to oxygenate until late in the disease process. This acyanotic, pursed-lip breather is referred to as a "pink puffer" (see the following table).

Clinical Manifestations of Emphysema Versus Chronic Bronchitis

Differential Feature	Emphysema "Pink Puffer"	Chronic Bronchitis "Blue Bloater"
Physical appearance	Thin, >60 years old	Obese, >50 years old
Mechanism	Lung parenchyma destruction; loss of elastic recoil	Narrowed airway lumen due to edema and mucus
Hematocrit	Normal	Elevated
Cor pulmonale	Late	Early
Airway resistance	Normal to slightly increased	Increased
Pao_2	Usually >60 mm Hg	Usually <60 mm Hg
$Paco_2$	Normal or <40 mm Hg	Elevated, >40 mm Hg
Sputum production	Increased	Markedly increased
Infection	Increased incidence	Markedly increased incidence
Residual volume	Markedly increased	Normal or slightly increased

Chronic bronchitis is characterized by proliferation and hypertrophy of bronchial goblet cells and hyperactivity of bronchial smooth muscle that results in increased mucus secretion and frequent airway occlusion. The copious secretions are often purulent with gram-positive and gram-negative bacteria present. These secretions and frequent airway occlusion usually cause pulmonary hypertension, right heart failure, and cor pulmonale. The cardiopulmonary dysfunction leads to a marked tendency toward decreased arterial oxygen saturation and carbon dioxide retention early in the disease process. The visual result is typically a cyanotic, plethoric, and edematous individual referred to as a "blue bloater."

8. How does an asthmatic patient compare with a patient with emphysema and chronic bronchitis?

Asthma is grouped with emphysema and chronic bronchitis as an obstructive respiratory disorder, but it has distinct features. Asthma is characterized by episodic bronchoconstriction, airway inflammation, and hypersecretion. During exacerbations, there is coughing, increased mucus production, dyspnea, and wheezing. Airflow obstruction is present, but it is partly reversible with bronchodilator therapy. During remissions, the patient is usually asymptomatic with normal or near-normal PFT data.

Bronchoconstriction associated with exacerbations of emphysema and chronic bronchitis is poorly responsive to bronchodilators. Vagal cholinergic tone may be a reversible component of airway narrowing in these two diseases.

Neutrophils are the major inflammatory cells activated in emphysema and chronic bronchitis. These white blood cells affect primarily peripheral airways, destroy lung parenchyma, and are largely unresponsive to corticosteroids. Airway hyperresponsiveness is associated with asthma and is in part the result of eosinophilic-mediated inflammation that affects airways, but does not involve lung parenchyma. In contrast to emphysema and chronic bronchitis, almost all aspects of this inflammatory process are markedly suppressed by corticosteroid therapy. Approximately 10% of patients with emphysema and chronic bronchitis also have asthma and share pathologic features. These patients are said to have "wheezy bronchitis" (see the figure on page 175).

9. What patients require preoperative PFTs?

The type of surgery and patient risk factors determine the need to perform PFTs preoperatively. PFTs may be indicated for the following reasons:
- Estimate lung function before pneumonectomy or lobectomy
- Determine perioperative interventions that may decrease complications
- Enhance risk assessment derived from the history and physical examination
- Assess significant physical risk factors, including
  - Symptomatic or severe lung disease
  - Heavy smoking history
  - Abnormal chest x-ray

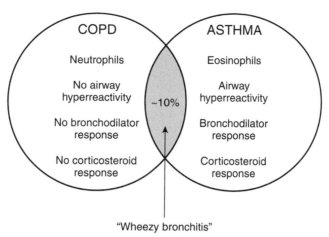

Overlap between chronic obstructive pulmonary disease (COPD) and asthma. Approximately 10% of patients with COPD also have asthma and share pathologic features ("wheezy bronchitis").

- Morbid obesity (>30% above ideal body weight)
- Presence of marked debilitation or malnourishment

10. What PFT values are predictive of increased postoperative risk?

No specific PFT absolutely identifies postoperative risk for complications, but some guidelines have been determined to help identify patients with higher perioperative risk and to identify patients who may be candidates for planned pneumonectomy. Patients with a predicted postoperative FEV_1 less than 800 mL typically are not considered surgical candidates except for patients being referred for lung reduction surgery (see the following table).

Preoperative Pulmonary Function Guidelines

Test*	Increased Postoperative Risk	Candidate for Pneumonectomy
FEV_1/FVC	<50% of predicted or <0.5	
FEV_1	<2 L or <50% of predicted	>2.0 L
FEF 25%–75%	<50% of predicted	
MVV	<50 L/min or <50% of predicted	>50 L/min or >50% of predicted
$Paco_2$	>50 mm Hg	
Predicted postoperative FEV_1		>0.8 L/min

11. Is regional anesthesia the preferred method to prevent pulmonary complications for a patient with respiratory disease?

In most cases, subarachnoid and epidural anesthetics are not superior for prevention of pulmonary complications. Regional blocks for peripheral extremities are associated, however, with lower pulmonary complication rates. Disease severity and anesthesia duration longer than 3.5 hours influence patient outcome more than the choice of a regional versus a general anesthetic.

12. Before anesthesia and surgery, what period of time is considered helpful for a patient to quit smoking?

Even 24 to 48 hours of smoking cessation is helpful to decrease the amount of carbon monoxide levels in the smoker's bloodstream. Carbon monoxide has an elimination half-life of 4 to 6 hours. It binds to hemoglobin at oxygen binding sites and shifts the oxyhemoglobin curve to the left. Preoperative smoking abstinence improves the patient's oxygenation during and after surgery. Patients derive more benefit if they refrain from smoking at least 6 to 8 weeks before surgery. This is the period of time required to increase mucociliary transport and to improve immune responsiveness.

13. How can intraoperative bronchospasm be prevented?

The first means of prevention is to perform a *careful history and physical examination* to assess current symptoms, medications, and patterns of self-care. Patients should have optimal preoperative inflammation reduction. Recent increases in medication use or signs of upper respiratory infection are reasons for concern in the perioperative period. Administration of an intravenous corticosteroid should be considered, especially for an asthmatic patient.

Patients with asthma, a smoking history, or a recent upper respiratory infection may benefit from a *preoperative inhaled bronchodilator, such as albuterol.* Anticholinergics are beneficial because of their mild bronchodilating effect. They are best administered prophylactically, 20 to 30 minutes before surgery. Patients already using inhalers should be encouraged to use them preoperatively, within 2 hours of surgery.

Propofol is the induction agent of choice in asthmatics, owing to its mild bronchodilating effects and its ability to blunt airway reflexes. Ketamine is a bronchodilator and is useful for patients with symptomatic asthma. All volatile agents cause bronchodilation. Sevoflurane, because of its low airway irritability, is a sensible choice when inhalation induction is necessary.

Airway provocation should be minimized. Lidocaine blunts airway reflexes; however, a study by Maslow reported that albuterol, but not intravenous lidocaine, prevented intubation-induced bronchoconstriction in asthmatic patients. A prudent approach may be to administer albuterol and lidocaine at induction and before extubation. Extubation should be performed at the earliest safe opportunity to prevent unnecessary mechanical bronchial stimulation by the endotracheal tube.

Drugs that cause histamine release, anticholinesterase agents, and histamine$_2$ receptor blocking agents have the potential to precipitate bronchoconstriction and should be avoided when possible.

14. Summarize ventilatory considerations for patients with obstructive and restrictive disorders.

Ventilatory considerations for patients with obstructive and restrictive disorders are compared in the following table.

Ventilatory Considerations in Obstructive Versus Restrictive Disease

Obstructive Disease	Restrictive Disease
Prolonged expiratory time to prevent gas trapping and inadvertent auto-PEEP	Prolonged inspiratory time to allow adequate time for gas exchange (inspiratory pause, addition of a sigh, or inverse I:E ratio)
Larger tidal volume (10–12 mL/kg) with slower respiratory rates to decrease turbulent airflow	Pressure-controlled ventilation allows adequate tidal volume delivery without exceeding alveolar pressures associated with barotrauma (35–40 cm H_2O).
Maintain preanesthetic carbon dioxide levels to prevent metabolic alkalosis and associated problems with acid-base balance.	Smaller tidal volumes (8–10 ml/Kg) with faster respiratory rates

I:E, inspiratory to expiratory; PEEP, positive end-expiratory pressure.

15. What do respiratory disease patients and gastroesophageal reflux disease patients have in common?

Patients with asthma, chronic bronchitis, and emphysema have a higher prevalence (39% to 70%) of reflux symptoms than the general U.S. adult population (14% to 19%). These patients are candidates for antacids and antireflux medications preoperatively. A rapid-sequence or modified rapid-sequence induction should be considered in this patient group.

Key Points

- Restrictive lung disease produces a decrease in lung volumes due to impaired expansion from lung or chest wall restriction.
- Obstructive disorders have impeded airflow out of the lungs from causes such as bronchoconstriction, excess mucus production, and collapsible airways.

Continued

Key Points   *continued*

- Chronic bronchitis results in copious, often purulent secretions that occlude the airways and cause pulmonary hypertension, right heart failure, and cor pulmonale. The visual result is typically a cyanotic, plethoric, and edematous individual referred to as a "blue bloater."
- Asthma is grouped with emphysema and chronic bronchitis as an obstructive respiratory disorder, but it has distinct features.
- Asthma is characterized by episodic bronchoconstriction, airway inflammation, and hypersecretion.
- Patients with a predicted postoperative FEV_1 less than 800 mL are typically not considered surgical candidates except for patients being referred for lung reduction surgery.
- Subarachnoid and epidural anesthesias are not superior for prevention of pulmonary complications.
- Patients derive more benefit if they refrain from smoking at least 6 to 8 weeks before surgery; however, stopping 24 to 48 hours before surgery decreases the amount of carbon monoxide in the blood.
- Propofol, ketamine, and all inhalational agents have bronchodilating effects, making them good choices in bronchospasm-susceptible patients.
- Patients with asthma, chronic bronchitis, and emphysema have a higher prevalence of reflux symptoms than the general U.S. adult population.

 Internet Resources

National Center for Biotechnology Information:
http://www.ncbi.nlm.nih.gov

Anesthesia.org: Evaluation and Perioperative Management of the Patient with Respiratory Disease:
http://www.anesthesia.org.cn/asa2002/rcl_source/253_Rock.pdf

Anesthesia.org: Bronchospasm: Successful Management:
http://www.anesthesia.org.cn/asa2002/rcl_source/411_Bishop.pdf

Update in Anaesthesia Practical Procedures Issue 12, Article 12 (2000): Anaesthesia for the Patient with Respiratory Disease:
http://www.nda.ox.ac.uk/wfsa/html/u12/u1212_01.htm

Nurse-Anesthesia.com:
http://www.nurse-anesthesia.com/

Virtual Anaesthesia Textbook:
http://www.virtual-anaesthesia-textbook.com/

Bibliography

Barnes PJ: Mechanisms in COPD: differences from asthma, *Chest* 117:10S-14S, 2000.

Benumof JL: Respiratory physiology and respiratory function during anesthesia. In Miller RD, editor: *Anesthesia,* ed 5, New York, 2000, Churchill Livingstone, pp 578-618.

Geer RT: Pulmonary complications of anesthesia. In Longernecker DE, Tinker JH, Morgan GE, editors: *Principles and practice of anesthesiology,* St. Louis, 1998, Mosby, pp 2353-2361.

Karlet M, Nagelhout J: Asthma: an anesthetic update, *AANA J* 69:317-324, 2001.

Kopp VJ, Boysen PG: Evaluation of the patient with pulmonary disease. In Longernecker DE, Tinker JH, Morgan GE, editors: *Principles and practice of anesthesiology,* St. Louis, 1998, Mosby, pp 232-241.

Maslow AD, et al: Inhaled albuterol, but not intravenous lidocaine, protects against intubation-induced bronchoconstriction in asthma, *Anesthesiology* 93:1198-1204, 2000.

Mokhlesi B, et al: Increased prevalence of gastroesophageal reflux symptoms in patients with COPD, *Chest* 119:1043-1048, 2001.

Morgan KC, Reger RB: Rise and fall of the FEV1, *Chest* 118:1639-1644, 2000.

Nakagawa N, et al: Relationship between the duration of the smoke-free period and the incidence of postoperative pulmonary complications after pulmonary surgery, *Chest* 120:705-710, 2001.

Patroniti' N, et al: Sigh improves gas exchange and lung volume in patients with acute respiratory distress syndrome undergoing pressure support ventilation, *Anesthesiology* 96:788-794, 2002.

Ruppel GL: *Manual of pulmonary function testing,* ed 7, St. Louis, 1998, Mosby.

West JB: *Pulmonary physiology and pathophysiology: an integrated, case-based approach,* ed 1, Philadelphia, 2001, Lippincott Williams & Wilkins

Chapter 20

Neurological Disorders

Steve L. Alves

1. Discuss the pathophysiology of spinal cord injury (SCI).

Most SCIs are traumatic and often result in partial or complete transection. Clinical manifestations depend on the level of the transection. Injuries above C3-5 (diaphragmatic innervation) require ventilatory support for survival. Transections above T1 result in quadriplegia, whereas transections above L4 result in paraplegia. The most common sites of injury are C5-6 and T12-L1.

Immediately after acute spinal cord transection, there is loss of sensation, flaccid paralysis, and loss of spinal reflexes below the level of injury. This period is referred to as the *spinal shock* phase of injury, and it typically lasts 1 to 3 weeks. During this time, spinal reflexes, muscle tone, and autonomic nervous system activity below the lesion gradually return. The following box identifies important manifestations of acute and chronic SCIs.

Manifestations of Acute and Chronic Spinal Cord Injury

Acute Spinal Cord Injury (Spinal Shock)
- Flaccid paralysis and complete loss of reflex and sensory activity at and below level of lesion
- Loss of vasomotor tone, cardiovascular instability, hypotension, bradycardia, venous pooling
- Paralytic ileus with distention
- Hypothermia

Chronic Spinal Cord Injury
- Proliferation of extrajunctional acetylcholine receptors
- Involuntary skeletal muscle spasms
- Risk for autonomic hyperreflexia
- Chronic pulmonary and genitourinary infections
- High risk for deep vein thromboses and pulmonary embolism
- Anemia
- Risk for hypothermia
- Mental depression
- Neuropathic pain
- Osteoporosis; prone to fractures

---

2. What is autonomic hyperreflexia?

Autonomic hyperreflexia is an unbridled sympathetic nervous system reflex response below the level of a spinal cord transection. It occurs most commonly with spinal cord transections at T5 and above and may appear anytime after the resolution of spinal shock.

Cutaneous (e.g., surgical incision, decubitus ulcer) or visceral (e.g., bladder or bowel distention) stimulation below the level of injury are common autonomic hyperreflexia triggers. Interruption of normal descending inhibitory impulses in the spinal cord allows an unmodulated sympathetic reflex response below the level of injury. The result is severe vasoconstriction below the transection. A baroreceptor-mediated reflex bradycardia and vasodilation occur above the transection. Cardiac dysrhythmias often accompany this phenomenon. Immediate interventions to lower the blood pressure are required. The following box lists manifestations and treatment of autonomic hyperreflexia.

Signs and Symptoms and Treatment of Autonomic Hyperreflexia

Signs and Symptoms
- Hypertension
- Reflex bradycardia
- Vasodilation and flushing above the transection; vasoconstriction and pallor below the transection
- Nasal and conjunctival congestion
- Headache
- Seizure activity
- Acute left ventricular failure (pulmonary edema)
- Subarachnoid hemorrhage

Treatment
- Remove the noxious stimulus
- Raise the head of bed (considering spine stability)
- Administer rapid-acting vasodilator drugs

---

3. What are the anesthesia implications for SCI patients?

Anesthesia management depends on the age of the injury. The primary focus immediately after an acute transection is preventing further damage, especially during patient positioning and airway manipulation. Anesthesia considerations for patients with nonacute transections include vigilant monitoring for autonomic hyperreflexia, avoiding hyperkalemia, and careful positioning. The following box outlines anesthesia management priorities for acute and chronic SCIs.

Anesthesia Considerations in the Presence of Spinal Cord Transection

Acute Spinal Cord Transection
- Maintain in-line stabilization of the neck with airway management; consider fiberoptic-guided intubation, especially if cervical spine injury is present or suspected.
- Prepare for cardiovascular instability. Position changes, mild blood loss, and positive-pressure ventilation may precipitate hypotension.
- Guard against hypothermia.
- Succinylcholine may be administered within the first 24 hours of an acute injury.

Chronic Spinal Cord Transection
- Monitor for autonomic hyperreflexia. Have rapid-acting vasodilators available.
- Use nondepolarizing muscle relaxants only. There is a risk of hyperkalemia with succinylcholine.
- Guard against hypothermia.
- Position carefully (osteoporosis).

---

4. Describe the pathophysiology of seizure disorders.

Seizures are an abnormal discharge of electrical activity in the brain. It is estimated that the disorder occurs in 2% to 5% of the population. Seizures may be a manifestation of an underlying central nervous system disease, a systemic disorder, or an idiopathic phenomenon. Partial seizure activity (focal) is clinically manifested by motor, sensory, autonomic, or psychic signs and symptoms that depend on the cortical area affected. Generalized seizures characteristically produce bilateral, symmetrical electrical activity without local onset. Grand mal seizures are most common and are characterized by a loss of consciousness followed by clonic and tonic motor activity.

5. Discuss the anesthesia considerations for patients with seizure disorders.

Preoperative evaluation of a patient with a seizure disorder should focus on the type of seizure activity, common precipitants, and pharmacological treatment. Seizures in adults usually are related to a structural brain lesion (e.g., head trauma, tumor, stroke) or systemic disorders (e.g., uremia, alkalosis, hypoxia, hypoglycemia, electrolyte imbalance, febrile illness, drug/alcohol overdose or withdrawal). Blood levels of antiepileptics should be measured preoperatively in patients with signs of toxicity and in patients with a recent seizure occurrence. At toxic levels, most medications cause ataxia, dizziness, confusion, and sedation.

If a seizure occurs, maintaining an open airway and adequate oxygenation are priorities. In adults, intravenous thiopental (50 to 100 mg), phenytoin (10 to 20 mg/kg), or diazepam (5 to 10 mg) may be used to treat seizure activity.

The intraoperative management of patients with seizure disorders should include the avoidance of anesthetic agents that may induce seizure activity. Methohexital and etomidate may activate seizure foci and should be used with caution in patients with focal epilepsy. In large doses, atracurium and cisatracurium may be contraindicated because of the reported epileptogenic potential of their metabolite laudanosine. Meperidine should be avoided because its metabolite normeperidine can precipitate seizure activity. Enflurane in concentrations greater than 2.5% and in combination with hyperventilation can precipitate electroencephalogram patterns resembling seizure activity.

Patients on long-term antiepileptic drug therapy may show hepatic microsomal enzyme (P-450) induction and may require increased doses of intravenous anesthetics and nondepolarizing neuromuscular blocking agents. The risk for hepatotoxicity from halothane may be increased with P-450 enzyme induction.

6. What are the characteristic features of Parkinson's disease?

Parkinson's disease is an adult-onset degenerative disorder of the extrapyramidal motor system, characterized by dopamine depletion and unopposed acetylcholine activity in the basal ganglia. This slowly progressive disease manifests as cogwheel rigidity, a resting (pill-rolling) tremor, postural instability, a fixed facial expression, shuffling gait, dementia, depression, akinesia, and diaphragmatic spasms.

A precursor of dopamine, levodopa, is the mainstay of Parkinson's disease therapy. Levodopa readily crosses the blood-brain barrier; dopamine does not. Side effects of levodopa treatment include nausea, vomiting, dyskinesia, cardiac irritability, and orthostatic hypotension. Drug preparations that combine levodopa with dopa decarboxylase inhibitor (carbidopa [Sinemet]) increase delivery and allow for lower dosing. Other dopamine agonists, bromocriptine (Parlodel) and pergolide (Permax), also may be employed.

7. Describe the anesthetic considerations for a patient with Parkinson's disease.

- Levodopa should be continued preoperatively, including the morning of surgery, because its duration is short. Abrupt withdrawal may lead to worsening of muscle rigidity and interfere with respiratory function.
- Return of airway reflexes and satisfactory respiratory effort should be evaluated carefully before extubation.
- Dopamine antagonists, such as phenothiazines, butyrophenones (droperidol), and metoclopramide, may exacerbate clinical symptoms and should be avoided. Anticholinergic drugs or antihistamines may be used to treat acute exacerbation of symptoms.
- Patients receiving long-term levodopa therapy may show either profound hypotension or hypertension with induction of anesthesia. Hypovolemia, catecholamine depletion, and autonomic instability may contribute to the cardiovascular dynamics.

- Cardiac irritability is associated with arrhythmias in some patients on levodopa therapy. Halothane, ketamine, and local anesthetics containing epinephrine should be used cautiously.
- Levodopa is associated with increased renal blood flow, and surgical patients on long-term levodopa therapy may require aggressive fluid replacement. Significant hypotension should be treated with fluid administration and small doses of a direct-acting vasopressor.
- Rare cases of hyperkalemia after succinylcholine have been reported in patients with Parkinson's disease.

8. Explain the characteristics of multiple sclerosis.

Multiple sclerosis is a disease of neuron demyelination that occurs at unpredictable and multiple sites in the central nervous system. Over time, chronic inflammation produces permanent axon scarring (gliosis). The disease is an autoimmune disorder of unknown etiology. It primarily affects patients during their 20s to 40s with a 2:1 female predominance. The disease typically follows an unpredictable course of exacerbations and remissions. Common signs and symptoms include fatigue, paresthesias, cold intolerance, visual disturbances, unsteady gait, muscle weakness and atrophy, respiratory insufficiency, dysphagia, and sleep apnea. Treatment is aimed at controlling symptoms and slowing the disease process. Glucocorticoids may lessen the severity and duration of acute attacks.

9. Summarize the anesthesia concerns when managing patients with multiple sclerosis.

- The stress of anesthesia and surgery may worsen symptoms of multiple sclerosis, but the effects are unpredictable. Elective surgery should be avoided during a relapse of the disease.
- Spinal anesthesia has been associated with worsening of symptoms and generally is avoided. Epidural and other regional techniques have been used, especially in obstetrical anesthesia, with no adverse effects.
- Autonomic nervous system dysfunction may lead to labile cardiovascular responses in some patients.
- Succinylcholine should be avoided because of the potential threat of hyperkalemia.
- The anesthetist should guard against increases in patient temperature. Temperature elevation intensifies symptoms by interfering with nerve conduction. A body temperature increase of 0.5° C may block conduction in demyelinated fibers.

10. Identify the clinical manifestations of amyotrophic lateral sclerosis.

Amyotrophic lateral sclerosis, also called *Lou Gehrig's disease,* is a progressive disease of upper and lower motor neurons. Patients typically present with muscle weakness, atrophy, fasciculations, and spasticity at age 50 to 60 years. The disease rapidly progresses; over 2 to 3 years, the symptoms become generalized, involving widespread skeletal and bulbar muscles.

11. What are the anesthetic implications in managing patients with amyotrophic lateral sclerosis?

- Progressive muscle weakness makes the patient susceptible to aspiration and ventilatory failure.
- Nondepolarizing neuromuscular blocking agents and respiratory depressant drugs should be titrated judiciously because patients often display enhanced sensitivity.
- Full return of muscle strength before extubation must be ascertained, and the adequacy of respiratory function should be monitored into the postoperative period.
- Succinylcholine is contraindicated because of the potential for exaggerated potassium release.

12. Discuss the pathophysiology of Guillain-Barré syndrome.

Guillain-Barré syndrome is characterized by a sudden onset of ascending motor paralysis. The disease typically begins in the legs and spreads cephalad over several days. Bulbar involvement and respiratory muscle paralysis are common manifestations. The disease is the result of an autoimmune reaction against the myelin sheath of peripheral nerves, and in most instances the syndrome follows a viral infection. Mortality (3% to 8%) is related to complications associated with cardiovascular instability, sepsis, ventilatory failure, or pulmonary embolism.

13. Summarize the important anesthetic concerns regarding Guillain-Barré syndrome.

- Respiratory complications are a main priority in managing Guillain-Barré syndrome patients.
- Autonomic nervous system instability may produce wide fluctuations in blood pressure, profuse diaphoresis, tachycardia, and cardiac conduction defects. The anesthetized patient may become hypotensive with changes in position, mild blood loss, or positive-pressure ventilation. Exaggerated hypertension may occur during laryngoscopy, surgical incision, and extubation.
- Succinylcholine should be avoided, owing to the potential for exaggerated potassium release.
- The use of regional anesthesia in these patients is controversial, but generally is not recommended.

 Key Points

- Clinical manifestations of SCI depend on the level of the transection. Injuries above C3-5 (diaphragmatic innervation) require ventilatory support for survival. Transections above T1 result in quadriplegia, whereas transections above L4 result in paraplegia. The most common sites of SCI are C5-6 and T12-L1.

Key Points   *continued*

- Autonomic hyperreflexia is an unbridled sympathetic nervous system reflex response below the level of a spinal cord transection. Interruption of normal descending inhibitory impulses in the spinal cord allow an unmodulated sympathetic reflex response below the level of injury.

- Preoperative evaluation of a patient with a seizure disorder should focus on the type of seizure activity, common precipitants, and pharmacological treatment.

- The intraoperative management of patients with seizure disorders should include the avoidance of anesthetic agents that may induce seizure activity.

- Patients on long-term antiepileptic drug therapy may show hepatic microsomal enzyme (P-450) induction and may require increased doses of intravenous anesthetics and nondepolarizing neuromuscular blocking agents.

- Parkinson's disease is an adult-onset degenerative disorder of the extrapyramidal motor system, characterized by dopamine depletion and unopposed acetylcholine activity in the basal ganglia.

- A precursor of dopamine, levodopa, is the mainstay of Parkinson's disease therapy and should be continued preoperatively, including the morning of surgery.

- The stress of anesthesia and surgery may worsen symptoms of multiple sclerosis, but the effects are unpredictable.

- Spinal anesthesia in multiple sclerosis has been associated with worsening of symptoms; however, epidural and other regional techniques have been used without adverse effects.

- Amyotrophic lateral sclerosis, also called *Lou Gehrig's disease,* is a progressive disease of upper and lower motor neurons.

- Guillain-Barré syndrome is the result of an autoimmune reaction against the myelin sheath of peripheral nerves, and in most instances the syndrome follows a viral infection.

- Respiratory complications are a main priority in managing patients with Guillain-Barré syndrome. Nervous system instability may produce wide fluctuations in blood pressure, profuse diaphoresis, tachycardia, and cardiac conduction defects. Succinylcholine should be avoided.

Internet Resources

GASNet: Seizures-Anesthesia:
http://gasnet.med.yale.edu/gta/chapters/seizures-anesthesia.php

Virtual Anaesthesia Textbook:
http://www.virtual-anaesthesia-textbook.com/

Nurse-Anesthesia.com:
http://www.nurse-anesthesia.com/

Continued

Internet Resources   *continued*

Manbit Technologies: Regional Blocks and Neurological Disease:
http://www.manbit.com/oa/C43.htm

Internet Handbook of Neurology: Demyelinating Diseases:
http://www.neuropat.dote.hu/myelin.htm

GASNet: Parkinson's:
http://gasnet.med.yale.edu/gta/chapters/parkinsons.php

Bibliography

Aker J: Neuroanatomy, physiology, and neuroanesthesia. In Nagelhout JJ, Zaglaniczny KL, editors: *Nurse anesthesia*, ed 2, Philadelphia, 2001, WB Saunders.

Albin M: *Textbook of neuroanesthesia with neurosurgical and neuroscience perspectives*, New York, 1997, McGraw-Hill.

Alves SL, Yermal SJ: Assessment of the neurologic system in the adult. In Waugaman, WR, Foster SD, Rigor BM, editors: *Principles and practice of nurse anesthesia*, ed 3, Stamford, Appleton & Lange, 1999.

Cottrell JE, Smith DS: *Anesthesia and neurosurgery*, ed 3, St. Louis, 1994, Mosby-Year Book.

Cucchiara RF, Black S, Michenfelder JD: *Clinical neuroanesthesia*, ed 2, New York, 1998, Churchill Livingstone.

Morgan GE, Mikhail MS, Murray MJ: *Clinical anesthesiology*, ed 3, New York, 2002, McGraw-Hill.

Newfield P, Cottrell JE: *Handbook of neuroanesthesia*, ed 3, Philadelphia, 1999, Lippincott Williams & Wilkins.

Neuromuscular and Musculoskeletal Diseases

Debra Rose Merritt

1. Define malignant hyperthermia (MH).

MH, first described by Denborough and Lorell in 1960, is an uncommon pharmacogenetic disease affecting skeletal muscle in humans, certain breeds of swine, horses, and other animals. When exposed to potent inhaled anesthetics or depolarizing muscle relaxants, susceptible individuals can experience fatal skeletal muscle hypermetabolism characterized by increased carbon dioxide production, oxygen consumption, and muscle membrane breakdown.

2. What is the pathophysiology of MH?

The final common pathway for the development of MH seems to be an uncontrolled increase in intracellular calcium in the muscle cell after exposure to triggering agents. This abnormal and sustained elevation in myoplasmic free calcium is controlled primarily by the calcium release channels of the sarcoplasmic reticulum by way of the ryanodine receptor.

3. What is the incidence of MH?

The exact incidence of the MH gene in the United States is unknown. Based on retrospective studies, the clinical incidence of MH is 1 in 15,000 pediatric anesthetics and 1 in 50,000 adult anesthetics. The incidence is higher when succinylcholine is used with other triggering agents. There are geographic variations in incidence. Areas in the United States with a higher occurrence include Wisconsin, West Virginia, and Michigan. MH has been observed in most races, in both sexes, and in all age groups. MH occurs most often in children, teenagers, and young adults, with teenagers having the highest incidence.

4. Identify the MH-triggering anesthetic agents.

All volatile *inhalational anesthetics* (e.g., halothane, isoflurane, enflurane, desflurane, sevoflurane, methoxyflurane, ether, cyclopropane) and the depolarizing muscle relaxant *succinylcholine* are capable of triggering MH in humans. An MH episode may not occur with each exposure in a susceptible patient. About half of all MH episodes have been preceded by one or more uneventful anesthetics.

5. List drugs that are considered safe for administration to MH-susceptible patients.

- Barbiturates, propofol, etomidate
- Benzodiazepines
- Opioids
- Droperidol
- Nitrous oxide
- Nondepolarizing muscle relaxants
- Anticholinesterase drugs
- Anticholinergic drugs
- Sympathomimetics
- Local anesthetics (esters and amides)

6. Identify other syndromes most commonly associated with MH susceptibility.

Central core disease, a rare, congenital myopathy characterized by neonatal hypotonia, proximal muscle weakness, decreased deep tendon reflexes, and skeletal abnormalities, is directly associated with MH susceptibility. There is a general "clinical" impression that patients with minor muscular abnormalities have an increased incidence of MH, and several groups have reported the association of susceptibility to MH and various myopathies, including central core disease, King Deborough syndrome, Duchenne muscular dystrophy (DMD), hyperkalemic periodic paralysis, and other myopathies. Only central core disease has been associated consistently with MH episodes, however, and shares the same genetic locus, the *RYR1* gene on chromosome 19, with MH.

7. Describe the clinical signs and symptoms of MH.

The clinical presentation of MH results from muscle hypermetabolism that leads to overproduction of carbon dioxide, lactate, and heat and causes sympathetic nervous system stimulation. Ultimately the body is unable to respond to the extraordinary increase in metabolic demand. When the metabolic demand no longer can be sustained, organ system failure ensues. Without prompt treatment, late complications and death are inevitable. Specific signs and symptoms are as follows:

- Hypercarbia; unexplained increase in end-tidal carbon dioxide during constant ventilation (earliest, most sensitive sign)
- Tachycardia, dysrhythmias
- Arterial hypoxemia, central venous oxygen desaturation
- Tachypnea (masked with controlled ventilation and neuromuscular blockade)
- Masseter muscle rigidity or trismus
- Muscle rigidity (variability in presentation; most specific sign)
- Metabolic and respiratory acidosis
- Skin mottling and cyanosis
- Core temperature elevation (late sign), diaphoresis
- Hyperkalemia, hypercalcemia, hyperphosphatemia
- Elevated serum creatinine phosphokinase (creatine kinase)
- Myoglobinuria

Late complications include the following:
- Disseminated intravascular coagulation
- Pulmonary edema
- Acute renal failure
- Blindness, seizures, coma, paralysis (central nervous system damage)

8. How should an episode of MH be managed?

The Malignant Hyperthermia Association of the United States (MHAUS) has outlined a protocol for the suggested therapy for MH. Successful treatment depends on early recognition and prompt administration of dantrolene. Symptomatic treatment is directed toward maintaining renal function and correcting hyperthermia, acidosis, and arterial hypoxemia.

ACUTE PHASE
Call for help, get dantrolene, MH cart—notify surgeon.
- Discontinue volatile agents and succinylcholine.
- Hyperventilate the lungs with 100% oxygen at flows of at least 10 L/min.
- Expedite or abort the surgical procedure; if emergent, use nontriggering agents.

Administer intravenous dantrolene, 2.5 mg/kg bolus.
- Be prepared to repeat the initial dose until signs of MH are controlled.
- A total dose of 10 mg/kg or more total may be required to control an episode.

Monitor and treat metabolic acidosis.
- Follow serial arterial blood gases, and administer sodium bicarbonate, 1 to 2 mEq/kg intravenously, as indicated.
- Consider central and intraarterial catheter placement for monitoring and blood sampling.

Institute active cooling measures.
- Cool patients with core temperatures greater than 39° C: use cold intravenous normal saline; cold lavage to open body cavities, stomach (via nasogastric tube), bladder, or rectum; surface cooling with ice packs to groin and axilla; and hypothermia blanket.
- Stop cooling at 38° C core temperature to prevent hypothermia.

DYSRHYTHMIAS
- Dysrhythmias usually respond to treatment of acidosis and hyperkalemia.
- Use standard antiarrhythmic drug therapy except calcium channel blockers, which can cause hyperkalemia or cardiac arrest in the presence of dantrolene sodium.

HYPERKALEMIA
- Treat with hyperventilation, sodium bicarbonate, glucose/insulin infusion, and calcium chloride.
- In adult patients, administer 10 units of regular insulin and 50 mL of 50% glucose intravenously.
- In pediatric patients, administer 0.15 units of insulin/kg and 1 mL/kg 50% glucose intravenously.

- Administer calcium chloride, 10 mg/kg, or calcium gluconate, 10 to 50 mg/kg, for life-threatening hyperkalemia.

MONITORING AND LABORATORY TESTS
- Perform blood studies (hemoglobin, myoglobin, electrolytes, creatine kinase, liver profile, blood urea nitrogen, lactate, glucose), coagulation studies (prothrombin time, fibrinogen, activated partial thromboplastin time, fibrinolytic split products, platelet count), and urine hemoglobin and myoglobin studies.
- Maintain urine output at greater than 2 mL/kg/hr with intravenous fluids, furosemide, and mannitol.
- Venous blood gas values may document hypermetabolism better than arterial values.

POST ACUTE PHASE
- Observe the patient in an intensive care unit for 24 to 36 hours due to the risk of recrudescence.
- Administer dantrolene, 1 mg/kg intravenously every 4 to 6 hours for at least 36 hours. Further doses may be indicated.
- Monitor arterial blood gases, serum creatine kinase, urine myoglobin, and coagulation parameters for at least 24 to 48 hours.
- Maintain urine output at greater than 2 mL/kg/hr with intravenous fluids, furosemide, and mannitol.
- Counsel the patient and family regarding MH and further precautions. Refer them to MHAUS for information and enrollment in the North American MH Registry. Send follow-up letter to the patient and his or her physician and refer them to the nearest biopsy center for biopsy. (MH hotline: 1-800-MH-HYPER [1-800-644-9737]; nonemergency information: MHAUS, 39 East State Street, PO Box 1069, Sherburne, NY 13460-1069; telephone: 1-800-986-4287 or 607-674-7901; e-mail: mhaus@norwich.net; website: www.mhaus.org).

9. Describe the method that can be used to facilitate the mixing and administration of dantrolene.

Dantrolene is packaged as 20 mg of lyophilized powder to be dissolved in 60 mL of sterile water. A 70-kg patient requires approximately 9 vials of dantrolene and 540 mL of sterile water to prepare the initial treatment dose. Reconstitution can be cumbersome and time-consuming. The following setup can facilitate this process: First, insert a secondary intravenous tubing set into 1 L of sterile water, and place a stopcock with an attached 60-mL syringe at the end. Next, insert a vented minispike dispensing pin into the vials of dantrolene. Attach and position the stopcock to withdraw sterile water, and inject into the dantrolene vial. Continue the process for each vial (see the figure on page 193).

10. Describe the mechanism of action of dantrolene and its possible side effects.

Dantrolene is a direct-acting skeletal muscle relaxant that blocks calcium release from myoplasmic sarcoplasmic reticulum. Although the precise mechanism is

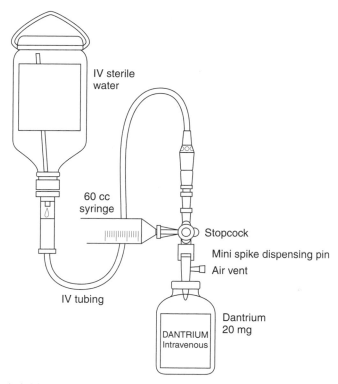

Setup for mixing and administration of dantrolene. *(Modified from Antil A: Anesthesia care provider worksheet. In Mashman D, Greenberg C, editors: Malignant hyperthermia procedure manual, Sherburne, NY, 2001, Malignant Hyperthermia Association of the United States.)*

unknown, dantrolene is believed to work by inhibiting the ryanodine receptor, the major calcium release channel of skeletal muscle sarcoplasmic reticulum. Side effects of treatment include drowsiness, dizziness, headache, hepatotoxicity, hyperkalemia, gastrointestinal upset, and local inflammatory phlebitis in small peripheral veins. The most serious complication after acute administration is generalized muscle weakness that may result in respiratory insufficiency or aspiration pneumonia, especially in patients with preexisting neuromuscular disease.

11. Discuss anesthetic preparation and management for a MH-susceptible patient.

- Check the MH cart and have it readily available.
- Prepare the anesthesia machine. Remove or seal vaporizers; apply a new carbon dioxide absorber, fresh gas hose, and disposable circuit. Flush the machine with a fresh gas flow of 10 L/min for 10 to 20 minutes.
- Schedule the MH-susceptible patient for first case of the day.
- Consider preoperative sedation. Routine dantrolene prophylaxis is not required.

- Implement an anesthetic with nontriggering agents.
- Inform postoperative care providers of the patient's MH status, and monitor the patient for 4 to 6 hours in the recovery room. If the clinical course is uneventful, additional laboratory tests are not necessary.

12. How is susceptibility to MH confirmed?

In vitro contracture tests, which measure the response of skeletal muscle strips to either halothane or caffeine, are the only reliable tests to diagnose suscepti-bility to MH. A muscle biopsy should be considered in all patients with a suspicious clinical history or a family history of MH or MH-related clinical signs. Based on guidelines established by the North American MH Registry, the halothane-caffeine contracture tests provide sensitivity of 100% and specificity of 78%.

13. Define masseter muscle rigidity (MMR), and describe strategies for managing a patient with MMR.

MMR is a rigidity of the jaw muscles that may be observed after the admini-stration of an intubating dose of succinylcholine. MMR occurs most commonly as a transient phenomenon in children, but it also may be a forewarning of MH. Controversy exists regarding the association of MMR with MH and appropriate management. MMR is reported to occur in 1% of children receiving halothane and succinylcholine. Although many of these cases do not progress to a fulminant MH episode, about 50% may prove to be MH susceptible by muscle biopsy.

When MMR develops, a decision must be made either to switch to a non-triggering anesthetic and continue the surgery or to stop the anesthetic and end the procedure. Strategies for managing a patient with MMR have been proposed, based on Kaplan's classification, which considers the degree of muscle rigidity. The following table presents a suggested treatment algorithm for MMR.

Treatment of Masseter Muscle Rigidity

Jaw Stiffness; Normal Response to Succinylcholine	Jaw Rigidity Interferes with Intubation	"Jaws of Steel" Makes Orotracheal Intubation Impossible
Continue with planned surgery	Stop inhalational agents and succinylcholine; ventilate with 100% oxygen	Stop inhalational agents and succinylcholine; ventilate with 100% oxygen
Monitor for MH	Continue surgery with nontrigger anesthetics; monitor for MH	

Treatment of Masseter Muscle Rigidity *continued*		
Jaw Stiffness; Normal Response to Succinylcholine	**Jaw Rigidity Interferes with Intubation**	**"Jaws of Steel" Makes Orotracheal Intubation Impossible**
No signs of MH; no further workup recommended	Observe in ICU for 24 hr; monitor serum creatine kinase and electrolytes, urine myoglobin; MH workup	Stop surgery; awaken patient Observe in ICU for 24 hr; monitor serum creatine kinase and electrolytes, urine myoglobin; MH workup

ICU, intensive care unit, MH, malignant hyperthermia

14. What is Duchenne muscular dystrophy?

DMD is one of the most common and severe forms of childhood muscular dystrophy. The disease is caused by an X-linked recessive gene mutation resulting in abnormal or absent dystrophin, a muscle membrane protein that provides mechanical stability to the sarcolemma. DMD has an incidence of 1 in 3500 live male births.

15. Describe the hallmark features of DMD.

DMD is characterized by painless degeneration and atrophy of skeletal, cardiac, and smooth muscle. Gait disturbances, difficulty climbing stairs, and frequent falling reflect skeletal muscle involvement. Increased sarcolemma permeability results in elevated serum creatine kinase concentrations. Degeneration of cardiac muscle can result in congestive cardiomyopathy and mitral regurgitation secondary to papillary muscle dysfunction and decreased myocardial contractility. Characteristic changes on the electrocardiogram include P-R interval prolongation, prominent R waves in V_1, deep Q waves in the limb leads, and atrial arrhythmias. Chronic weakness of the respiratory muscles results in loss of pulmonary reserve and retention of secretions. As DMD progresses, muscle wasting and skeletal deformities produce kyphoscoliosis, causing a restrictive ventilatory impairment. Death usually occurs by 15 to 25 years of age as a result of cardiorespiratory failure.

16. What are the anesthetic considerations for patients with DMD?

Patients with DMD are at increased risk for pulmonary aspiration due to weak laryngeal reflexes and gastrointestinal hypomotility. A prophylactic nasogastric tube should be placed to avoid gastric dilation. Succinylcholine is contraindicated in these patients because of the associated risk of rhabdomyolysis, hyperkalemia, and cardiac arrest. When muscle weakness is prominent, nondepolarizing muscle relaxants have an exaggerated effect. Sedatives and narcotics should be avoided or administered with extreme caution. The use of regional anesthesia may diminish the risk of postoperative pulmonary dysfunction in DMD patients.

17. Define myasthenia gravis.

Myasthenia gravis is an acquired, chronic IgG antibody–mediated disease of the neuromuscular junction. Autoimmune destruction or inactivation of post-synaptic acetylcholine receptors at the neuromuscular junction produces weakness and rapid fatigability of voluntary skeletal muscles with repetitive use. Women frequently are affected between age 20 and 30 years; men commonly present with the disease at age older than 60 years. The disease frequently is associated with abnormalities of the thymus gland.

18. Describe the clinical course of myasthenia gravis.

The clinical course is marked by periods of exacerbations and remissions. Extra-ocular muscles often are affected causing ptosis and diplopia. Bulbar muscle weakness may produce dysphagia, dysarthria, and difficulty handling oral secretions. Arm, leg, and truncal weakness is common. Patients with myasthenia gravis have a higher incidence of other autoimmune diseases, including thyroid disorders, rheumatoid arthritis, and systemic lupus erythematosus. Infection, electrolyte abnormalities, pregnancy, emotional stress, and surgery can worsen myasthenic symptoms. Aminoglycoside antibiotics, magnesium, lithium, calcium channel blockers, and antiarrhythmics have the potential to exacerbate muscle weakness.

19. Name the treatment modalities that are available for patients with myasthenia gravis.

Treatment modalities include anticholinesterase drugs, immunosuppression, plasmapheresis, and thymectomy.

20. Identify risk factors that may indicate the need for postoperative ventilation after a thymectomy?

Disease duration of more than 6 years, the presence of chronic obstructive pulmonary disease, and a pyridostigmine dose greater than 750 mg/day in association with significant bulbar weakness may be predictive of the need for postoperative ventilation after thymectomy.

21. What are the anesthetic considerations for patients with myasthenia gravis?

Anesthetic considerations include the following:
- Increased risk of aspiration
- Unpredictable response to succinylcholine (relative resistance, prolonged effect, or phase II block)
- Volatile anesthetics alone may provide adequate muscle relaxation for intubation and surgery

- Profound sensitivity to nondepolarizing muscle relaxants (if required, decrease initial dose by one half to two thirds; monitor with a peripheral nerve stimulator)
- Sensitive to respiratory depressant drugs
- Potential problems with anticholinesterase therapy ("cholinergic crisis"; enhanced vagal reflexes; hyperperistalsis; prolonged duration of ester-type local anesthetics, succinylcholine, and mivacurium)
- Anticipate postoperative respiratory failure

 Key Points

- MH is a fatal skeletal muscle hypermetabolism characterized by increased carbon dioxide production, oxygen consumption, and muscle membrane breakdown that occurs when susceptible individuals are exposed to potent inhalational anesthetics or depolarizing muscle relaxants or both.

- The pathophysiology of MH seems to be an uncontrolled increase in intracellular calcium in the muscle cell after exposure to triggering agents. This abnormal and sustained elevation in myoplasmic free calcium is controlled primarily by the calcium release channels of the sarcoplasmic reticulum by way of the ryanodine receptor.

- All volatile inhalational anesthetics (e.g., halothane, isoflurane, enflurane, desflurane, sevoflurane, methoxyflurane, ether, cyclopropane) and the depolarizing muscle relaxant succinylcholine are capable of triggering MH in humans.

- Barbiturates, propofol, etomidate, benzodiazepines, opioids, droperidol, nitrous oxide, nondepolarizing muscle relaxants, anticholinesterase drugs, anticholinergic drugs, sympathomimetics, and local anesthetics are safe for MH-susceptible patients.

- The association of susceptibility of MH and various myopathies has been reported, including central core disease, King Deborough syndrome, DMD, hyperkalemic periodic paralysis, and other myopathies.

- Dantrolene is a direct-acting skeletal muscle relaxant that blocks calcium release from myoplasmic sarcoplasmic reticulum.

- In vitro contracture tests, which measure the response of skeletal muscle strips to either halothane or caffeine, are the only reliable tests to diagnose susceptibility to MH.

- DMD is characterized by painless degeneration and atrophy of skeletal, cardiac, and smooth muscle.

- Patients with DMD are at increased risk for pulmonary aspiration due to weak laryngeal reflexes and gastrointestinal hypomotility. Succinylcholine is contraindicated in these patients because of the associated risk of rhabdomyolysis, hyperkalemia, and cardiac arrest.

- Myasthenia gravis is an acquired, chronic IgG antibody–mediated disease of the neuromuscular junction. Autoimmune destruction or inactivation of postsynaptic acetylcholine receptors at the neuromuscular junction produces weakness and rapid fatigability of voluntary skeletal muscles with repetitive use.

Internet Resources

Malignant Hyperthermia Tutorial: Created by the Department of Anaesthesia, University of Basel, Switzerland:
http://www.medana.unibas.ch/eng/mh/mhtutori.htm

MHAUS (Malignant Hyperthermia Association of the United States):
http://www.mhaus.org/index.cfm/fuseaction/Content.Display/PagePK/Home.cfm

Medstudents.com: Anesthesiology—Malignant Hyperthermia:
http://www.medstudents.com.br/anest/anest1.htm

Myasthenia Gravis Association of America, Inc.: Myasthenia Gravis—A Summary:
http://www.myasthenia.org/information/summary.htm

Myasthenia Gravis Links:
http://pages.prodigy.net/stanley.way/myasthenia/

Virtual Anaesthesia Textbook:
http://www.virtual-anaesthesia-textbook.com/

GASNet Index:
http://www.gasnet.org/gta/index.php

Bibliography

Antil A: Anesthesia care provider worksheet. In Mashman D, Greenberg C, editors: *Malignant hyperthermia procedure manual*, Sherburne, NY, 2001, Malignant Hyperthermia Association of the United States.

Baraka A: Anaesthesia and myasthenia gravis, *Can J Anaesth* 39:476-486, 1992.

Gronert GA, Antognini JF, Pessah IN: Malignant hyperthermia. In Miller RD, editor: *Anesthesia,* ed 5, New York, 2000, Churchill Livingstone, pp 1033-1051.

Hopkins PM: Malignant hyperthermia: advances in clinical management and diagnosis, *Br J Anaesth* 85:118-128, 2000.

Karen SM, Lojeski EW, Muldoon SM: Malignant hyperthermia. In Miller RD, Tremper KK, editors: *Atlas of anesthesia: principles of anesthetic techniques and anesthetic emergencies,* Philadelphia, 1998, Churchill Livingstone, pp 9.1-9.13.

Naguib M, Flood P, McArdle J, et al: Advances in neurobiology of the neuromuscular junction, *Anesthesiology* 96:202-231, 2002.

Roizen MF: Anesthetic implications of concurrent diseases. In Miller RD, editor: *Anesthesia,* ed 5, New York, 2000, Churchill Livingstone, pp 903-999.

Rosenberg H: Malignant hyperthermia: the disease of anesthesia, *ASA Refresher Course* 151:1-6, 2001.

Schulte am Esch J, Scholz J, Wappler F: *Malignant hyperthermia,* Lengerich, 2000, Pabst Science Publishers.

Stoelting RK, Dierdorf SF: *Anesthesia and co-existing disease,* ed 4, New York, 2002, Churchill Livingstone, pp 517-527, 716-721.

Fluid and Electrolyte Disturbances

Christopher G. Rutledge

1. What is an electrolyte?

An electrolyte is any substance that when dissolved in a solvent (H_2O) conducts electricity. Electrolytes dissociate into ions—either cations (positively charged) or anions (negatively charged).

2. Define osmolality, osmolarity, and tonicity.

Osmolality is the number of milliosmoles per kilogram of water. *Osmolarity* is the number of milliosmoles per liter of solution. Osmolality and osmolarity refer to the concentration of solute per weight (osmolality) and volume (osmolarity). *Tonicity* refers to the effect the osmolality has on cell volume.

3. Is normal saline hypotonic, isotonic, or hypertonic? Is 5% dextrose in water hypotonic, isotonic, or hypertonic?

Normal saline is an isotonic, 0.9% sodium chloride solution. This means that there are 9 g of sodium chloride per 1 L of fluid. If the molecular weight of sodium chloride is known, the osmolarity of the solution can be calculated:

One gram molecular weight (GMW) of a substance exerts 1 osmole of pressure. Na^+ and Cl^- have molecular weights of 23 and 35. The GMW of sodium chloride is 58. Normal saline contains 9 g per 1 L of fluid and exerts a fraction of an osmole. Mathematically this works out to be 9/58, which equals 0.15 Osm, or 150 mOsm. This may appear hypotonic, but sodium chloride actually has two ions (Na^+ and Cl^-), and each exerts its own osmotic force. This results in 300 mOsm ($150 \times 2 = 300$). Normal serum osmolarity is approximately 280 to 290 mOsm.

D5W can be calculated in a similar fashion. There is 50 g or 5% dextrose per 1 L of fluid. The GMW of dextrose is 180; 50/180 = 0.277 Osm or 277mOsm. This is close to serum osmolarity. Although dextrose exerts an osmotic force, it also is metabolized leaving only H_2O, making it a hypotonic fluid.

4. Name common causes of hyponatremia.

Hyponatremia may be caused by absorption of solute-free irrigation fluids (hysteroscopy, TURP), Addison's disease, syndrome of inappropriate antidiuretic hormone, cirrhosis, and nephrotic syndrome. Certain drugs also have the potential to cause hyponatremia, including chlorpropamide, vincristine, carbamazepine, mannitol, and loop diuretics.

5. What signs and symptoms might the hyponatremic patient exhibit?

Signs and symptoms of hyponatremia are usually evident at serum Na^+ less than 120 mEq/L and include mental status changes (apprehension, combativeness, lethargy), hypertension, nausea and vomiting, bradycardia, and pulmonary edema. Seizures and coma are associated with serum sodium levels < 115 mEq/L.

6. Why must hyponatremia be corrected slowly?

Treatment of hyponatremia includes fluid restriction and administration of normal saline and loop diuretics (furosemide [Lasix], 10 to 40 mg intravenously). Hypertonic saline (3% sodium chloride) may be used to treat severe hyponatremia. Rapid correction of hyponatremia can cause central pontine myelinolysis and can result in permanent neurologic damage or death. Correction of serum Na^+ levels should not exceed 1 to 1.5 mEq/L/hr, and treatment should be discontinued when serum Na^+ reaches 130 mEq/L.

7. What is the normal range for serum calcium and for ionized calcium?

Normal values for serum calcium are 8.5 to 10.5 mg/dL. Normal values for ionized calcium are 4 to 5 mg/dL.

8. Why are serum and ionized Ca^{2+} levels measured?

Calcium is a divalent cation that is 40% protein bound, 10% chelated (with bicarbonate, citrate, and phosphate), and 50% ionized. Ionized Ca^{2+} is active in physiological processes.

9. How are serum Ca^{2+} levels, serum citrate levels, and serum phosphate levels affected by pH?

Acid-base changes can alter *serum Ca^{2+}* levels. A decrease in serum pH (acidemia) causes a decrease in the protein binding of Ca^{2+} and an increase in serum ionized Ca^{2+}. Just the opposite occurs with alkalemia. An increase in pH (alkalemia) decreases serum ionized Ca^{2+} levels.

Citrate and *phosphate* chelate Ca^{2+} and cause decreases in ionized Ca^{2+} levels. Citrate is a preservative in stored blood, and administration of large amounts of packed red blood cells can cause decreased levels of ionized Ca^{2+}, owing to citrate binding. High serum phosphate levels may accompany cellular destruction from cancer, chemotherapy, or rhabdomyolysis. Patients with chronic renal failure commonly have hyperphosphatemia and hypocalcemia.

10. Describe common signs and symptoms associated with hypocalcemia.

Calcium is responsible for controlling the threshold potentials of cell membranes. Hypocalcemia lowers the threshold and increases cell excitability; this may result in enhanced neuromuscular irritability and tetany. Tetany can result in spasm of the laryngeal muscles (laryngospasm). Symptomatic patients may be stridorous or have complete airway obstruction. Chvostek's and Trousseau's signs are classic manifestations of hypocalcemia. Chvostek's sign is elicited by tapping the facial nerve with the index finger, resulting in repeated contractions of the facial muscle. Trousseau's sign is the contraction of the fingers and wrist after transient limb ischemia (induced by inflation of a blood pressure cuff or application of a tourniquet). The electrocardiogram of patients with hypocalcemia may show a prolonged Q-T interval. Other clinical manifestations of hypocalcemia include circumoral paresthesias, skeletal muscle cramps, and hypotension.

11. An otherwise healthy 44-year-old woman, American Society of Anesthesiologists level I, is 48 hours postsurgical parathyroidectomy. What electrolyte disturbance is she at risk for?

This patient is at risk for *hypocalcemia*. Parathyroid hormone is the primary regulator of serum calcium. Parathyroid hormone increases serum Ca^{2+} levels, primarily by resorbing calcium salts from the bone. The sudden decrease in parathyroid hormone levels after parathyroidectomy, inadvertent removal of all four parathyroid glands, and the "hungry bone syndrome" (rapid absorption of Ca^{2+} by calcium-depleted bones) may account for postsurgical hypocalcemia.

12. List common causes of hypercalcemia.

Common causes of hypercalcemia include the following:
- Hyperparathyroidism
- Sarcoidosis
- Cancer
- Prolonged immobilization
- Thiazide diuretics
- Milk-alkali syndrome
- Paget's disease

13. How is acute hyperkalemia treated?

Hyperkalemia is a potentially life threatening situation and is considered a medical emergency at levels greater than 7 mEq/L. Early recognition and treatment is integral to preventing serious sequelae. Cardiac muscles become irritable in the presence of hyperkalemia, owing to the cell resting membrane potential moving closer to the threshold potential. Administration of calcium raises the threshold and decreases the irritability of myocardial cells. To counteract the effects of hyperkalemia in adults, 5 to 10 mL of 10% calcium chloride is given intravenously over 10 minutes. Calcium administration does not change serum potassium concentrations.

Other mechanisms for reducing serum potassium concentrations include administration of insulin (2 units of regular insulin in 100 mL D5W, administered at a rate of 2 to 5 mL/min), administration of beta$_2$ adrenergic agonists, and inducing alkalosis (hyperventilation or sodium bicarbonate administration). Useful estimations are as follows:

- For every 10 mm Hg decrease in PaCO_2, the serum K^+ decreases by 0.5 mEq/L.
- For every 0.1 increase in pH, the serum K^+ decreases by 0.6 mEq/L.

14. Describe the electrocardiogram changes associated with hyperkalemia and hypokalemia.

A patient with marked *hyperkalemia* ($K^+ > 6$ mEq/L) may present with peaked T waves, a widened QRS complex, and loss of P waves. With increasing serum K^+ concentrations, ventricular tachycardia, ventricular fibrillation, or asystole may occur.

A patient with *hypokalemia* ($K^+ < 3.5$ mEq/L) may have shallow or inverted T waves, prominent U waves, and a prolonged P-R interval.

15. List seven causes of hyperkalemia.

Causes of hyperkalemia include the following:
- Acidosis
- Administration of potassium-containing fluids
- Addison's disease
- Massive blood transfusion
- Tissue trauma
- Rhabdomyolysis
- Renal failure

Medications that may precipitate hyperkalemia include the following:
- Cyclosporine
- Beta adrenergic blocking agents
- Succinylcholine
- Spironolactone
- Penicillin
- Angiotensin-converting enzyme inhibitors

16. What physiological responses are associated with changes in serum magnesium levels?

Magnesium has varied physiological functions, including vasodilation, positive inotropism, adenosine triphosphate formation, inhibition of Ca^{2+} influx in sarcolemma channels, and immunological functions. Elevated serum Mg^{2+} levels can have deleterious effects ranging from muscle weakness to cardiovascular collapse (see the following table).

Serum Magnesium Levels And Physiological Responses

Mg^{2+} (mEq/L)	Physiological Response
1.7–2.4	Normal range
4–6	Therapeutic
10	Loss of deep tendon reflexes
15	Respiratory muscle paralysis
>25	Cardiovascular collapse

17. How are neuromuscular blocking agents affected by magnesium levels?

Elevations in serum Mg^{2+} inhibit the entry of Ca^{2+} into presynaptic nerve terminals and inhibit acetylcholine release at the neuromuscular junction. High Mg^{2+} levels may enhance and prolong the effects of nondepolarizing muscle relaxants.

18. How is acute hypermagnesemia treated?

Calcium chloride or calcium gluconate can be used to treat hypermagnesemia. If applicable, removal of the causative agent (e.g., magnesium sulfate, antacids) must be implemented.

Key Points

- Severe hyponatremia (Na^+ <120 mEq/L) is evidenced by mental status changes, hypertension, nausea and vomiting, bradycardia, and pulmonary edema.
- Correction of serum Na^+ levels should not exceed 1 to 1.5 mEq/L/hr, and treatment should be discontinued when serum sodium reaches 130 mEq/L.
- Normal values for serum calcium are 8.5 to 10.5 mg/dL. Normal values for ionized calcium are 4 to 5 mg/dL.
- Hypercalcemia can be caused by hyperparathyroidism, sarcoidosis, cancer, prolonged immobilization, thiazide diuretics, milk-alkali syndrome, and Paget's disease.
- Hyperkalemia is considered a medical emergency at levels greater than 7 mEq/L.
- To counteract the effects of hyperkalemia, 5 to 10 mL of 10% calcium chloride is administered intravenously over 10 minutes.
- Administration of insulin (2 units of regular insulin in 100 mL D5W, administered at a rate of 2 to 5 mL/min), administration of $beta_2$ adrenergic agonists, and inducing alkalosis (hyperventilation or sodium bicarbonate administration) are other mechanisms for reducing serum potassium.

Continued

Key Points *continued*

- A patient with marked hyperkalemia ($K^+ > 6$ mEq/L) may present with peaked T waves, a widened QRS complex, and loss of P waves; ventricular tachycardia; ventricular fibrillation; or asystole.
- The electrocardiogram of a hypokalemic patient ($K^+ < 3.5$ mEq/L) may show shallow or inverted T waves, prominent U waves, and a prolonged P-R interval.
- Elevated serum Mg^{2+} levels can have deleterious effects ranging from muscle weakness to cardiovascular collapse.
- High Mg^{2+} levels may enhance and prolong the effects of nondepolarizing muscle relaxants.

Internet Resources

Georgetown University Community and Family WebServer: Fluids and Electrolytes:
http://gucfm.georgetown.edu/welchjj/netscut/fen/fluids.html

Indiana State University School of Nursing: Fluids and Electrolytes:
http://www.indstate.edu/nurs/mary/Fluidlytecf/

Virtual Anaesthesia Textbook:
http://www.virtual-anaesthesia-textbook.com/

Nurse-Anesthesia.com:
http://www.nurse-anesthesia.com/

Update in Anesthesia:
http://www.nda.ox.ac.uk/wfsa/html/pages/up_srch.htm

Bibliography

Estes CM, Maye JP: Severe intraoperative hyponatremia in a patient scheduled for elective hysteroscopy: a case report, *AANA J* 71:203-205, 2003.

Hoekelman RA: The physical examination of infants and children. In Bates B, editor: *A guide to physical examination and history taking,* ed 7, Philadelphia, 1997, JB Lippincott, pp 654-655.

McCance KL: Cellular biology. In McCance KL, Huether SE, editors: *Pathophysiology,* ed 3, St. Louis, 1998, Mosby, pp 20-22.

Roizen MF: Diseases of the endocrine system. In Benumof JL, editor: *Anesthesia and uncommon diseases,* ed 4, Philadelphia, 1998, WB Saunders, pp 225-231.

Schwartz JJ, Rosenbaum SH, Graf GJ: Anesthesia and the endocrine system. In Barash PG, Cullen BF, Stoelting RK, editors: *Clinical anesthesia,* ed 3, Philadelphia, 1996, Lippincott-Raven, pp 1045-1046.

Wicks TC: Magnesium homeostasis and deficiency. *AANA J* 67:171-179, 1999.

Coagulation and Hematologic Disorders

Richard G. Ouellette and Sandra M. Ouellette

1. **List three mechanisms responsible for hemostasis or prevention of blood loss.**

   Three mechanisms responsible for hemostasis are:
   * Vascular spasm
   * Formation of a platelet plug
   * Formation of a blood clot

2. **How do platelets contribute to vascular constriction?**

   Platelets release vasoconstrictor substances, including thromboxane A_2.

3. **What is a normal platelet count?**

   A normal platelet count ranges from 150,000 to 300,000 cells/mm^3.

4. **How long do platelets last in the blood?**

   Platelets have a life span of 8 to 12 days. They are eliminated from the circulation by the tissue macrophage system, particularly the spleen.

5. **List the clotting factors and their names.**

Factor I	Fibrinogen
Factor II	Prothrombin
Factor III (tissue thromboplastin)	Tissue factor
Factor IV	Calcium
Factor V	Proaccelerin; labile factor
Factor VII	Serum prothrombin conversion accelerator
Factor VIII	Antihemophilic factor; antihemophilic factor
Factor IX	Christmas factor; antihemophilic factor B
Factor X	Stuart factor
Factor XI	Plasma thromboplastin antecedent
Factor XII	Hageman factor
Factor XIII	Fibrin stabilizing factor

   See also the figure on page 206.

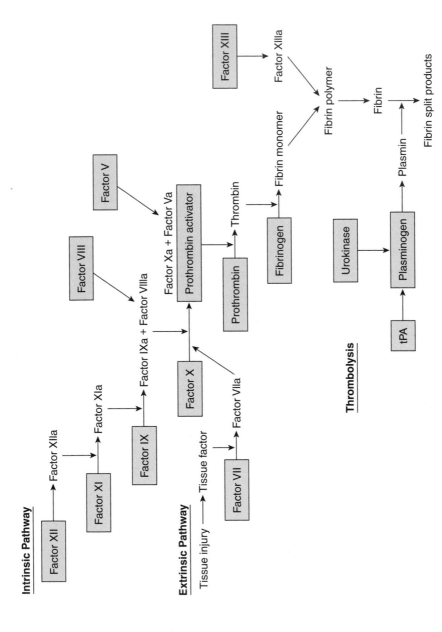

Blood clotting cascade and thrombolysis. *(Copyright 2002, Gladstone Institutes.)*

6. **What role does vitamin K play in coagulation?**

Vitamin K is required by the liver for formation of factors II (prothrombin), VII, IX, and X and the anticoagulant protein C.

7. **What causes clot retraction?**

Platelets cause clot retraction.

8. **List the events that are responsible for the formation of prothrombin activator and the initiation of coagulation.**

The following events are responsible for the formation of prothrombin activator:
- Trauma to the vascular wall or tissue
- Trauma to blood
- Contact of the blood with damaged endothelial cells or collagen

9. **What role does calcium play in coagulation?**

Except for the first two steps in the intrinsic pathway, calcium ions are required for promotion or acceleration of all the blood clotting reactions.

10. **What physiological factors prevent blood clotting?**

- Smoothness of the endothelial surface prevents activation of the intrinsic system.
- A layer of glycocalyx on the endothelium repels clotting factors and platelets.
- Thrombomodulin binds the procoagulant thrombin.
- Circulating antithrombin III and heparin complex prevents coagulation.

11. **How does heparin prevent coagulation?**

Heparin combines with antithrombin III and increases the anticoagulant effect of antithrombin III by 100-fold to 1000-fold. This powerful complex inhibits coagulation by inactivating factors II, IX, X, XI, and XII.

12. **Where in the body is heparin synthesized?**

Heparin is synthesized in basophilic mast cells, especially in the lung.

13. **What is the role of plasmin?**

Plasma proteins contain a euglobulin called *plasminogen*. When activated, plasminogen becomes plasmin or fibrinolysin. Plasmin digests fibrin and fibrinogen; prothrombin; and factors V, VIII, and XII.

14. Name three laboratory tests used to evaluate primary hemostasis.

- *Platelet count* determines the circulating platelet number, but not the functional quality of the platelet.
- *Bleeding time* evaluates platelet function; a normal bleeding time requires a sufficient number of platelets that can adhere and aggregate.
- *Clot retraction* reflects normal platelet function; the clot should retract in 2 to 4 hours.

15. What bleeding time is acceptable for elective surgery?

The upper limit of the bleeding time acceptable for elective surgery is 10 minutes.

16. What does the prothrombin time (PT) measure?

The PT measures the extrinsic and common pathways. The PT is prolonged when there is a deficiency, abnormality, or inhibition of factors I, II, V, VII, or X.

17. What does the partial thromboplastin time (PTT) measure?

The PTT measures the intrinsic and common pathways. The PTT is prolonged if there is a deficiency, abnormality, or inhibition of factors I, II, V, VIII, IX, X, XI, or XII.

18. What is the international normalized ratio (INR)?

The INR was introduced to address inconsistencies between the PT and clinical anticoagulant effects. The INR is the ratio of the patient's PT to a reference PT. It is based on the result that would have been obtained if international reference reagents had been used in the PT test.

19. What is the activated clotting time (ACT)?

The ACT evaluates the intrinsic and final common pathways of the coagulation cascade. Normal values are 90 to 120 seconds. The ACT is widely used to monitor heparin effects in the perioperative period.

20. Define thromboelastography.

Thromboelastography evaluates clot formation from initial procoagulant activation and fibrin formation to eventual clot lysis. Diagnosis of coagulation factor activity deficiency, platelet abnormalities, and disseminated intravascular coagulopathy is possible from a single blood sample.

21. List the three most common hereditary coagulation disorders.

- Hemophilia A (classic hemophilia)—factor VIII deficiency
- Hemophilia B (Christmas disease)—factor IX deficiency
- von Willebrand's disease—von Willebrand factor deficiency

22. Describe von Willebrand's disease.

Von Willebrand factor is necessary for the proper adherence of platelets to exposed endothelium. Von Willebrand's disease is an inherited disorder that affects both sexes. It is due to defective or deficient von Willebrand factor. Patients have a prolonged bleeding time but normal platelet count. Treatment consists of replacing von Willebrand factor with cryoprecipitate or the administration of desmopressin to stimulate release of von Willebrand factor.

23. Name three deficiencies associated with a hypercoagulable state.

Deficiencies associated with a hypercoagulable state include deficiencies of:
• Antithrombin III
• Protein C
• Protein S

Deficiencies of these proteins are associated with an increased risk of thromboembolism. In normal concentrations, protein C and its cofactor protein S inhibit factors V and VIII and stimulate fibrinolysis.

24. What patients are candidates for long-term anticoagulation therapy?

Patients with multiple episodes of venous thromboembolism, hereditary hyper-coagulable states, cancer, mechanical heart valves, and atrial fibrillation may be on long-term anticoagulation therapy.

25. How do warfarin drugs block coagulation?

Warfarin derivatives interfere with the synthesis of vitamin K–dependent clotting factors, factors II, VII, IX, and X. At low doses, factor VII is inhibited, and the PT is prolonged, but the PTT is normal. At high doses, factors II, VII, IX, and X are inhibited, and the PT and the PTT are prolonged.

26. How should a patient being treated preoperatively with warfarin be managed for elective surgery?

Patients on long-term oral anticoagulation therapy often require temporary correction of anticoagulation before a surgical procedure. Most patients who need temporary correction can be managed safely by stopping oral anticoagulant treatment 4 to 5 days before surgery and resuming it as soon as practical after surgery. Patients at risk for thromboembolism may require concurrent heparin therapy.

More specific guidelines recommend withholding four doses of warfarin if the INR is between 2.0 and 3.0. If the INR is greater than 1.8 1 day before surgery, vitamin K, 1 mg, may be given subcutaneously. Surgery can be performed safely when the INR is 1.5 or less.

Rarely, factor replacement therapy (e.g., fresh frozen plasma or prothrombin complex concentrate) is required when anticoagulation must be corrected rapidly before urgent surgery.

27. State the treatment of acute hemorrhage associated with warfarin overdose.

Fresh frozen plasma, 10 to 20 mL/kg, or phytonadione (vitamin K_1), 5 to 10 mg orally or subcutaneously, is administered to treat acute hemorrhage.

28. Discuss common causes of vitamin K deficiency.

Vitamin K is a fat-soluble vitamin that is continually synthesized in the intestinal tract by bacteria. Malnutrition, gastrointestinal malabsorption, antibiotic-induced elimination of intestinal flora, and bile duct obstruction all are potential causes of vitamin K deficiency. Neonates have undeveloped intestinal bacterial flora and lack stores of vitamin K and can become deficient in the absence of supplemental therapy.

29. What causes sickle cell disease?

Sickle cell disease is an inherited autosomal recessive disorder produced by the substitution of the amino acid valine for glutamic acid on the beta globin chain of hemoglobin. The amino acid substitution results in the formation of an abnormal hemoglobin, hemoglobin S. Hemoglobin S responds to hypoxemia (P_{O_2} < 40 mm Hg), acidosis, hypothermia, and dehydration by elongating and solidifying into a sickle shape. Sickled erythrocytes are stiff and can result in vascular occlusion, organ infarction, sequestration of blood in the liver and spleen, and pain.

30. Explain the difference between sickle cell anemia and sickle cell trait.

Sickle cell anemia is a homozygous form of the disease; the patient receives the abnormal gene from each parent. Patients with sickle cell trait inherit hemoglobin S from one parent and normal hemoglobin (hemoglobin A) from the other. Patients with sickle cell trait are carriers of the abnormal gene, but they rarely have clinical manifestations.

31. What can the anesthetist do to prevent a sickle cell crisis in a surgical patient?

- Keep the patient warm.
- Hydrate the patient well.
- Avoid hypotension and low-flow conditions.
- Avoid hypoxemia.

32. What is the P50 for a patient with sickle cell disease?

Sickle cell anemia shifts the oxyhemoglobin curve to the right and is associated with a P50 of 31.

33. What is methemoglobin?

Methemoglobinemia is an unstable form of hemoglobin that carries oxidized ferric iron (Fe^{3+}), instead of the reduced ferrous form (Fe^{2+}) that is capable of binding oxygen. The ferric form of hemoglobin is unable to bind oxygen. Additionally, methemoglobin shifts the oxyhemoglobin dissociation curve to the left, prohibiting the release of hemoglobin to tissues. Nitrate-containing compounds (nitroglycerin, nitroprusside, benzocaine) can produce methemoglobinemia. Pulse oximetry readings are unreliable estimates of hemoglobin oxygenation in patients with methemoglobinemia because the SpO_2 is read as 85% regardless of the PaO_2.

34. Summarize treatment for methemoglobinemia.

- Remove the inciting drug or toxin.
- Give oxygen.
- Administer methylene blue, 1 to 2 mg/kg, intravenously over 5 minutes (paradoxically, methylene blue doses >7 mg/kg can cause methemoglobinemia).

35. What is the most common cause of intraoperative coagulopathy?

Dilutional thrombocytopenia is the most common intraoperative coagulation disturbance. Dilutional thrombocytopenia is observed especially in trauma patients with massive transfusion. Eighty percent of the patient's estimated blood volume may have to be replaced before clinically significant thrombocytopenia occurs if the preoperative platelet count was normal. Each unit of administered platelets increases the platelet count an estimated 5000 to 10,000 cells/mm^3.

36. Define idiopathic thrombocytopenia purpura.

Idiopathic thrombocytopenia purpura, or autoimmune thrombocytopenia purpura, is characterized by persistent thrombocytopenia attributable to antiplatelet immunoglobulins that bind to platelet membranes and cause premature rupture. Treatment is usually with corticosteroids, which interfere with the immune attack on platelets. If treatment with corticosteroids is inadequate, a splenectomy may be indicated.

37. Explain the hematologic significance of glucose-6-phosphate dehydrogenase (G6PD) deficiency.

G6PD deficiency is an inheritable, X-linked recessive disorder whose primary effect is the reduction in the enzyme G6PD in red blood cells. G6PD protects against red blood cell oxidation, and deficiency can result in hemolysis and anemia when the patient is exposed to oxidant stresses, such as bacterial or viral infections or certain drugs.

Drugs that can precipitate hemolysis and should be avoided in these patients include the following:
- Antimalarial agents
- Sulfonamides (antibiotic)
- Aspirin

- Nonsteroidal anti-inflammatory drugs
- Nitrofurantoin
- Quinidine
- Quinine
- Methylene blue
- Vitamin K, vitamin C
- Others

Abnormalities in G6PD are relatively common, especially in blacks and individuals of eastern Mediterranean or Chinese ancestry. In the United States, approximately 10% to 14% of black men are affected.

38. How does hypothermia alter coagulation?

All coagulation factors work best within a narrow temperature range. Temperatures less than 34° C cause prolongation of the PT, the PTT, and thrombin time. Platelet function also is impaired in hypothermic patients.

 Key Points

- Platelets have a lifespan of 8 to 12 days. They are eliminated from the circulation by the tissue macrophage system, particularly the spleen.
- Vitamin K is required by the liver for the formation (γ-carboxylation) of Factors II, VII, IX, and X.
- Protamine is a positively charged protein commercially prepared from the sperm of salmon and other species of fish. It produces its effect by combining with negatively charged heparin to form a stable complex that lacks anticoagulant activity. Each milligram of protamine neutralizes approximately 100 USP units of heparin.
- The PT measures the extrinsic and common pathways.
- The APTT measures the intrinsic and common pathways.
- Sickle cell disease is an inherited autosomal recessive disorder resulting from the substitution of the amino acid valine for glutamic acid on the beta globin chain of hemoglobin. The amino acid substitution produces an abnormal hemoglobin, *hemoglobin S (Hb S)*.
- Methemoglobinemia is an unstable form of hemoglobin that carries oxidized ferric iron (Fe^{+3}) instead of the reduced ferrous form (Fe^{+2}) that is capable of binding oxygen. The ferric form of hemoglobin is unable to bind oxygen.

Internet Resources

Genes and Disease:
http://www.ncbi.nlm.nih.gov/books/bv.fcgi?call=bv.View..ShowSection&rid=gnd.section.98

Mayo Clinic.com—Sickle Cell:
http://www.mayoclinic.com/invoke.cfm?id=DS00324

Hardin MD. Blood Disease and Hematology:
http://www.lib.uiowa.edu/hardin/md/hem.html

Puget Sound Blood Center Online:
http://www.psbc.org

Bibliography

Gerbasi FR: Hematology and anesthesia. In Nagelhout JJ, Zaglaniczny KL, editors: *Nurse anesthesia,* Philadelphia, 2002, WB Saunders, pp 804-813.

Guyton AC, Hall JE: Hemostasis and blood coagulation. In: *Textbook of medical physiology,* ed 10. Philadelphia, 2000, WB Saunders, pp 419-429.

Lake CL, Moore RA: *Blood: hemostasis, transfusion, and alternative in the perioperative period,* New York, 1995, Raven Press.

Murray DJ: Monitoring of hemostasis. In Longnecker DE, Tinker JH, Morgan GE, editors: *Principles and practices of anesthesiology,* ed 2, St. Louis, 2001, Mosby, pp 923-941.

Murray DJ: Evaluation of the patient with anemia and coagulation disorders. In Longnecker DE, Tinker JH, Morgan GE, editors: *Principles and practices of anesthesiology,* ed 2, St. Louis, 2001, Mosby, pp 360-378.

Nuttall GA, Ereth MH, Oliver WC, et al: Monitoring coagulation and hemostasis: perioperative assessment of coagulation and platelet function. In Lake CL, Hines RL, Blitt CD, editors: *Clinical monitoring,* Philadelphia, 2001, WB Saunders, pp 389-419.

Petrovitch CT, Drummon JC: Hemotherapy and hemostasis. In Barash PG, Cullen FB, Stoelting RK, editors: *Clinical anesthesia,* ed 4, Philadelphia, 2001, Lippincott Williams & Wilkins, pp 201-236.

Salem RM: *Blood: conservation in the surgical patient,* Baltimore, 1996, Williams & Wilkins.

Spiess BD: Normal and abnormal blood coagulation patterns. In Prys-Roberts C, Brown BR, editors: *International practice of anesthesia,* Oxford, 2002, Butterworth-Heinemann, pp 1:43:1-1:43:17.

Fluid Management and Transfusion

Michael J. Kremer

1. Discuss the important considerations of intraoperative fluid therapy.

Intraoperative fluid therapy provides fluid for maintenance requirements and deficits caused by hemorrhage and insensible losses. Because fluid requirements vary based on different patient and surgical needs, guidelines have been developed regarding intraoperative fluid therapy, as follows:

- Infuse a maintenance-type fluid to replace insensible losses for the interval since the last oral intake, 2 mL/kg/hr.
- Administer replacement-type fluids for intraoperative insensible losses, 2 mL/kg/hr.
- Estimate surgical trauma, and infuse appropriate replacement:
  - Minimal trauma—add 4 mL/kg/hr
  - Moderate trauma—add 6 mL/kg/hr
  - Severe trauma—add 8 mL/kg/hr
- Infuse colloid solution to replace blood loss exceeding 20% of the patient's circulating volume.
- Monitor vital signs and urine output, adjusting fluid to maintain urine output of 1 mL/kg/hr or greater.

2. How are fluid infusion rates calculated?

Maintenance fluid requirements are calculated based on body weight and age:
- Adults generally require 2 mL/kg/hr.
- Children generally require 2 to 4 mL/kg/hr, respectively.
- Infants generally require 4 to 6 mL/kg/hr.

3. Describe the composition of parenteral fluids.

Maintenance fluids provide replacement for normal fluid loss, such as loss via the lungs, urine, and skin. Replacement fluids are administered to correct a loss of isotonic fluid from the body, including ascites and interstitial edema.

Crystalloid solutions contain electrolytes dissolved in water or in dextrose and water. Commonly used crystalloid solutions are saline solutions and lactated Ringer's (Hartman's) solutions.

Colloid solutions (e.g., 5% albumin, 6% hydroxyethyl starch) contain natural or synthetic molecules that are impermeable to the vascular membrane. Colloids determine the colloid osmotic pressure that balances the distribution of water between the intravascular and the intersititial spaces. Colloid solutions may be used to replace blood loss or to restore intravascular volume. To replace blood loss, colloid solutions should be administered in a ratio of volume to estimated blood loss of approximately 1:1.

4. Discuss the indications for blood transfusion therapy.

The main indication for intraoperative blood transfusion is to *maintain intravascular volume and oxygen-carrying capacity to the tissues.* A blood transfusion may be indicated if acute blood loss is greater than 30% of the total blood volume in a normal healthy patient or greater than 15% to 20% in an elderly patient. Healthy individuals or individuals with chronic anemia usually can tolerate a hematocrit (Hct) of 20% to 25%, assuming normal intravascular volume. Elderly patients and patients with coronary artery disease or peripheral vascular disease may require minimal Hct values of 28% or greater.

5. Describe the estimation of blood volume.

Estimated allowable blood loss (EABL) is calculated as follows:

$$EABL = (Hct_{starting} - Hct_{allowable}) \times blood\ volume \div Hct_{starting}$$

Blood volume in an adult is approximately 7% of lean body mass, or about 70 mL of blood/kg of body weight.

6. Show how the volume of blood to transfuse is calculated.

$$Volume\ to\ transfuse = (Hct_{desired} - Hct_{present}) \times blood\ volume \div Hct_{transfused\ blood}$$

7. How are blood losses replaced intraoperatively?

If blood loss is less than the amount calculated to require transfusion, the loss can be replaced with a crystalloid solution to maintain adequate fluid balance in the patient. Guidelines for replacing fluid due to blood loss are as follows:
- 2 mL of crystalloid solution for each 1 mL of blood loss without a Foley catheter
- 3 mL of crystalloid solution for each 1 mL of blood loss with a Foley catheter in place

Blood or blood components or both are indicated when losses are greater than the calculated acceptable blood loss.

8. How is blood compatibility determined?

Because of the presence of red blood cell (RBC) antigens and antibodies, only specific blood types can be given to an individual. The following table shows the type of blood that can be administered on the basis of ABO and Rh blood types.

Blood Groups, Antigens, Antibodies, and Blood Compatibility			
Blood Group	Antigen on Red Blood Cells	Antibodies in Serum	Blood Group Compatibility
A	A	Anti-B	A, O
B	B	Anti-A	B, O
AB	A and B	—	AB, A, B, O
O	—	Anti-A and Anti-B	O only
Rh-positive	D	—	Rh-positive and Rh-negative
Rh-negative	—	Anti-D if sensitized	Rh-negative

An individual with type AB blood is termed a *universal recipient,* and an individual with type O blood is termed a *universal donor.*

Laboratory tests are routinely performed to detect harmful antigen/antibody interactions before transfusion. The most important test is *ABO/Rh blood typing.* This test identifies the RBC antigens and major plasma antibodies in the blood of the donor and recipient. Another commonly used test is the *antibody screen,* which detects the presence of various antibodies in the blood of the recipient and donor. Normally the final compatibility test is the *crossmatch,* which simulates a trial transfusion. The blood of the donor and the recipient is mixed and checked for signs of incompatibility.

9. How can blood be administered in life-threatening situations?

If an emergency blood transfusion is needed, type-specific (A, B, AB, or O) RBCs usually can be obtained quickly if the blood type of the patient is known. If type-specific blood is unavailable or if the blood type of the patient is unknown, type O Rh-negative RBCs should be transfused. If 2 or more units of type O-negative blood (which contains anti-A and anti-B antibodies) have been given, it is recommended that the blood of the recipient be screened for antibodies before the recipient is given blood of his or her own type.

10. Discuss potential complications of blood transfusion therapy.

The blood preservation process accounts for some of the potential complications associated with transfusion. Citrate intoxication from the addition of citrate-phosphate-dextrose preservative to stored blood can occur with rapid transfusion. Citrate normally is metabolized efficiently by the liver. If the rate of blood transfusion exceeds approximately 1 unit of blood per minute in an average-sized adult, however, decreased ionized calcium may result, as the accumulating citrate chelates serum Ca^{2+}. Acid-base changes also can occur with blood transfusion. The pH of stored blood decreases due to the addition of citrate-phosphate-dextrose preservative and metabolism of glucose to lactate.

Other possible adverse effects associated with transfusion therapy include decreased blood 2,3-diphosphoglycerate with an associated leftward shift of the oxygen-hemoglobin dissociation curve, hyperkalemia, volume overload, hypothermia, microaggregate delivery, and dilutional coagulopathy. Sufficient concentrations of coagulation factors V and VIII may remain in banked whole blood, but not in packed RBCs.

11. Describe the roles of specific components in transfusion therapy.

Whole blood is not readily available because of the increased use of components. It contains 450 mL of blood and 63 mL of anticoagulant. Generally, 1 unit of whole blood increases the Hct 3% to 4% and the hemoglobin level by 1 g/dL (see the table below).

Packed RBCs contain approximately 200 mL of RBCs and differ from whole blood in that they contain only 50 mL of plasma. One unit of packed RBCs has a Hct of about 70% and can raise the Hct of a euvolemic adult by 2% to 3%. Packed RBCs restore oxygen-carrying capacity but do not provide coagulation

Specific Components in Transfusion Therapy

Component	Composition	Volume (mL)	Indications
Whole blood	RBCs, WBCs, platelets, plasma	500	Deceased RBCs and plasma volume; deficient factors V, VIII
Packed RBCs	RBCs, WBCs, platelets, reduced plasma	250	Decreased RBCs; symptomatic anemia
Leukocyte-reduced RBCs	RBCs; $<5 \times 10^8$ WBCs; no platelets or plasma	200	History of febrile reactions due to leukocyte antibodies
Saline-washed packed RBCs	RBCs; $<5 \times 10^8$ WBCs; no platelets or plasma	180	History of allergic reactions to plasma proteins
Platelet concentrate	$>5 \times 10^{10}$ platelets; RBCs; WBCs; plasma	50	Thrombocytopenia, thrombocytopathy
Fresh frozen plasma	Plasma with all coagulation factors; no platelets	220	Coagulation factor deficiency or disorders
Cryoprecipitate	Fibrinogen; factors VIII, XIII; von Willebrand's factor	15	Deficiencies of factors VIII and XIII, fibrinogen, von Willebrand's disease

RBCs, red blood cells; WBCs, white blood cells

factors. Because of the increased viscosity of packed RBCs, they should be diluted with at least 100 mL of normal saline to decrease hemolysis and increase flow rate. The decision to transfuse must be related to specific patient needs rather than a preestablished laboratory value. The following table shows suggested trigger levels for transfusion and associated clinical findings.

Indications for Transfusion of Red Blood Cells, Fresh Frozen Plasma, and Platelets

Component	Trigger Level	Specific Indications/Considerations
Packed RBCs	Hgb 10 g/dL	Patients with increased oxygen demand, pulmonary disease, or decreased cardiac reserve; elderly patients; patients with coronary artery disease or peripheral vascular disease; patients on sustained mechanical ventilation
	Hgb 8 g/dL	If >500 mL blood loss anticipated during surgery; postoperative cardiac surgery; ASA II-III patients in postoperative period
	Hgb 6 g/dL	Well-compensated, chronically anemic patients; healthy ASA I-II patients undergoing planned hemodilution
Fresh frozen plasma	PT > 1.5× control APTT > 1.5× control Coagulation factor assay: <25% activity	Clinical course suggests coagulopathy; massive blood transfusion; reversal of warfarin effect; congenital coagulation factor deficiency
Platelet concentrates	Platelet count <20,000 mm^3 Platelet count <50,000 mm^3	Even if no indication of bleeding; if active bleeding or before surgery

APTT, activated partial thromboplastin time; ASA, American Society of Anesthesiologists; Hgb, hemoglobin; PT, prothrombin time; RBCs, red blood cells.

12. List recommended safety practices for blood administration.

- A blood warmer should always been used when blood is administered during surgery.
- The American Association of Blood Banks and the American Red Cross recommend that all blood be filtered to extract particles potentially harmful to the recipient. The standard filter has pores measuring 170 to 230 μ and removes degenerated platelets, leukocytes, and fibrin.
- Blood products should not be infused with glucose-containing solutions because these solutions can cause RBC hemolysis, or with lactated Ringer's solution, which contains calcium and may induce clot formation. Normal saline, 5% albumin, and fresh frozen plasma all are compatible with banked blood.

13. What are the indications for plasma administration?

Plasma is used primarily to restore coagulation factors. Two sources of plasma include *fresh frozen plasma* and *single donor plasma*. Fresh frozen plasma is separated from whole blood and frozen within 6 hours of collection. It can be stored for 1 year. Fresh frozen plasma is indicated to treat bleeding or a documented coagulopathy. It replaces labile (factors V and VIII) and stable coagulation factors. The need for fresh frozen plasma may be established based on prolonged prothrombin time and partial thromboplastin time.

14. What are the indications for platelet replacement?

Platelets may be administered via fresh whole blood, platelet-rich plasma, or platelet concentrates. A single unit of platelet concentrate has approximately 50 mL of plasma for suspension. One unit of platelet concentrate increases the recipient's platelet concentration by 5000 to $10,000/mm^3$ in an adult. Intraoperative platelet administration, 6 to 8 units or 1 unit per 10 kg of body weight, may be indicated for thrombocytopenic bleeding associated with massive transfusion.

15. Describe the indications for cryoprecipitate administration.

Cryoprecipitate is used for the replacement of specific coagulation factors. It is produced by thawing fresh frozen plasma and collecting the precipitate, a volume of 5 to 10 mL. The supernatant is used as single donor plasma. It can be frozen and stored for 1 year. Cryoprecipitate is used primarily for controlling bleeding associated with deficiencies in factor VIII, von Willebrand's factor, factor XIII, fibrinogen, or fibronectin.

16. When should albumin and other plasma derivatives be considered for fluid replacement?

Albumin and other plasma derivatives (e.g., plasma protein fraction) are used for acute volume expansion. These derivatives contain no cellular elements and are given without regard to ABO or Rh compatibility. Albumin is heat treated at 60° C for 10 hours, which eliminates the possibility of transmission of blood-borne disease. Albumin is available as a 5% or 25% solution in saline and has an intravascular half-life of more than 24 hours.

17. What are synthetic plasma expanders, and what are their mechanisms of action?

Volume expansion also can be accomplished with synthetic colloid solutions, such as dextrans and hetastarch. Dextran is composed of polymerized glucose molecules. The half-life of dextran is approximately 6 hours. Hetastarch (hydroxyethyl starch) is a synthetic polymer composed mainly of amylopectin, with an intravascular half-life of greater than 24 hours. Alterations in the coagulation system have been identified with hetastarch use. Hetastarch and dextran contain no coagulation factors. Anaphylactoid reactions have been reported with their use.

18. Describe the assessment and treatment of hemolytic transfusion reactions.

Hemolytic transfusion reactions are estimated to occur at a rate of 1 in 30,000 transfusions, and most are due to blood incompatibility from clerical errors. Symptoms of anxiety, agitation, chest pain, flank pain, headache, dyspnea, chills, or fever may indicate an acute hemolytic transfusion reaction. In patients under general anesthesia, signs may include fever, hypotension, tachycardia, unexplained bleeding (disseminated intravascular coagulation), and hemoglobinuria. If a transfusion reaction is suspected, the following steps should be taken:

- Stop the transfusion.
- Treat hypotension with fluids and vasopressors as indicated. Consider corticosteroids.
- Send unused donor blood and a fresh patient blood sample to the blood bank to be recrossmatched.
- Send patient blood samples for determination of free hemoglobin, haptoglobin, Coombs' test, and disseminated intravascular coagulation screening.
- Preserve renal function by maintaining brisk urine output (intravenous fluid, furosemide, mannitol).

 Key Points

- Intraoperative fluid therapy provides fluid for maintenance requirements and deficits caused by hemorrhage and insensible losses.
- A maintenance-type fluid is infused to replace insensible losses for the interval since the last oral intake, 2 mL/kg/hr.
- Replacement-type fluids are administered for intraoperative insensible losses, 2 mL/kg/hr.
- The anesthetist should estimate surgical trauma and infuse appropriate replacement, as follows:
  - Minimal trauma—add 4 mL/kg/hr
  - Moderate trauma—add 6 mL/kg/hr
  - Severe trauma—add 8 mL/kg/hr
- Colloid solutions (e.g., 5% albumin, 6% hydroxyethyl starch) contain natural or synthetic molecules that are impermeable to the vascular membrane and may be used to replace blood loss or to restore intravascular volume.
- The main indication for intraoperative blood transfusion is to maintain intravascular volume and oxygen-carrying capacity to the tissues.
- A blood transfusion may be indicated if acute blood loss is greater than 30% of the total blood volume in a normal healthy patient or greater than 15% to 20% in an elderly patient.
- EABL is calculated as follows:
  - $EABL = (Hct_{starting} - Hct_{allowable}) \times blood\ volume \div Hct_{starting}$
- Volume to transfuse is calculated as follows:
  - $Volume\ to\ transfuse = (Hct_{desired} - Hct_{present}) \times blood\ volume \div Hct_{transfused\ blood}$

Continued

Key Points   *continued*

- Blood group to be infused is based on ABO and Rh types. An individual with type AB blood is termed a *universal recipient,* and an individual with type O blood is termed a *universal donor.*
- If an emergency blood transfusion is needed, type-specific (A, B, AB, or O) RBCs usually can be obtained quickly if the blood type of the patient is known.
- If type-specific blood is unavailable or if the blood type of the patient is unknown, type O Rh-negative RBCs should be transfused.
- Blood components are used in transfusion therapy rather than whole blood (see table in Question 11).
- All blood should be filtered through a 170-mc to 230-mc filter.
- Blood should not be infused with glucose-containing solutions or lactated Ringer's solution.
- One unit of platelet concentrate increases the recipient's platelet concentration by 5000 to 10,000/mm^3 in an adult.
- Cryoprecipitate is used for the replacement of specific coagulation factors, primarily for controlling bleeding associated with deficiencies in factor VIII, von Willebrand's factor, factor XIII, fibrinogen, or fibronectin.
- Hemolytic transfusion reactions are most likely due to blood incompatibility from clerical errors.

 Internet Resources

Department of Reproductive Health and Research (RHR), World Health Organization: Managing Complications in Pregnancy and Childbirth: A guide for midwives and doctors:
http://www.who.int/reproductive-health/impac/Clinical_Principles/
Clinical_use_blood_C23_C33.html

Surgical-tutor.org: Blood products:
http://www.surgical-tutor.org.uk/default-home.htm?core/preop2/blood.htm~right

The University of Virginia Health System Department of Anesthesiology: Blood, Fluid, and Electrolyte Replacement:
http://www.healthsystem.virginia.edu/internet/anesthesiology/Dept-Info/Education/
Lectures/blood.cfm

The University of Tennessee Health Science Center, Dept. of Family Medicine: Volume, Electrolyte, and Blood Product Replacement:
www.utmem.edu/FPSA/Fluidslecture.ppt

Bibliography

Deisering LF: Fluid therapy. In Waugaman WR, Foster SD, Rigor BM, editors: *Principles and practice of nurse anesthesia*, ed 3, Stamford, CT, 1999, Appleton & Lange, pp 593-608.

Garcia A, Veillon DM, McCaskill D: Universal leukoreduction of cellular blood components in 2001? *Am J Clin Pathol* 116:778-780, 2001.

Goodnough LT, Brecher ME, Kanter MH, et al: Transfusion medicine: second of two parts—blood conservation, *N Engl J Med* 340:525-533, 1999.

Hansell DM, Allain RM: Transfusion therapy. In Hurford WE, et al, editors: *Clinical anesthesia procedures of the Massachusetts General Hospital,* ed 5, Philadelphia, 1998, Lippincott Williams & Wilkins, pp 583-600.

Reeves-Viets JL: Blood and blood component therapy. In Waugaman WR, Foster SD, Rigor BM, editors: *Principles and practice of nurse anesthesia,* ed 3, Stamford, CT, 1999, Appleton & Lange, pp 609-638.

Rossetto CL, McMahon JE: Current and future trends in transfusion therapy, *J Pediatr Oncol Nurs* 17:160-173, 2000.

Solheim BG, Wesenberg F: Rational use of blood products, *Eur J Cancer* 37:2421-2425, 2001.

Stehling L, Doherty DC, Faust RJ, et al: Practice guidelines for blood component therapy, *Anesthesiology* 84:732-746, 1996.

Swendner K, Gerbasi FR: Fluids, electrolytes, and blood component therapy. In Nagelhout JJ, Zaglaniczny KL, editors: *Nurse anesthesia,* ed 2, Philadelphia, 2001, WB Saunders, pp 349-364.

Chapter 25

Acid-Base Balance

Kathleen Carl

1. Describe how the body maintains acid-base balance.

Acids are continually produced by cellular metabolism of carbohydrates, fats, and protein. Major by-products of metabolism include carbonic acid (H_2CO_3) and carbon dioxide (CO_2). CO_2 reacts with water according to the following equation to produce H_2CO_3:

$$CO_2 + H_2O \leftrightarrow H_2CO_3 \leftrightarrow H^+ + HCO_3^-$$

The hydration of CO_2 is catalyzed by the enzyme carbonic anhydrase, which is present in high concentration in red blood cells. An increase in extracellular hydrogen ion concentration drives this reaction to the left. Conversely, a decrease in extracellular hydrogen ion concentration drives this reaction to the right.

The lungs regulate carbonic acid production ($CO_2 + H_2O \leftrightarrow H_2CO_3$) by regulating CO_2. High P_{CO_2} produces respiratory acidosis by driving the reaction to the right. The kidneys regulate bicarbonate (HCO_3^-) production and excretion.

2. What role do the kidneys play in regulating acid-base balance?

The kidneys maintain acid-base balance by regulating the excretion or reabsorption of acids and bases, primarily:
- Reabsorption of bicarbonate
- Excretion of acids

3. List normal arterial blood gas values.

pH	7.4 (7.35–7.45)
Pa_{CO_2}	40 mm Hg (35–45 mm Hg)
Pa_{O_2}	80 to 100 mm Hg
Sa_{O_2}	90% to 97%
HCO_3^-	24 mEq/L (22–26 mEq/L)
Base excess	0 mEq/L (–3 to +3)

4. Describe the physiological effects of acidosis.

The physiological effects of acidosis represent a balance between its direct neuromuscular depressant effects and an associated sympathoadrenal stimulation. The depressant effects are most apparent at an arterial pH less than 7.20.

The physiological effects of acidosis are as follows:
- Rightward shift of the oxygen (O_2) hemoglobin (Hgb) dissociation curve, facilitating Hgb unloading of O_2
- Hyperkalemia
- Myocardial depression
- Vasodilation
- Decreased myocardial and vascular smooth muscle responsiveness to catecholamines

5. List the physiological effects of alkalosis.

The physiological effects of alkalosis are as follows:
- Leftward shift of the O_2 Hgb dissociation curve, increasing O_2 binding to Hgb
- Hypokalemia
- Decreased plasma ionized calcium $[Ca^{2+}]$
- Vasoconstriction (cerebral, coronary, systemic)
- Bronchoconstriction

6. List causes of metabolic acidosis.

Causes of metabolic acidosis are listed in the following table.

Causes of Metabolic Acidosis

Loss of Bicarbonate	Addition of Acid
Gastrointestinal loss (vomiting, nasogastric suction, diarrhea)	Lactic acid (shock, local ischemia, cardiopulmonary bypass)
Depressed renal function (kidney regulates the reabsorption of bicarbonate)	Ketoacidosis (starvation, diabetes)
	Exogenous (salicylic acid, methanol, ethylene glycol)
	Renal failure (inability to excrete acid)
	Hypoaldosteronism

7. What are some causes of respiratory acidosis?

Respiratory acidosis results from the following:
- Conditions that decrease respiratory drive—oversedation, anesthesia, lesions of the medulla

- Conditions that obstruct the airway—asthma, soft tissue edema, bronchitis
- Conditions that interfere with gas exchange at the capillary/alveolar level—pulmonary edema, emphysema
- Conditions that impair chest wall expansion—abdominal distention, obesity, myasthenia gravis, Guillain-Barré syndrome, kyphoscoliosis
- Conditions that increase CO_2 production—malignant hyperthermia, thyroid storm

In each of the above-listed examples, accumulation of CO_2 leads to an increase in $[H^+]$ and a decrease in pH.

8. Describe the physiological compensatory responses to metabolic acidosis.

Acid excretion mechanisms are necessary to maintain acid-base balance. The primary acute response to metabolic acid-base disturbances is respiratory control of CO_2. Increases in H^+, associated with metabolic acidosis, stimulate central chemoreceptors, increasing alveolar ventilation, in an attempt to lower the P_{CO_2}. As a general rule, a Pa_{CO_2} change of 10 mm Hg corresponds to a pH change of 0.08. Renal compensation during metabolic acidosis may include the following:

- Increased excretion of titratable acids
- Increased reabsorption of HCO_3^-
- Increased production of ammonia

As a general rule, respiratory compensatory responses occur immediately in response to acute metabolic acidosis, but take 12 to 24 hours to reach steady state. Renal compensatory responses occur in 12 to 24 hours and take 5 days for maximal response.

9. A 57-year-old trauma patient arrives in the operating room cold and hypotensive from blood loss. Intraoperative arterial blood gas results show a profound metabolic acidosis with pH 7.1. How is this treated?

Acute metabolic acidosis during anesthesia is usually the result of hypovolemia or myocardial depression, both producing inadequate tissue perfusion. Other indicators suggesting tissue O_2 deprivation are high serum lactate levels and a base deficit. Restoring the blood volume and cardiac output and warming the patient usually adjusts the pH back toward normal. Severe metabolic acidosis (pH < 7.2) may be treated with sodium bicarbonate according to the following equation:

Patient weight (kg) × 0.3 × base deficit = sodium bicarbonate dose (mEq)

Usually, about half of the calculated dose is administered intravenously, and the arterial blood gas determinations are repeated in 20 minutes.

Example: **70 kg × 0.3 × base deficit 15 = 315 mEq**

The administered dose would be 150 mEq.

10. What is a pulmonary shunt?

A *right-to-left pulmonary shunt* describes the fraction of the cardiac output from the right side of the heart that bypasses lung units to enter the left side of the heart and systemic arteries without being oxygenated. The pulmonary shunt fraction (Q_S/Q_T) is normally less than 5%. Increased shunt is associated with hypoxemia and an increase in the alveolar-to-arterial O_2 difference. Left-to-right shunts are not common and are usually due to congenital heart disease.

11. Define physiological dead space.

Dead space is "wasted ventilation" or ventilation that does not participate in gas exchange. Normally, *physiological dead space* (V_D) is about one third of each tidal volume (V_T), or about 2 mL/kg. Physiological dead space is a combination of anatomical and alveolar dead space:
- *Anatomical dead space* is the volume of the conducting airways that does not participate in gas exchange. Normal anatomical dead space includes the pharynx, trachea, and bronchial tree down to the respiratory zone.
- *Alveolar dead space* is the alveolar volume that does not receive perfusion. Factors that restrict perfusion to ventilated alveoli contribute to alveolar dead space.

The Bohr equation calculates the total physiological dead space as a fraction of the V_T:

$$V_D/V_T = P_{A_{CO_2}} - P_{E_{CO_2}}/P_{A_{CO_2}} \text{ (E = mixed expired, A = alveolar)}$$

12. Name perianesthetic causes that can increase alveolar dead space.

PHYSIOLOGICAL BLOCKAGE OF PULMONARY BLOOD FLOW
- Pulmonary thromboembolism
- Pulmonary air embolism
- Amniotic embolism
- Fat embolism

LOW PULMONARY PERFUSION PRESSURE
- Decreased cardiac output
- West zone 1

HIGH ALVEOLAR GAS PRESSURE
- Positive end-expiratory pressure
- Large tidal volumes

13. What effect does dead space have on end-tidal CO_2 ($P_{ET_{CO_2}}$)?

Increased dead space dilutes and lowers $P_{ET_{CO_2}}$ and acutely increases the $P_{a_{CO_2}}/P_{ET_{CO_2}}$ difference.

14. Summarize the information venous blood O_2 saturation (Svo_2) provides.

The normal Svo_2 is 75%. A 5% to 10% increase or decrease is considered significant. A decrease in Svo_2 may be due to the following:
- A decrease in cardiac output with a higher tissue extraction ratio
- An increase in tissue metabolism and increased O_2 extraction
- Decreased arterial O_2 saturation due to decreased O_2 supply

15. How is blood O_2 content calculated?

Blood O_2 content is the sum total of O_2 bound to Hgb and O_2 in solution in the plasma:

$$O_2 \text{ content (mL/dL blood)} = [\text{Hgb(g/dL blood)} \times 1.34 \times \% \text{ saturation of Hgb}] + [Po_2 \times 0.003 \text{ mL } O_2/\text{dL blood/mm Hg}]$$

where 1.34 = the amount of O_2 (mL) bound to each gram of Hgb and 0.003 = the blood solubility of O_2. Normal arterial O_2 content = 20 mL/dL; normal venous O_2 content = 15 mL/dL. For each 100 mL of blood, 5 mL of O_2 are delivered to the tissue; the arterial-venous O_2 difference = 5 mL/dL.

16. What are ketoacids?

Ketoacids are the by-products of fat metabolism. They include beta-hydroxybutyric acid, acetoacetic acid, and acetone (volatile). Ketoacids are metabolized in the liver. Under conditions of unbridled fat breakdown (starvation, diabetic ketoacidosis), ketoacids overwhelm the metabolic capacity of the liver, accumulate, and produce metabolic acidosis.

17. Explain what is meant by base excess on an arterial blood gas report.

The *base excess* is a calculated value, derived from the *Henderson-Hasselbalch equation*. It is the amount of base that would have to be added to, or removed from, oxygenated blood to achieve a pH of 7.40, given a temperature of 37° C and a $Paco_2$ of 40 mm Hg. A positive base excess is associated with metabolic alkalosis, and a negative base excess (base deficit) is associated with metabolic acidosis.

18. List nonrenal and renal causes of metabolic alkalosis.

The table on page 230 lists nonrenal versus renal causes of metabolic alkalosis.

19. Describe the effects pH changes have on serum potassium.

Serum K^+ increases with acidosis. Elevated extracellular H^+ diffuses into the cell to be buffered, and to maintain electrochemical equilibrium, K^+ exits the cell. With alkalosis, H^+ diffuses out of the cell, and K^+ enters, decreasing the extracellular K^+ concentration. As a general rule, serum K^+ increases by 0.6 mEq/L for each 0.10 decrease in pH.

Nonrenal and Renal Causes of Metabolic Alkalosis

Nonrenal	Renal
Vomiting	↑ Extracellular volume
Excess sodium bicarbonate administration	Hyperaldosteronism
Metabolism of salts of organic acids	K⁺ depletion
	Cl⁻ depletion

---

20. **Identify the two most common acid-base disturbances seen in a postoperative patient.**

    The two most common acid-base disturbances seen in a postoperative patient are:
    - *Metabolic acidosis* due to blood loss and third-space losses with inadequate volume replacement
    - *Respiratory acidosis* due to ventilatory depression by muscle relaxants, opioids, and residual anesthetics

21. **Name the acid-base disorder commonly seen in a cold and hypoxic neonate.**

    A cold and hypoxic neonate commonly has *metabolic acidosis.*

22. **A premature infant has which acid-base disorder?**

    A premature infant has respiratory acidosis.

23. **Which acid-base disorder depicts the following values?**

↑ pH, ↑ P_{CO_2}, ↑ HCO_3	Partially compensated metabolic alkalosis
↓ pH, ↑ P_{CO_2}, ↑ HCO_3	Partially compensated respiratory acidosis
↓ pH, ↓ P_{CO_2}, ↓ HCO_3	Partially compensated metabolic acidosis
↑ pH, ↓ P_{CO_2}, ↓ HCO_3	Partially compensated respiratory alkalosis

24. **A patient post cardiopulmonary resuscitation has a $Paco_2$ of 40 mm Hg, pH 7.62, and base excess of 15 mEq/L. What could explain this acid-base disorder?**

    This patient has metabolic alkalosis; this could be due to an overzealous administration of sodium bicarbonate.

25. A patient with chronic obstructive pulmonary disease has a $Paco_2$ of 55 mm Hg and a pH of 7.35. What could explain this acid-base result?

This acid-base result likely represents respiratory acidosis due to CO_2 retention and a compensatory metabolic alkalosis. The physiological compensatory response to chronic respiratory acidosis is bicarbonate retention by the kidneys. Over time, the retained bicarbonate crosses the blood-brain barrier and buffers H^+ bathing the respiratory control center. With these circumstances, the patient's central chemoreceptor response is blunted, and the patient may rely only on the peripheral chemoreceptor hypoxic drive for stimulating ventilation.

 Key Points

- The physiological effects of acidosis are:
  - Right shift of O_2 Hgb dissociation curve
  - Hyperkalemia
  - Myocardial depression
  - Vasodilation
  - Decreased responsiveness to catecholamines
- The physiological effects of alkalosis are:
  - Left shift of O_2 Hgb dissociation curve
  - Hypokalemia
  - Decreased plasma ionized calcium
  - Vasoconstriction
  - Bronchoconstriction
- Respiratory acidosis results from conditions that decrease respiratory drive, obstruct the airway, interfere with gas exchange at the capillary level, impair chest wall expansion, or increase CO_2 production.
- Blood O_2 content is the sum total of O_2 bound to Hgb and O_2 in solution in the plasma.
  - O_2 content (mL/dL blood) = [Hgb(g/dL blood) × 1.34 × % saturation of Hgb] + [Po_2 × 0.003 mL O_2/dL blood/mm Hg]
- Ketoacids are the by-products of fat metabolism.
- The base excess is a calculated value, derived from the Henderson-Hasselbalch equation. It is the amount of base that would have to be added to, or removed from, oxygenated blood to achieve a pH of 7.40, given a temperature of 37° C and a $Paco_2$ of 40 mm Hg.
- The two most common acid-base disturbances seen in postoperative patients are metabolic acidosis and respiratory acidosis.

Internet Resources

GASNet: Acid Base:
http://www.gasnet.org/acid-base/

Nurse-Anesthesia.com:
http://www.nurse-anesthesia.com/

Acid base balance. Update in Anaesthesia: Pharmacology Issue, vol 13, 2001:
http://www.nda.ox.ac.uk/wfsa/html/u13/u1312_01.htm

Virtual Anaesthesia Textbook:
http://www.virtual-anaesthesia-textbook.com/

Tulane University School of Medicine, Department of Anesthesiology: Acid Base Tutorial:
http://www.acid-base.com/

Martin L: Acid-base balance. In: Pulmonary Physiology in Clinical Practice: The Essentials for Patient Care and Evaluation:
http://www.mtsinai.org/pulmonary/books/physiology/chap7_1.htm

Bibliography

Breen PH: Arterial blood gas and pH analysis: clinical approach and interpretation, *Anesth Clin North Am* 19:885-905, 2001.

Grogono AW: Acid-base balance. Available online: http://www.gasnet.org/acid-base/. Accessed May 12, 2003.

Guyton AC, Hall JE: Regulation of acid-base balance. In: *Textbook of medical physiology,* ed 10, Philadelphia, 2000, WB Saunders.

Renal Disease

Sandra M. Ouellette

1. What percentage of the cardiac output is normally directed toward the kidneys?

The percentage of cardiac output directed toward the kidneys is 20% to 25%. A normal renal blood flow (RBF) is about 1200 mL/min.

2. What is a normal glomerular filtration rate (GFR)?

A normal GFR is 125 mL/min, or 180 L/day.

3. Discuss the role of renin.

Renin is released from the kidneys (juxtaglomerular cells) in response to beta adrenergic receptor stimulation or decreased renal perfusion. It catalyzes the conversion of angiotensinogen to angiotensin I, which is then converted to angiotensin II by a angiotensin-converting enzyme in the lungs. Angiotensin II causes vasoconstriction and stimulates the release of aldosterone. Aldosterone causes the distal segments of the renal nephron to reabsorb sodium and water.

4. Define acute renal failure.

Acute renal failure is the loss of renal function over hours or days. It usually is associated with an increase in the serum creatinine (SCR) level of greater than 0.5 mg/dL, an increase in SCR of more than 50% of baseline level, or a decrease in renal function sufficient to require dialysis. Perioperative acute renal failure accounts for approximately half of all patients requiring acute hemodialysis.

5. List the classifications of acute renal failure, and state which type is most common.

The classifications of acute renal failure are as follows:
- *Prerenal (70%, most common):* hypovolemia, hemorrhage, third-space losses (trauma, sepsis, burns), decreased left ventricular function (poor ejection fraction, cardiomyopathy), acute renal artery obstruction (thrombosis, dissecting aortic aneurysm, intraoperative aortic surgical clamp)
- *Renal (25%):* acute tubular necrosis, vasculitis, acute glomerulonephritis, interstitial nephritis
- *Postrenal (5%):* ureter obstruction

6. **List conditions that place patients at high risk for acute renal failure.**

The following conditions place patients at high risk for acute renal failure:
- Hepatic insufficiency
- Sepsis
- Volume depletion
- Renal trauma or preexisting renal insufficiency
- Hemorrhagic shock
- Abdominal tamponade
- Multiple organ dysfunction
- Advanced age
- Myoglobinuria
- Scleroderma
- Diabetes
- Cardiovascular disease

Although there are many causes of perioperative acute renal failure, 90% of cases are due to hypovolemia and poor renal perfusion.

7. **What is the mortality rate associated with perioperative acute renal failure?**

Perioperative acute renal failure is associated with a 50% mortality rate.

8. **Describe the renal responses to anesthesia and surgery.**

The physiological stress of trauma and surgery is associated with a reversible decrease in RBF and GFR and reduced urinary excretion of sodium and water. These changes are usually due to alterations in intravascular and extravascular volume and the neuroendocrine effects of antidiuretic hormone, aldosterone, and catecholamines. These renal responses are generally less marked during regional anesthesia. Positive-pressure ventilation and positive end-expiratory pressure also reduce RBF and urinary output. This condition improves with volume expansion.

9. **What type of antibiotic is the most nephrotoxic?**

Aminoglycosides are the most nephrotoxic. Neomycin is the most nephrotoxic aminoglycoside. Other potentially nephrotoxic antibiotics include vancomycin, cephalosporins (especially with aminoglycosides), penicillins, and sulfonamides. In the setting of hypovolemia or sepsis, the nephrotoxic effect of these drugs is enhanced.

10. **Describe conditions that increase the risk of contrast media–induced renal failure.**

The risk of contrast media–induced renal failure may be increased under certain conditions. Preexisting renal insufficiency is the most important risk factor. If the patient's SCR is less than 1.5 mg/dL, the risk is 0.6%. The risk increases to 3% if the SCR is 1.5 to 4.5 mg/dL. Other risk factors include diabetes mellitus, dehydration, congestive heart failure, multiple myeloma, liver disease, and vascular disease. The combination of diabetes mellitus and renal insufficiency increases the risk of contrast media–induced acute renal failure to 9%. Vigorous hydration, as appropriate, should accompany the administration of radiocontrast agents.

11. Identify the most important strategies for prevention of acute renal failure.

- Maintenance of an adequate intravascular volume
- Maintenance of oxygen transport (cardiac output, renal blood flow, arterial oxygen content)
- Pharmacological therapy (mannitol, dopamine, furosemide)

12. List surgical procedures that place the patient at particular risk for acute renal failure.

The following procedures place the patient at particular risk for acute renal failure:
- Biliary surgery
- Burns
- Cardiac surgery
- Transplant
- Trauma
- Vascular surgery (especially suprarenal cross-clamp)

13. Compare the effects of dopamine and fenoldopam on renal function.

Both drugs are D_1 receptor agonists. *Dopamine* at low doses (0.5 to 3 mcg/kg/min) acts as a nonselective agonist at dopamine receptors, causing renal vasodilation and increasing GFR and urinary flow. *Fenoldopam* is a specific D_1 agonist that dilates renal and mesenteric vasculature and increases RBF at doses that do not influence blood pressure. Higher doses reduce blood pressure but maintain renal perfusion.

14. Name and identify normal values for three tests used to evaluate GFR.

Three tests used to evaluate GFR are:
- Blood urea nitrogen (BUN)—10 to 20 mg/dL
- SCR—0.7 to 1.5 mg/dL
- Creatinine clearance—110 to 150 mL/min

15. Is BUN a sensitive indicator of renal function?

No. BUN levels are highly dependent on extrarenal factors. Production is increased with a high-protein diet or gastrointestinal bleeding. BUN levels are elevated with dehydration and reduced with overhydration. Despite extrarenal influences, a BUN level greater than 50 mg/dL almost always reflects a decreased GFR.

16. **Name common renal function tests that evaluate renal tubular function.**

Urine specific gravity (1.003 to 1.030) and *urine osmolarity* (38 to 1400 mOsm/L) evaluate renal tubular function.

17. **Is plasma creatinine a reliable measure of renal function?**

Plasma creatinine is a specific indicator of GFR. When skeletal muscle is constant, the plasma concentration of creatinine depends on GFR. In general, a 50% increase in plasma creatinine reflects a 50% reduction in GFR.

18. **What is the most reliable clinical estimate of GFR?**

Creatinine clearance. It is independent of age or whether a steady state exists. Moderate renal dysfunction is present when creatinine clearance values are less than 25 mL/min. Patients with creatinine clearance less than 10 mL/min are anephric and hemodialysis dependent.

19. **List the five most significant physiological changes associated with chronic renal failure.**

Physiological changes associated with chronic renal failure are:
- Chronic anemia
- Coagulopathies
- Electrolyte imbalances
- Metabolic acidosis
- Systemic hypertension

20. **Why are patients with end-stage renal disease (ESRD) anemic?**

The anemia associated with ESRD is primarily the result of decreased renal production of erythropoietin. Erythropoietin stimulates maturation and release of erythrocytes from the bone marrow. Additional factors may include decreased red blood cell survival, gastrointestinal blood loss, bone marrow suppression, and hemodilution.

21. **What bleeding disorder is common in patients with ESRD?**

ESRD is associated with the release of *defective von Willebrand factor,* which causes abnormal platelet adhesion. Patients with ESRD exhibit a bleeding tendency despite a normal platelet count, prothrombin time, or partial thromboplastin time. A bleeding time best correlates with a bleeding tendency. Preoperative treatment may include administration of desmopressin (0.3 to 0.4 mg/kg intravenously over 30 minutes) or cryoprecipitate.

22. What is the most serious electrolyte abnormality associated with ESRD, and how should it be treated in an emergency.

Hyperkalemia is the most serious electrolyte abnormality associated with ESRD. Treatment includes administration of calcium to restore normal cardiac conduction, inducing alkalosis (sodium bicarbonate, hyperventilation), or administration of glucose and insulin to move potassium into the cell. Elective surgery should be postponed if the serum potassium is greater than 5.5 mEq/L. Potassium should be monitored immediately before surgery, even when dialysis has been performed in the previous 6 to 8 hours.

23. In what way is mild metabolic acidosis a benefit to a patient with ESRD?

Acidosis shifts the oxygen-hemoglobin dissociation curve to the right and places an anemic patient in a more favorable position for tissue oxygenation.

24. At what plasma level might inorganic fluoride ion be harmful and to what organ?

Inorganic fluoride may be harmful at 50 mcmol/L to the *kidneys*.

25. Metabolism of which volatile agents is associated with inorganic fluoride ion release?

Methoxyflurane, enflurane, and sevoflurane should be avoided in patients with renal disease because their metabolism is associated with inorganic fluoride ion release.

26. What other nephrotoxic substance may be associated with sevoflurane anesthesia?

Sevoflurane degradation by alkali, such as soda lime, produces a nephrotoxic product, *compound A*. Concern has been expressed that more compound A accumulates with prolonged anesthesia or when fresh gas flows are less than 2 L/min.

27. What changes in blood volume can be expected in a dialysis-dependent patient?

Blood volume depends on when the patient was last dialyzed. It is low soon after dialysis and high right before the next dialysis is due. Estimates of blood volume may be made by comparison of body weight before and after hemodialysis and assessment of vital signs. Regardless of the blood volume status, these patients often respond to induction of anesthesia as if they are hypovolemic. A goal preoperatively is to have the adult patient 2.5 kg greater than dry weight.

28. How do patients with ESRD respond to anesthetic drugs?

ESRD patients have an exaggerated response to anesthetic drugs. Uremia causes disruption of the blood-brain barrier. Also, decreased protein binding of drugs may result in more free drug available at receptor sites.

29. How does a patient with ESRD respond to succinylcholine?

Potassium release is not exaggerated, but there is a theoretical concern that patients with extensive uremia and neuropathies might be at increased risk. Small doses of a nondepolarizing agent before succinylcholine do not reliably attenuate the succinylcholine-induced release of potassium. The nurse anesthetist should use caution if the potassium is already high. Succinylcholine may be used, provided that the serum potassium is not greater than 5 mEq/L.

30. How does acidosis contribute to increased drug effect from sedatives and hypnotics?

Acidosis may favor a more rapid entry of drug into the brain by increasing the nonionized fraction of the drug.

31. Identify the muscle relaxants of choice for patients with ESRD.

Atracurium, cisatracurium, and mivacurium are the muscle relaxants of choice. Minor prolongation of the effects of mivacurium may be due to reduced plasma pseudocholinesterase. Atracurium and cisatracurium have non–organ-dependent pathways of elimination, enzymatic ester hydrolysis, and Hoffmann elimination.

32. How does a patient with renal impairment respond to reversal agents?

Renal excretion is the primary route of elimination for anticholinesterases (edrophonium, neostigmine, pyridostigmine). The half-lives of these drugs are prolonged. Although 50% of atropine and glycopyrrolate is excreted by the kidneys, they are safe to use. Scopolamine is less dependent on renal excretion, but its central effects are enhanced by azotemia.

 Key Points

- The percentage of cardiac output directed toward the kidneys is 20% to 25%. The normal RBF is about 1200 mL/min, and a normal GFR is 125 mL/min, or 180 L/day.
- Renin release is the first step in a complex physiological process that ultimately causes the nephron to reabsorb sodium and water.
- Acute renal failure is the loss of renal function over hours or days. Perioperative acute renal failure accounts for approximately half of all patients requiring acute hemodialysis.
- There are three classes of renal failure: prerenal (70%), renal (25%), and postrenal (5%).
- Conditions posing a high risk for acute renal failure include sepsis, volume depletion, renal trauma, preexisting renal insufficiency, hemorrhagic shock, multiple organ dysfunction, diabetes, and cardiovascular disease.
- Of perioperative acute renal failure cases, 90% are due to hypovolemia and poor renal perfusion.

Key Points   *continued*

- The most nephrotoxic class of antibiotics is the aminoglycosides. The most nephrotoxic aminoglycoside is neomycin. Other potentially nephrotoxic antibiotics include vancomycin, cephalosporins (especially with aminoglycosides), penicillins, and sulfonamides.
- The most important strategies for prevention of acute renal failure are maintenance of adequate intravascular volume, maintenance of oxygen transport, and pharmacological therapy.
- The most reliable clinical test for renal function is creatinine clearance.
- The five most significant physiological changes associated with chronic renal failure are:
  - Chronic anemia
  - Coagulopathies
  - Electrolyte imbalances
  - Metabolic acidosis
  - Systemic hypertension
- Patients with end-stage renal disease (ESRD) are anemic because of decreased renal production of erythropoietin, which stimulates maturation and release of erythryocytes from bone marrow.
- Hyperkalemia is the most serious electrolyte abnormality associated with ESRD.
- Sevoflurane degradation by alkali, such as soda lime, produces a nephrotoxic product, compound A, and inorganic fluoride.
- Patients with ESRD could be at increased risk for exaggerated release of potassium in response to the use of succinylcholine.
- Acidosis may favor a more rapid entry of drug into the brain by increasing the nonionized fraction of the drug.
- Mivacurium, atracurium, and cisatracurium are muscle relaxants of choice in renal failure patients.

Internet Resources

GASNet: Renal Function and Anesthesia:
http://www.gasnet.org/about/search.php?p1=renal+function+and+anesthesia

Virtual Anaesthesia Textbook:
http://www.virtual-anaesthesia-textbook.com/

Nurse-Anesthesia.com:
http://www.nurse-anesthesia.com/

Continued

Internet Resources   *continued*

Anesthesia and Chronic Renal Failure, Update in Anaesthesia, Issue 11, 2000:
http://www.nda.ox.ac.uk/wfsa/html/u11/u1103_01.htm

American Society of Anesthesiologists: Syllabus on Geriatric Anesthesiology: Perioperative
Renal Insufficiency and Failure in Elderly Patients:
http://www.asahq.org/clinical/geriatrics/perio.htm

Bibliography

Bolsin SN: Anesthesia and patients with renal disease. In Prys-Robert C, Brown BR, editors: *International practice of anesthesia*, Oxford, 2002, Butterworth-Heinemann, pp 1-6.

Guyton AC, Hall JE: The kidneys and body fluid. In: *Textbook of medical physiology*, ed 9, Philadelphia, 2001, WB Saunders, pp 264-344.

Isna JR: The kidneys and anesthesia: renal structure and function, renal effects of anesthetics. In Prys-Robert C, Brown BR, editors: *International practice of anesthesia*, Oxford, 2002, Butterworth-Heinemann, pp 1-9.

Lowes RJ, Prough DS: Renal dysfunction. In Benumof JL, Saidman LJ, editors: *Anesthesia and perioperative complications*, ed 2, St. Louis, 1999, Mosby, pp 471-502.

Morgan EG, Mikhail MS: Anesthesia for patients with renal disease. In: *Clinical anesthesiology*, ed 3, Stamford, CT, 2002, Appleton & Lange, pp 679-691.

Morgan EG, Mikhail MS: Renal physiology and anesthesia. In: *Clinical anesthesiology*, ed 3, Stamford, CT, 2002, Appleton & Lange, pp 662-678.

Ouellette SM, Owens SH: Renal anatomy, physiology, and pathophysiology. In Nagelhout J, Zaglaniczny K, editors: *Nurse anesthesia*, ed 2, Philadelphia, 2001, WB Saunders, pp 634-667.

Stoelting RK, Dierdorf SF: Renal disease. In: *Anesthesia and co-existing disease*, ed 4, New York, 2002, Churchill Livingstone, pp 341-372.

Wilson WC, Aronson S: Oliguria: a sign of renal success or impending renal failure? *Anesthesiol Clin North Am* 19:841–843, 2001.

Gastrointestinal Disorders

Rebecca L. M. Gombkoto

1. Describe the characteristics of gastric secretions.

The body and the fundus of the stomach are lined by *gastric glands,* which secrete hydrochloric acid, pepsinogen, intrinsic factor, and mucus. Pepsinogen is activated by hydrochloric acid, within the stomach, to form the proteolytic enzyme pepsin.

The antrum of the stomach is lined by *pyloric glands.* Pyloric glands secrete gastrin and mucus. The release of gastrin is stimulated by protein-rich foods. Gastrin induces the release of histamine, which stimulates the secretion of hydrochloric acid.

The entire stomach is covered by a layer of *mucus-secreting cells.* Mucus forms a thick lining over the gastric mucosa, establishing a barrier of protection against the digestive activity of the gastric acids and proteolytic enzymes.

2. What prevents reflux of gastric contents into the esophagus?

The last 3 cm of the esophagus, just before its communication with the stomach, consists of circular muscle that forms the lower esophageal sphincter (LES). In contrast to musculature in the midportion of the esophagus, which is typically relaxed, the LES remains contracted, preventing the reflux of gastric contents. The intraluminal pressure at the level of the LES is approximately 30 mm Hg. Swallowing stimulates peristalsis of the midportion of the esophagus followed by relaxation of the LES, permitting food to enter the stomach.

3. Define gastroesophageal reflux disease (GERD).

GERD refers to mucosal damage to the esophagus that results from the chronic reflux of gastric contents. It is estimated that 40% of adults in the United States have GERD. Reflux may cause inflammation of the esophageal mucosa, referred to as *reflux esophagitis,* or ulcerations of the mucosa, referred to as *erosive esophagitis.* Chronic reflux has the potential to damage the squamous epithelial cells that line the esophagus. The damaged squamous cells are replaced with metaplastic columnar epithelial cells. This process results in *Barrett's metaplasia* or Barrett's esophagus. Barrett's metaplasia is associated with an increased risk of esophageal adenocarcinoma.

4. Discuss causes of gastroesophageal reflux.

Delayed gastric emptying and increased gastric acidity may cause reflux, but the primary cause of gastroesophageal reflux is a reduction in LES tone. LES tone decreases with increasing age. Certain foods and medications also relax the LES. Foods or beverages containing alcohol, coffee, chocolate, fat, and peppermint cause a reduction in LES pressure. Drugs that decrease LES tone include alpha adrenergic antagonists, beta$_2$ adrenergic agonists, anticholinergics, calcium channel blockers, benzodiazepines, barbiturates, propofol, opioids, inhalational agents, dopamine, estrogen, progesterone, nitrates, theophylline, and tricyclic antidepressants. Mechanical devices, such as a nasogastric tube, interfere with the competence of the LES.

5. Describe the symptoms associated with GERD.

Heartburn is the most common symptom associated with GERD. Approximately 10% of adults in the United States have heartburn every day. Regurgitation, causing a sour taste in the mouth, is also common. Difficulty swallowing and painful swallowing are symptoms of advanced GERD. Extraesophageal symptoms often occur and can mimic other disease processes. Patients with GERD may present with noncardiac chest pain, chronic cough, hoarseness, respiratory symptoms, anemia, weight loss, or damage to the dental enamel and gums.

6. Discuss pharmacological agents used to treat GERD.

Pharmacological treatment of GERD is summarized in the table on page 243. Patients with mild and infrequent symptoms of GERD are treated initially with *antacids*. The reaction between antacids and hydrochloric acid results in the formation of less acidic or poorly soluble salts. Antacids increase gastric pH and increase LES tone. Alginic acid–containing antacids also form a protective barrier layer that coats gastric contents. Side effects are associated with antacid use. Long-term use may cause hypophosphatemia. Diarrhea is common with magnesium-containing antacids. Constipation is seen with antacids containing aluminum or calcium. Nonparticulate antacids include sodium citrate (Bicitra) and Alka-Seltzer Gold. Maalox and Mylanta are examples of particulate antacids.

Patients whose reflux is not managed with antacids are usually treated with *histamine-2 receptor antagonists (H2RAs)*. The H2RAs block histamine-2 receptors on the gastric parietal cells, inhibiting the secretion of hydrochloric acid. Gastric fluid secretion also is reduced, resulting in decreased gastric volume. Commonly used H2RAs include ranitidine, cimetidine, famotidine, and nizatidine.

Proton-pump inhibitors (PPIs) are used extensively for the treatment of GERD. By inhibiting the H^+,K^+-ATPase in gastric parietal cells, PPIs suppress gastric acid secretion. Five PPIs currently are used: lansoprazole, pantoprazole, rabeprazole, omeprazole, and its optical isomer esomeprazole.

Metoclopramide, a prokinetic agent, produces cholinergic-mediated stimulation of the gastrointestinal tract, resulting in an increase in LES tone, relaxation of

Pharmacological Treatment of Gastroesophageal Reflux Disease			
Drug Class	**Mechanism of Action**	**Generic Name**	**Trade Name**
Antacids	Increase LES tone. React with hydrochloric acid to increase gastric pH	Sodium citrate	Bicitra Alka-Seltzer, Gold Mylanta Maalox
Histamine receptor blockers	Antagonize histamine$_2$ receptors on gastric parietal cells, inhibiting the secretion of hydrochloric acid	Ranitidine Cimetidine Famotidine Nizatidine	Zantac Tagamet Pepcid Axid
Proton-pump inhibitors	Inhibit H^+/K^+, ATPase in gastric parietal cells suppressing gastric acid secretion	Lansoprazole Pantoprazole Rabeprazole Omeprazole Esomeprazole	Prevacid Protonix Aciphex Prilosec Nexium
Prokinetic agents	Stimulate gastrointestinal cholinergic receptors, producing increased LES tone, relaxation of the pylorus, and improved gastric emptying	Metoclopramide	Reglan

the pylorus, and improved gastric emptying. As such, gastric volume and the incidence of reflux are reduced. Metoclopramide antagonizes dopamine receptors in the central nervous system. With long-term use, extrapyramidal symptoms may occur.

7. Discuss preoperative considerations for patients with GERD.

Patients with gastroesophageal reflux are at risk for aspiration. An adequate period of preoperative fasting is necessary to minimize the chance of regurgitation. Supplemental medications aimed at increasing gastric pH, lowering gastric volume, and increasing LES tone should be considered. Clear, nonparticulate antacids effectively increase gastric pH when administered 15 to 30 minutes before induction of anesthesia. The H2RAs ranitidine, administered 1 hour before induction, and cimetidine, administered 1 to 1.5 hours before induction, increase gastric pH. The PPIs are more effective when repeated doses are administered. If a single dose is to be administered on the day of surgery, rabeprazole and lansoprazole effectively increase gastric pH. Omeprazole is not effective when given as a single dose on the day of surgery. Although prokinetic agents such as metoclopramide do not alter gastric pH, they effectively reduce gastric fluid volume, increase LES tone, and produce an antiemetic effect. Metoclopramide should be administered 15 to 30 minutes before induction.

A careful review of the patient's history is prudent. Patients with GERD frequently have concomitant disease processes, such as obesity, that require special attention. A history of alcohol use or tobacco use or both is common in these patients.

8. Discuss considerations for the anesthetic management of a patient with GERD.

If a general anesthetic is chosen, the airway must be secured with a cuffed endotracheal tube. Before induction, the patient should be preoxygenated. Cricoid pressure should be applied and maintained during induction and intubation. Positive-pressure ventilation may inflate the stomach and should be avoided until the airway is secured. At the conclusion of the surgical procedure, the patient must be fully awake and in control of his or her reflexes before extubation.

Consideration should be given to drug interactions that may occur when patients are receiving pharmacological treatment for GERD. Antacids may bind with other medications, resulting in an increase or a decrease in their pharmacological effect. Cimetidine and, to a lesser extent, ranitidine bind to cytochrome P-450 and may prolong the effect of drugs that are metabolized by the cytochrome P-450 system. PPIs may alter the bioavailability of drugs dependent on gastric pH for absorption. PPIs also have the potential to inhibit or induce the cytochrome P-450 enzyme system. Omeprazole inhibits enzymes responsible for the metabolism of benzodiazepines, cyclosporines, phenytoin, and warfarin. It also induces the metabolism of caffeine. Esomeprazole inhibits diazepam, and lansoprazole induces theophylline metabolism. Pantoprazole and rabeprazole are least likely to cause interactions involving the cytochrome P-450 system.

9. Describe the anatomy of the biliary ducts.

Bile, formed in the liver, drains into the right and left hepatic ducts. From there, most bile flows up the cystic duct and is stored in the gallbladder until it is required to aid in the absorption and digestion of fats and fat-soluble vitamins. The confluence of the hepatic duct and the cystic duct forms the common bile duct.

Pancreatic secretions drain into the pancreatic duct. The pancreatic duct joins the common bile duct to form the ampulla of Vater. Bile and pancreatic juices empty into the duodenum. The terminal portion of the ampulla of Vater is surrounded by smooth muscle that forms the sphincter of Oddi. The sphincter of Oddi controls the release of secretions into the duodenum. Two preampullary sphincters, the sphincter choleduchus and the sphincter pancreaticus, control the release of secretions from the common bile duct and the pancreatic duct.

10. What causes gallstones?

More than 75% of gallstones are composed of cholesterol. Most cholesterol is converted to bile acids in the liver. Some cholesterol is solubilized in micelles, however, and secreted in the bile unchanged. Bile is concentrated (5 to 20 times) in the gallbladder. Several factors may lead to the formation of gallstones. Reabsorption of excess amounts of water, electrolytes, or bile acids by the mucosa of the gallbladder may concentrate cholesterol, causing it to precipitate out of solution. Stasis, resulting from reduced motility of the gallbladder, also may cause precipitation. When cholesterol precipitates, gallstones are formed.

11. Describe clinical manifestations associated with gallstones.

If a gallstone is small, it may pass down the cystic duct into the common bile duct and be expelled into the duodenum, without symptoms. Larger stones may migrate, become trapped in the ductal system, and produce clinical manifestations.

Biliary colic refers to the pain that develops from spasms that occur when the cystic duct is obstructed by a stone. The pain associated with biliary colic is intense, develops suddenly, and is usually located in the epigastrium. Biliary colic also may be precipitated by opioid-induced sphincter of Oddi spasm.

Acute cholecystitis results when obstruction of the cystic duct causes an inflammatory reaction within the wall of the gallbladder. Pain, frequently lasting longer than 3 hours, is caused by the inflammation. Vomiting and fever are common.

Choledocholithiasis refers to gallstones that have migrated into the common bile duct. Patients may experience biliary colic. Ductal obstruction prevents the forward flow of bile. Pressure within the common bile duct increases, causing ductal distention and a reflux of bile into the liver. Hepatocellular damage may result in biliary cirrhosis or jaundice. A common symptom of biliary obstruction is pruritus. Cholangitis, bacteremia resulting from choledocholithiasis, may cause septic shock.

12. Discuss the indications for a cholecystectomy.

Although stones may form within the ductal system, most stones found in the cystic duct and the common bile duct are gallstones that form in the gallbladder. The primary indication for a cholecystectomy is symptomatic gallstones because removal of the gallbladder prevents the formation of gallstones. Elective cholecystectomies are commonly performed laparoscopically. An open cholecystectomy is indicated if scarring or inflammation would prevent laparoscopic identification of the anatomy or if peritonitis has developed. Discovery of choledocholithiasis during a laparoscopic procedure may require conversion to an open procedure so that the common bile duct may be explored and stones removed.

13. Name the advantages of laparoscopic cholecystectomy.

The laparoscopic cholecystectomy is associated with less postoperative pain than the open procedure. Infiltration of local anesthesia at the trocar site, before trocar insertion, may reduce postoperative pain further and decrease the need for postoperative analgesics and antiemetics. The use of a selective serotonin receptor antagonist, such as ondansetron, may reduce the incidence of post-operative nausea and vomiting, which are common after laparoscopic procedures.

14. Explain the function of the pancreas.

The pancreas is an endocrine and an exocrine gland. As an *exocrine organ,* the pancreas secretes enzymes responsible for the digestion of fats, proteins, and carbohydrates. Pancreatic secretions also contain significant quantities of bicarbonate ions, which help neutralize the acidic contents of the stomach when they enter the duodenum. As an *endocrine organ,* the pancreas secretes insulin and glucagon to control blood glucose levels.

15. Describe acute pancreatitis.

Of cases of acute pancreatitis, 80% are caused by gallstones or alcohol consumption. Other causes include sphincter of Oddi dysfunction, trauma, toxins, infection, hyperlipidemia, and hypercalcemia. Acute pancreatitis results when pancreatic enzymes, which normally remain inactive until they enter the duodenum, are prematurely activated and erode the pancreas. If liberated, digestive enzymes and vasoactive substances cause inflammation and ischemia of structures within the peritoneal cavity and retroperitoneal spaces.

The most common symptom of acute pancreatitis is *pain,* which typically is located in the epigastrium, umbilical area, or lower back. Nausea and vomiting are common. Most patients experience a low-grade fever. High-grade fever is associated with infection and bacteremia. Third spacing of fluid may result in tachycardia and hypotension. Fluid replacement is necessary to prevent intravascular volume depletion. Laboratory findings may reveal hyperglycemia, hypocalcemia, and acidosis. Serum amylase and lipase levels increase within hours of disease onset.

Mild episodes of acute pancreatitis may be self-limiting. Severe forms may be fatal, however, if diagnosis and treatment are delayed.

16. Describe the causes and manifestations of chronic pancreatitis.

Chronic pancreatitis is characterized by permanent parenchymal and functional damage. Clinically, chronic pancreatitis may be difficult to diagnose because recurrent attacks of chronic pancreatitis resemble acute pancreatitis. Of cases of chronic pancreatitis, 70% are caused by *chronic alcohol consumption.* Other causes include obstruction, trauma, malnutrition, and hereditary pancreatitis. Most patients with chronic pancreatitis present with *pain.* Nausea, vomiting, and weight loss are commonly seen. When the diseased pancreas is unable to secrete enzymes to meet the digestive requirements, malabsorption results in diarrhea, steatorrhea, and azotorrhea. Endocrine insufficiency results in diabetes. Approximately 25% of patients develop pancreatic pseudocysts.

17. Define endoscopic retrograde cholangiopancreatography (ERCP).

ERCP is performed by advancing an endoscope into the duodenum. The major papilla, the intraduodenal opening to the ductal system, is identified and cannulated. Contrast medium, injected under fluoroscopy, allows for the visualization of portions of the ductal system. Complete pancreatography or cholangiography also may be performed.

18. Why is ERCP performed?

ERCP is used for diagnosis and treatment of pancreatic, hepatic, and biliary diseases. Radiographic evaluation may identify structural abnormalities or obstruction of the ductal system. Manometry may be performed during an ERCP. Manometry is used to evaluate the function of the pancreatic duct, the biliary ducts, and the ductal sphincters, in particular the sphincter of Oddi.

As a diagnostic tool, the use of ERCP is declining in favor of less invasive techniques. ERCP is frequently used for therapeutic interventions, however. ERCP may be used to extract gallstones in patients with jaundice or pancreatitis due to ductal obstruction. A sphincterotomy may be performed to aid in the removal of stones or treatment of sphincter of Oddi dysfunction. Stents may be placed to allow for biliary or pancreatic drainage. Balloon dilation may be used to alleviate strictures.

19. What complications are associated with ERCP?

Complications occur in 12.7% of patients undergoing ERCP. If a sphincterotomy is performed, the complication rate increases to 29%. The most common complication after ERCP is pancreatitis.

20. Discuss the physiology and pharmacology associated with the sphincter of Oddi.

The terminal portion of the ampulla of Vater is surrounded by smooth muscle that forms the sphincter of Oddi. The sphincter of Oddi controls the flow of secretions into the duodenum. Parasympathetic stimulation relaxes and sympathetic stimulation enhances sphincter tone.

Relaxation of the sphincter of Oddi may ease cannulation of the major papilla during an ERCP or allow for the extraction of ductal stones. Drugs that relax the sphincter include glucagon, nitroglycerin, anticholinergics, calcium channel blockers, naloxone, cholecystokinin octapeptide, and prostaglandin E_1. Sphincter contraction may prevent accurate evaluation of intraoperative cholangiograms. Contraction of the sphincter may be precipitated by the administration of opioids. It is essential that drugs that relax or contract the sphincter be avoided during sphincter manometry so that accurate pressures and function may be evaluated. Drugs that do not affect sphincter tone include diazepam, midazolam, and propofol.

CONTROVERSY

21. Who should administer propofol in the endoscopy suite?

Endoscopists and gastrointestinal assistants have routinely used opioids, benzo-diazepines, and droperidol to sedate patients undergoing endoscopy. Technically advanced procedures, such as ERCP, pose unique challenges for the endoscopist. Most ERCP patients are medically compromised. The procedure requires that the patient remain still in a left lateral, semiprone position for an extended period. Many endoscopists have found that patients are more cooperative during an ERCP when sedated with propofol, rather than midazolam.

Propofol is a cardiovascular and respiratory depressant. The short duration of action mandates that propofol be continuously titrated or administered by infusion. Propofol has a narrow therapeutic index. Patients can progress rapidly from the intended level of moderate sedation/analgesia (conscious sedation) to deep sedation/analgesia or even general anesthesia. The manufacturer's warning label states that propofol "should be administered only by persons trained in the administration of general anesthesia and not involved in the conduct of the surgical/diagnostic procedure." Who should administer propofol in the endo-scopy suite is controversial even among gastrointestinal endoscopists. From a patient safety perspective, however, it seems essential that an anesthesia provider administer propofol in the endoscopy suite.

 Key Points

- The primary cause of gastroesophageal reflux is a reduction in LES tone.
- Drugs that decrease LES tone include alpha adrenergic antagonists, beta$_2$ adrenergic agonists, anticholinergics, calcium channel blockers, benzodiazepines, barbiturates, propofol, opioids, inhalational agents, dopamine, estrogen, progesterone, nitrates, theophylline, and tricyclic antidepressants.
- Heartburn is the most common symptom associated with GERD. Regurgitation, chronic cough, hoarseness, respiratory symptoms, anemia, and weight loss also can be symptoms.
- The sphincter of Oddi controls the flow of secretions into the duodenum. Parasympathetic stimulation relaxes and sympathetic stimulation enhances sphincter tone.
- Acute cholecystitis results when obstruction of the cystic duct causes an inflammatory reaction within the wall of the gallbladder.
- Choledocholithiasis refers to gallstones that have migrated into the common bile duct.
- Laparoscopic cholecystectomy is associated with less postoperative pain than the open procedure.
- Acute pancreatitis is caused by gallstones, alcohol consumption, sphincter of Oddi dysfunction, trauma, toxins, infection, hyperlipidemia, or hypercalcemia.
- Chronic pancreatitis is characterized by permanent parenchymal and functional damage. The most common cause is chronic alcohol consumption. Other causes include obstruction, trauma, malnutrition, and hereditary pancreatitis.

Internet Resources

GERD Information Resource Center:
http://www.gerd.com/

International Foundation for Functional Gastrointestinal Disorders: Gastrointestinal
functional and motility disorders:
http://www.iffgd.org/GIDisorders/GImain.html

Emedicine.com: Pancreatitis:
http://www.emedicine.com/EMERG/topic354.htm

The Merck Manual of Diagnosis and Therapy, Section 3. Gastrointestinal Disorders:
Chapter 26. Pancreatitis:
http://www.merck.com/mrkshared/mmanual/section3/chapter26/26a.jsp

Omni: Cholelithiasis:
http://omni.ac.uk/browse/mesh/detail/C0008350L0008350.html

Bibliography

Fazel A, Burton FR: The effect of midazolam on the normal sphincter of Oddi: a controlled study, *Endoscopy* 34:78-81, 2002.

Freeman ML, et al: Risk factors for post-ERCP pancreatitis: a prospective, multicenter study, *Gastrointest Endosc* 54:425-434, 2001.

Hasaniya NW, Zayed FF, Faiz H, et al: Preinsertion local anesthesia at the trocar site improves perioperative pain and decreases costs of laparoscopic cholecystectomy, *Surg Endosc* 15:962-964, 2001.

Lee SP, Ko CW: Gallstones. In Yamada T, Alpers DH, Laine L, et al, editors: *Textbook of gastroenterology*, ed 3, Philadelphia, 1999, Lippincott Williams & Wilkins, pp 2258-2280.

Ng A, Smith G: Gastroesophageal reflux and aspiration of gastric contents in anesthesia practice, *Anesth Analg* 93:494-513, 2001.

Orlando RC: Reflux esophagitis. In Yamada T, Alpers DH, Laine L, et al, editors: *Textbook of gastroenterology*, ed 3, Philadelphia, 1999, Lippincott Williams & Wilkins, pp 1235-1263.

Pennachio DL: The latest approaches to pancreatic disease, *Patient Care* 35:55-70, 2001.

Shaheen N: Gastroesophageal reflux, Barrett esophagus, and esophageal cancer: clinical applications, *JAMA* 287:1982-1986, 2002.

Spechler SJ, et al: Long-term outcome of medical and surgical therapies for gastroesophageal reflux disease: follow-up of a randomized controlled trial, *JAMA* 285:2331-2338, 2001.

Wolfe D, Brull SJ: Anesthesia for ERCP: clinical practice and safety aspects, *Same Day Surg* 26:1-6, 2002.

Liver Disease

Tim Palmer

1. Name the essential physiological functions of the liver.

Important physiological functions of the liver are bile production, protein synthesis and metabolism, glycogen storage, insulin clearance, gluconeogenesis, and drug and toxin metabolism. The liver also functions as a filter and degrader of toxins, hormones, and minerals and as a potential reservoir of blood.

2. Describe the physiological function of bile.

Bile is the primary secretory substance produced by the liver. It is formed at a rate of approximately 1 L/day. Bile is concentrated and stored in the gallbladder and released in response to the hormone cholecystokinin, in response to the presence of fat or protein in the duodenum. Bile is an important emulsifier of fat and aids in the absorption of fat and fat-soluble vitamins (vitamins A, D, E, K) across the gastrointestinal tract.

3. What proteins are synthesized by the liver?

Almost all proteins are synthesized in the liver, with a notable exception being immunoglobulins. Decreased serum oncotic pressure and impaired protein binding of drugs are associated with liver failure.

4. How much albumin is synthesized by the liver every day?

The healthy liver synthesizes 10 to 15 g of albumin every day. Normal serum albumin is 3.5 to 5.5 g/dL.

5. Is serum albumin an accurate indicator of acute hepatic dysfunction?

Serum albumin is not an accurate indicator of acute hepatic dysfunction due to its long half-life (20 days). Significant liver disease should be suspected, however, if the serum albumin is less than 3 g/dL.

6. Describe hematological effects associated with liver disease.

The liver is responsible for the production of all clotting proteins except factor VIII, which is produced by endothelial cells. A deficiency in vitamin K (secondary to impaired bile production or activity) may result in further deficiencies in vitamin K–dependent factors II, VII, IX, and X. Normal coagulation occurs as long as 20% to 30% of normal clotting factors are present. A clinical coagulopathy manifests only after significant hepatic disease. An elevated prothrombin time is an important and sensitive indicator of impaired hepatic synthesis capacity.

7. Name hormones, vitamins, and minerals that are dependent on hepatic metabolism and storage.

The liver degrades insulin, steroid hormones, antidiuretic hormone, thyroid hormone, and glucagon. The hepatocytes also are responsible for the storage of vitamins A, B_{12}, E, and D. Iron metabolism is aided by the hepatic synthesis of transferrin and heptoglobin.

8. Why is a patient with hepatic disease more likely to develop hypoglycemia perioperatrively?

Gluconeogenesis, an important source of glucose production from lactate, glycerol, and amino acids, is impaired with liver disease. Increased circulating insulin and decreased liver glycogen stores also may contribute to hypoglycemia.

9. Describe the blood supply to the liver.

The liver receives approximately 30% of the cardiac output. This averages 1500 mL/min. Of this, approximately 25% comes from the hepatic artery, and 75% comes from the portal vein.

10. Does anesthesia impair hepatic blood flow?

General and regional anesthesias are associated with reduced hepatic perfusion. Abdominal surgery, especially liver surgery, profoundly reduces hepatic perfusion.

11. How does the liver function as a reservoir for blood?

The liver is innervated by the sympathetic and parasympathetic nervous systems. Sympathetic stimulation is capable of displacing 80% of liver blood volume, approximately 500 mL, into the general circulation.

12. Describe the effects volatile anesthetics have on hepatic blood flow.

Volatile anesthetics decrease hepatic blood flow in proportion to decreased cardiac output and blood pressure. Of the volatile anesthetic agents, isoflurane, desflurane, and sevoflurane best preserve the intrinsic autoregulatory capability of the liver to maintain its blood supply. Halothane impairs hepatic autoregulatory activity most.

13. What laboratory tests are useful in determining the magnitude of hepatic disease?

No single laboratory test is reliable in determining the degree of hepatic disease. The large capacity and functional reserve of the liver permits substantial disease before overt clinical signs of insufficiency. Hepatocyte injury and death release alkaline phosphatase and transaminases into the serum. Elevated serum glutamic pyruvic transaminase (or alanine aminotransferase [ALT]) and serum glutamic oxaloacetic transaminase (or aspartate aminotransferase [AST]) are nonspecific indicators of hepatic insult. The enzyme most reflective of hepatic disease is serum ALT due to its primary location in the liver. Normal levels of ALT and AST are less than 35 to 45 IU/L. Serum bilirubin levels (normal 0.3 to 1.1 mg/dL) are elevated with hepatic disease but also are nonsensitive indicators.

14. What causes portal hypertension and ascites?

PORTAL HYPERTENSION

The most common cause of portal hypertension is cirrhosis secondary to chronic alcoholism (Laennec's cirrhosis). Cirrhosis also may be caused by biliary obstruction, chronic hepatitis, right heart failure, alpha$_1$-antitrypsin deficiency, Wilson's disease, and hemochromatosis. Anatomic alterations occur within the liver parenchyma secondary to hepatocyte necrosis and inflammation. As a result, fibrous nodular tissue replaces normal parenchymal tissue, causing obstruction, compression, and ultimately interruption of hepatic function and portal blood flow. Engorgement of vessels within the portal system and back pressure transmitted to the splanchnic circulation result in splenomegaly and esophageal, gastric, and rectal varices.

ASCITES

Ascites develops secondary to decreased plasma oncotic pressure, increased hydrostatic pressure within the hepatic sinusoids, and sodium retention. The increased intraabdominal pressure creates a restrictive type of ventilatory impairment by decreasing the functional residual capacity and impairing diaphragmatic function.

15. How does severe liver disease affect the cardiovascular system?

Patients with severe liver disease have a hyperdynamic circulatory state due to increased levels of nonmetabolized endogenous vasodilatory substances, dilutional anemia, and decreased blood viscosity. High cardiac output and decreased systemic vascular resistance are present. If chronic alcohol abuse is the causative factor of hepatic disease, cardiomyopathy also may develop.

16. How does severe liver disease affect renal function?

The hypoalbuminemia and decreased intravascular volume associated with liver disease can cause a progressive decline in renal perfusion resulting in renal insufficiency and ultimately renal failure. *Hepatorenal syndrome* is associated with progressive ascites, azotemia, oliguria, and multiple organ system failure. Development of hepatorenal syndrome carries a significant mortality. Treatment is supportive until definitive therapy (i.e. hepatic transplantation) is undertaken.

17. What is Child's classification system?

Child's classification is a three-tiered evaluation tool that provides a clinical appraisal of a patient's hepatic reserve (see the following table).

Child's Classification System

Risk Group	Type A	Type B	Type C
Bilirubin (mg/dL)	<2	2–3	>3
Serum albumin (g/dL)	>3.5	3–3.6	<3
Ascites	None	Controlled	Poorly controlled
Encephalopathy	Absent	Minimal	Coma
Nutrition	Excellent	Good	Poor
Mortality rate	2–5%	10%	50%

Adapted from Palmer T: Hepatobiliary and gastrointestinal disorders. In Nagelhout J, Zaglaniczny K, editors: Nurse anesthesia, ed 2, Philadelphia, 2001, WB Saunders, pp 668-704.

18. Discuss causes of hepatitis.

Hepatitis is an inflammatory hepatic disease that is the result of viral infection, drug reaction, or exposure to hepatotoxins. Hepatitis A (HAV), B (HBV), C (HCV), and D (HDV); Epstein-Barr virus; and cytomegalovirus are viral causes of hepatic inflammation and injury. Despite the sharp decline in HBV infection, it remains the number one hepatitis risk for health care workers. End-stage liver disease secondary to HCV is a common indication for liver transplantation in the United States. Intravenous drug abusers, immunosuppressed patients, health care workers, and patients residing in group homes or long-term care facilities are at risk for developing infectious hepatitis. The following table outlines features of HAV, HBV, HCV, and HDV.

Characteristic Features of Viral Hepatitis

	Type A	Type B	Type C (Blood-Borne non-A, non-B)	Type D
Transmission	Fecal-oral (ingestion of contaminated food or water, person-to-person contact)	Contact with infected blood or body fluid; sexual contact; mother to fetus	Contact with infected blood or body fluid; mother to fetus	Contact with infected blood or body fluid; sexual contact

Characteristic Features of Viral Hepatitis *continued*

	Type A	Type B	Type C (Blood-Borne non-A, non-B)	Type D
Course	Does not progress to chronic liver disease. Most patients recover without treatment	Progresses to chronic liver disease in 1-10% patients. Can progress to cirrhosis and cancer	Progresses to chronic liver disease in 50-70% patients. Can progress to cirrhosis and cancer	Coinfection with HBV. Often results in fulminant hepatitis
HCW implications	Careful attention to hygiene required. Vaccine available. Post-exposure I available.	High HCW risk. Vaccine recommended for all children and high-risk groups. Post-exposure I available	No vaccine. Post-exposure I effect uncertain	High HCW risk. HBV prevents HDV infection
Mortality	0.2%	0.3–1.5%	1%	2–30%

HBV; hepatitis B virus; HCW, health care worker; HVC; hepatitis D virus; I, immunoglobulin.
Adapted from Palmer T: Hepatobiliary and gastrointestinal disorders. In Nagelhout J, Zaglaniczny K, editors: Nurse anesthesia, ed 2, Philadelphia, 2001, WB Saunders, pp 668-704.

19. What are important anesthetic considerations for the patient with hepatitis?

Only urgent surgery to correct life-threatening disease should be performed on a patient with acute symptomatic hepatitis. For a patient with chronic stable hepatitis, liver function tests, measures of coagulation status, serum glucose and electrolyte levels, and renal function tests should be assessed before surgery.

20. Describe halothane hepatitis; what are the most commonly recognized risk factors?

Exposure to halothane may result in variable degrees of hepatic impairment. An estimated 1 in 10,000 patients develops postoperative jaundice subsequent to halothane exposure. Fulminant hepatic failure occurs with an incidence of 1 in 30,000 patients after halothane exposure. Metabolic breakdown of halothane in the liver results in the formation of a membrane hapten antigen (trifluoro-acetylated protein), which induces an immune-mediated inflammatory process. Contributory factors include intraoperative liver hypoxia and increased cyto-chrome P-450 activity. Additional risk factors are being a woman of childbearing age, obesity, and prior exposure to halothane (within 28 days). Postoperative hepatitis also may occur after exposure to enflurane, isoflurane, or desflurane, but because these agents undergo limited metabolism in the liver, the incidence is rare.

21. List some general pharmacological considerations for a patient with hepatic disease.

- Highly protein bound drugs, such as benzodiazepines and barbiturates, may show prolonged or exaggerated effects.
- Drugs dependent on plasma esterases (produced in the liver) for their metabolism, including succinylcholine, ester local anesthetics, and esmolol, may have prolonged effects.
- Nondepolarizing neuromuscular relaxants that are metabolized in the liver (pancuronium, vecuronium, rocuronium) may have prolonged activity. Cisatracurium is an attractive alternative.
- Opioids that undergo hepatic metabolism should be titrated judiciously to avoid prolonged respiratory depression.
- Nitrous oxide may cause sympathomimetic-induced hepatic vasoconstriction, limiting its utility in patients with hepatic disease.
- Halothane should be avoided because it undergoes the greatest degree of reductive hepatic metabolism and is implicated in causing the greatest decrease in hepatic perfusion.

22. What is carcinoid syndrome, and where are carcinoid tumors found?

Carcinoid tumors are rare, slow-growing neoplasms derived from neuro-ectodermal stem cells. These tumors secrete bioactive substances, such as serotonin, histamine, and bradykinin, which cause aberrant effects on cardio-vascular, gastrointestinal, and respiratory systems. Normally the liver is effective in metabolizing the tumor by-products before they reach the general circulation. In the presence of primary hepatic insufficiency or hepatic neoplastic disease, these substances bypass the liver, resulting in signs and symptoms of carcinoid syndrome. Common manifestations include cutaneous flushing, intestinal hypermotility, bronchospasm, labile blood pressure, right-sided heart failure, tricuspid regurgitation, and tachycardia.

23. What is octreotide acetate?

Octreotide is an analogue of somatostatin (growth hormone inhibitory hormone) that inhibits the release of carcinoid tumor products. A typical dose of octreotide is 50 mcg given intravenously or subcutaneously.

24. Summarize anesthetic considerations for a patient with carcinoid syndrome.

- Provocation of carcinoid symptoms may be induced by sympathetic nervous system activation (anxiety, pain, hypotension, hypercarbia) and by direct manipulation of the carcinoid tumor. Drugs that cause histamine release also are capable of precipitating release of tumor products.

- Medical preparation for a patient with known carcinoid tumor may include preoperative administration of octreotide (Sandostatin), corticosteroids, bradykinin antagonists (D-ARG bradykinin), and histamine receptor (H_1 and H_2) antagonists.
- A stress-free anesthetic, including optimal preoperative sedation and intraoperative analgesia, is an important goal for patients undergoing resection of a carcinoid tumor. Anesthetic management should employ intraarterial blood pressure, urine output, and central venous pressure monitoring.
- Intraoperative hypotension may be treated with direct-acting vasopressors, such as phenylephrine, intravenous fluids, and octreotide. Catecholamines and indirect-acting adrenergic receptor agonist drugs are best avoided. Hypertension may be treated with deepening the anesthetic, beta adrenergic receptor blockers, nitroprusside, and serotonin antagonists such as ketanserin.

Key Points

- Important physiological functions of the liver include bile production, protein synthesis and metabolism, glycogen storage, insulin clearance, gluconeogenesis, and drug and toxin metabolism. The liver also functions as a filter and degrader of toxins, hormones, and minerals and as a potential reservoir of blood.
- Bile is an important emulsifier of fat and aids in the absorption of fat and fat-soluble vitamins (vitamins A, D, E, K) across the gastrointestinal tract.
- The healthy liver synthesizes 10 to 15 g of albumin every day.
- Significant liver disease should be suspected if the serum albumin is less than 3 g/dL.
- The liver is responsible for the production of all clotting proteins except factor VIII.
- The liver degrades insulin, steroid hormones, antidiuretic hormone, thyroid hormone, and glucagon. The hepatocytes are also responsible for the storage of vitamins A, B_{12}, E, and D. Iron metabolism is aided by the hepatic synthesis of transferrin and heptoglobin.
- The liver receives approximately 30% of the cardiac output. This averages 1500 mL/min. Of this, approximately 25% comes from the hepatic artery, and 75% comes from the portal vein.
- General and regional anesthesias are associated with reduced hepatic perfusion.
- Sympathetic stimulation is capable of displacing 80% of liver blood volume, approximately 500 mL, into the general circulation.
- Elevated serum glutamic pyruvic transaminase (or ALT) and serum glutamic oxaloacetic transaminase (or AST) are nonspecific indicators of hepatic insult.
- The enzyme most reflective of hepatic disease is serum ALT due to its primary location in the liver.
- The most common cause of portal hypertension is cirrhosis secondary to chronic alcoholism (Laennec's cirrhosis).
- Cirrhosis causes interruption of hepatic function and portal blood flow. Engorgement of vessels within the portal system and back pressure transmitted to the splanchnic circulation result in splenomegaly and esophageal, gastric, and rectal varices.

Continued

Key Points   *continued*

- Ascites develops secondary to decreased plasma oncotic pressure, increased hydrostatic pressure within the hepatic sinusoids, and sodium retention.

- Patients with severe liver disease have a hyperdynamic circulatory state due to increased levels of endogenous vasodilatory substances, anemia, and decreased blood viscosity. High cardiac output and decreased systemic vascular resistance are present.

- Child's classification is a three-tiered evaluation tool that provides a clinical appraisal of a patient's hepatic reserve (see table in Question 17).

- Hepatitis is an inflammatory hepatic disease that is the result of viral infection, drug reaction, or exposure to hepatotoxins. HAV, HBV, HCV, and HDV; Epstein-Barr virus; and cytomegalovirus are viral causes of hepatic inflammation and injury.

- Only urgent surgery to correct life-threatening disease should be performed on a patient with acute symptomatic hepatitis. For a patient with chronic stable hepatitis, liver function tests, measures of coagulation status, serum glucose and electrolyte levels, and renal function tests should be assessed before surgery.

- Carcinoid tumor manifestations include cutaneous flushing, intestinal hypermotility, bronchospasm, labile blood pressure, right-sided heart failure, tricuspid regurgitation, and tachycardia.

Internet Resources

Anesthesiologyinfo.com: Hepatic Disease and Biliary Tract Problems in Anesthesia—Part 1 of 3: Normal Physiology, Laboratory Tests:
http://anesthesiologyinfo.com/articles/04212002.php

Anaesthesia and the Liver, Update in Anaesthesia, Issue 10, 1999:
http://www.nda.ox.ac.uk/wfsa/html/u10/u1005_01.htm

Virtual Anesthesia Textbook:
http://www.virtual-anaesthesia-textbook.com/

Nurse-Anesthesia.com:
http://www.nurse-anesthesia.com/

Bibliography

Babineau TJ, Bothe A, Steele G: The liver. In Sabiston DC, Lyerly HK, editors: *Sabiston's essentials of surgery*, ed 2, Philadelphia, 1994, WB Saunders, pp 362-363.

Conn HO: Transjugular intrahepatic portal systemic shunts: the state of the art, *Hepatology* 17:148-158, 1993.

Hawker F: Liver function tests. In Hawker F, editor: *The liver*, Philadelphia, 1993, WB Saunders, pp 43-70.

Jenset RT, Norton JA: Carcinoid tumors and the carcinoid syndrome. In Devita VT, Hellman S, Rosenberg SA, editors: *Cancer principles and practice of oncology*, ed 5, Philadelphia, 1997, Lippincott-Raven.

Morgan GE, Mikhail MS: *Clinical anesthesiology,* ed 2. Stamford, CT, 1996, Appleton & Lange, pp 625-635.

Palmer T: Hepatobiliary and gastrointestinal disorders. In Nagelhout J, Zaglaniczny K, editors: *Nurse anesthesia,* ed 2, Philadelphia, 2001, WB Saunders, pp 668-704.

Redai I, Emond J, Brentjens T: Anesthetic considerations during liver surgery, *Surg Clin North Am* 84:401-412, 2004.

Stoelting RK, Dierdorf SF: Diseases of the gastrointestinal system. In Stoelting RK, Dierdorf SF, editors: *Anesthesia and co-existing disease,* ed 4, New York, 2004, Churchill-Livingstone, pp 299-324.

Endocrine Disorders

Anne Marie Hranchook

1. **Identify the major hypothalamic releasing and inhibitory hormones that control the anterior pituitary function.**

   - *Prolactin-inhibitory factor*—now identified as *dopamine*; maintains tonic inhibitory control over prolactin release
   - *Prolactin-releasing hormone*—stimulates the release of prolactin by the anterior pituitary
   - *Growth hormone–releasing hormone*—promotes the release of growth hormone by the anterior pituitary
   - *Growth hormone–inhibitory hormone (somatostatin)*—inhibits growth hormone release
   - *Thyroid-releasing hormone*—stimulates the production and release of thyroid-stimulating hormone by the anterior pituitary
   - *Corticotropin-releasing hormone*—stimulates the release of adrenocorticotropic hormone by the anterior pituitary
   - *Gonadotropin-releasing hormone*—causes the release of the two gonadotropic hormones, follicle-stimulating hormone and luteinizing hormone

2. **What is the cause of acromegaly, and what signs and symptoms may be manifested by individuals with this disorder?**

   Excess secretion of *growth hormone* before puberty produces *gigantism,* and excess secretion after puberty produces *acromegaly.* The secretion of excess growth hormone in adults is most often due to an *adenoma* of the anterior pituitary gland. The onset of clinical manifestations is insidious. Symptoms are the result of parasellar extension of the adenoma and the systemic effects of excess growth hormone (see the following table).

Signs and Symptoms of Acromegaly	
Parasellar Manifestations	**Peripheral Effects of Excess Growth Hormone**
Enlarged sella turcica	Skeletal overgrowth (large hands and feet, prognathism)
Headache	Visceromegaly (heart, lungs, thyroid) and soft tissue overgrowth (lips, tongue, epiglottis, vocal cords)

Continued

Signs and Symptoms of Acromegaly   *continued*

Parasellar Manifestations	Peripheral Effects of Excess Growth Hormone
Visual field defects	Connective tissue overgrowth (recurrent laryngeal nerve paralysis)
Rhinorrhea	Peripheral neuropathy (carpal tunnel syndrome)
	Osteoarthritis, osteoporosis
	Skeletal muscle weakness
	Diabetes mellitus

---

3. Identify the main anesthetic considerations for a patient with acromegaly.

AIRWAY

A difficult airway may be present due to facial deformities, subglottic narrowing, and vocal cord enlargement. A goiter also may distort the airway. Careful airway assessment preoperatively is essential, and indirect laryngoscopy has been recommended to assess fully the degree of airway pathology. The presence of hoarseness, stridor, or dyspnea indicates airway involvement. The incidence of difficult intubation in this patient population is approximately 10% to 13% versus 2% to 5% for the general population. Larger sized masks, large blades for laryngoscopy, and smaller internal diameter endotracheal tubes should be available. An awake fiberoptic intubation may be considered for patients with known glottic stenosis or vocal cord paresis. Additional airway adjuncts, such as an intubating laryngeal mask airway, and equipment for emergency tracheostomy may be needed.

CARDIOVASCULAR

Acromegalic patients have a 28% incidence of hypertension due to accelerated atherosclerosis. Myocardial hypertrophy with reduced left ventricular function may be present. These patients should be questioned about exercise tolerance, history of congestive heart failure, or angina pectoris. A preoperative electrocardiogram should be assessed for the presence of ST-segment elevation or depression, T-wave inversion, and Q waves. An echocardiogram may be useful to assess left ventricular function and determine the patient's ejection fraction. An Allen's test should be performed before radial artery catheter insertion because inadequate ulnar artery collateral circulation is common.

METABOLIC

Glucose intolerance is encountered frequently, and overt diabetes occurs in 25% of acromegalic patients. Perioperative monitoring of plasma glucose levels and electrolytes is recommended.

4. Define neurogenic diabetes insipidus (DI), and discuss its management.

Neurogenic DI is associated with decreased circulating antidiuretic hormone (ADH) or decreased response to ADH at the renal collecting tubules. It is often the result of destruction or disruption of pituitary neurons responsible for the synthesis of ADH. DI that develops after pituitary gland surgery usually occurs within the first 24 hours and usually is reversible. The following criteria suggest a diagnosis of DI:

- Increased plasma osmolality (>295 mOsm)
- Hypotonic urine (<300 mOsm)
- High urine output (>2 mL/kg/hr)

TREATMENT

DI is treated with oral or intravenous fluid replacement and synthetic ADH analogues. DDAVP (1-desamino-8-D-arginine-vasopressin) can be given as a nasal spray or by injection. Most cases of DI resolve spontaneously over a few days.

5. Define the syndrome of inappropriate antidiuretic hormone secretion (SIADH), and discuss its management.

SIADH is the result of excess ADH. Common causes include intracranial trauma, infection, tumors, and bronchial carcinoma (especially small cell type). Drugs that may cause SIADH include chlorpropamide, clofibrate, and carbamazepine. Excess ADH leads to water retention, increased intravascular volume, and dilutional hyponatremia. The syndrome is usually transient and rarely lasts for more than 7 to 10 days.

TREATMENT

An initial approach to treatment is restriction of free water intake. Demeclocycline may be administered to antagonize the effects of ADH on the renal tubules. In severe cases, hypertonic saline may be used to correct the hyponatremia. Correction of low serum Na^+ concentrations should proceed slowly and cautiously, over 24 to 48 hours, at a rate not to exceed raising the serum Na^+ concentration faster than 1.0–1.5 mEq/L/hr. Rapid correction of serum sodium can result in central pontine myelinolysis and permanent neurologic injury.

6. Discuss criteria that must be met before elective surgery for patients with known hyperthyroid disease.

Elective surgery should not be performed until a hyperthyroid patient is rendered euthyroid and the resting heart rate is less than 85 to 90 beats/min. This may be accomplished with antithyroid drugs, commonly carbimazole and propylthiouracil. Effective treatment with these drugs may require 6 to 8 weeks. Beta adrenergic antagonist drugs are used to control the symptoms of excessive sympathetic nervous system activity. If emergency surgery is required for a patient with uncontrolled hyperthyroidism, the patient should be treated with intravenous propranolol, 1 mg per minute, up to 10 mg, and monitored assiduously in the perioperative period for signs and symptoms of thyroid storm (fever, tachycardia, agitation, systolic hypertension, wide pulse pressure). Thyroid storm is a medical emergency and should be treated aggressively with hydration, cooling, intravenous beta adrenergic antagonists (propranolol is the beta-adrenergic blocker of choice because it also prevents the peripheral conversion of thyroxine to triiodothyronine), propylthiouracil (250 mg every 6 hours orally or by nasogastric tube), and correction of any precipitating cause.

7. **Compare common clinical features associated with hyperthyroidism and hypothyroidism.**

Clinical features of hyperthyroidism and hypothyroidism are compared in the following table.

Clinical Features of Hyperthyrodism and Hypothyroidism

Clinical System	Hyperthyroidism	Hypothyroidism
Cardiovascular	Tachycardia, cardiac arrhythmias, wide pulse pressure, heart failure, vasodilation	Bradycardia, cardiomegaly, cardiac failure, vasoconstriction, reduced plasma volume
General	Weight loss, tremor, heat intolerance, sweating, goiter	Cold intolerance, arthralgia, alopecia, goiter
Respiratory	Increased respiratory rate, dyspnea on exertion, reduced respiratory muscle strength	Hypoventilation, decreased ventilatory response to hypoxia and hypercapnia, sleep apnea
Gastrointestinal	Diarrhea, nausea, vomiting	Constipation, delayed gastric emptying
Neurological	Anxiety, irritability, insomnia	Fatigue, lethargy, slow mentation
Ophthalmic	Proptosis, lid retraction, reduced blinking	—

8. **Describe the primary role of parathyroid hormone (PTH).**

PTH plays a central role in calcium homeostasis. It acts on bone, kidney, and the intestine, increasing the concentration of calcium in the blood and lowering serum phosphate.
- *Bone:* PTH inhibits osteoblasts and stimulates osteoclast-mediated bone resorption. This results in increased extracellular calcium.
- *Intestine:* PTH enhances calcium and phosphate absorption from the gut by promoting the formation of active vitamin D.
- *Kidney:* PTH enhances calcium reabsorption from the renal tubules. It also increases phosphate excretion. Vitamin D is converted to an active form, 1,25-dihydroxycholecalciferol, in the kidney under the influence of PTH.

9. **Damage to the recurrent laryngeal nerves is a potential complication of thyroid and parathyroid surgery. Discuss the implications of unilateral versus bilateral damage.**

The recurrent laryngeal nerves supply all of the muscles of the larynx except the cricothyroid muscle and the mucous membranes below the vocal cords. Permanent recurrent laryngeal nerve injury is rare. Transient nerve injury may occur as a result of nerve stretching or compression during surgery.

Unilateral recurrent laryngeal nerve injury most commonly causes hoarseness, but may be asymptomatic in some patients, owing to the opposite cord undergoing compensatory hyperabduction. Bilateral nerve paralysis is evident immediately after extubation. Unopposed adduction of the vocal cords causes stridor, aphonia, or complete airway obstruction. Failure of both cords to move requires immediate reintubation.

10. What are the most common long-term complications associated with diabetes mellitus that are of special concern to the nurse anesthetist?

CORONARY HEART DISEASE

Diabetics are four to five times more likely to have coronary heart disease than nondiabetics. Patients may have myocardial ischemia or myocardial infarction without typical symptoms due to associated neuropathy. Diabetic autonomic neuropathy may contribute to ventricular arrhythmias and sudden death in these patients.

HYPERTENSION

Elevated blood pressure is especially prevalent in type 2 diabetes. Angiotensin-converting enzyme inhibitors are considered the first-line drug for treatment of hypertension in patients with diabetes due to their renal protective properties.

NEUROPATHY

Diabetics develop nerve damage, in part associated with chronic hyperglycemia. The neuropathy is most often a distal sensory or sensorimotor polyneuropathy with a variable amount of autonomic involvement. Autonomic dysfunction occurs in 40% of type 1 and 17% of type 2 diabetics. Manifestations of autonomic dysfunction include gastroparesis, postural hypotension, a labile blood pressure, tachycardia, a blunted ventilatory response to hypoxemia, diarrhea, and bladder paresis. Diabetic gastroparesis enhances the risk of acid aspiration during anesthetic induction.

DIABETIC NEPHROPATHY

Diabetic nephropathy and end-stage renal failure develop in 30% to 40% of patients with type 1 diabetes. Ensuring adequate hydration and renal perfusion reduces the risk of postoperative renal dysfunction in these patients.

11. Describe a method for continuous intravenous insulin infusion during the perioperative period.

A continuous infusion protocol using regular insulin can be adjusted to control blood glucose levels using the following formula:

Regular insulin administration (units/hr) = plasma glucose (mg/dL) ÷ 150

The denominator is reduced to 100 for patients taking corticosteroids equivalent to prednisone, 100 mg/day. With this formula, the plasma glucose usually is maintained in the range of 120 to 180 mg/dL. The insulin drip can be prepared by placing 50 units of regular insulin into 250 mL of 0.9% sodium chloride.

Approximately 60 mL of the insulin solution can be used to purge the tubing, saturating insulin-binding sites in the plastic tubing. The insulin drip should be placed on an intravenous infusion pump at the calculated infusion rate and piggybacked into a 5% dextrose solution. The glucose-containing intravenous infusion is begun at 100 to 150 mL/h per 70 kg. A separate intravenous line is established for routine fluid replacement. Potassium chloride, 20 to 30 mEq, is often added to each 1 L infused in the primary intravenous site. "Tight" blood glucose control increases the risk of hypoglycemia. Frequent blood glucose determinations (at least every hour) are mandatory with this method.

12. What oral agents are available to treat type 2 diabetes, and how do these agents work?

SULFONYLUREAS

The sulfonylureas were the first oral agents used to treat diabetes. These agents work by stimulating insulin release from pancreatic beta cells. The sulfonylureas are divided into two groups: first generation (acetohexamide, tolazamide, tolbutamide, chlorpropamide) and second generation (glipizide, glyburide, glimepiride). Hypoglycemia is a potentially serious problem that must be monitored, especially with longer acting agents, such as chlorpropamide and glyburide.

BIGUANIDES

Biguanides work by decreasing hepatic glucose production and increasing peripheral glucose uptake. Lactic acidosis, a rare but potentially fatal problem, has been reported with biguanides. Lactic acidosis is precipitated by drug accumulation; even mild renal impairment is a contraindication to biguanide therapy.

ALPHA-GLUCOSIDASE INHIBITORS

Alpha-glucosidase inhibitors block the intestinal enzymes (maltase, sucrase, glucoamylase) that digest starches into absorbable monosaccharides, resulting in a slower and lower rise in plasma glucose.

THIAZOLIDINEDIONES

Thiazolidinediones decrease hepatic glucose output by inhibiting gluconeogenesis. They also decrease plasma glucose by increasing the insulin sensitivity of skeletal muscle, liver, and adipose tissue. Liver enzymes must be monitored closely with these agents.

NONSULFONYLUREA SECRETAGOGUES

Nonsulfonylurea secretagogues have a mechanism of action similar to the sulfonylureas and increase insulin production by pancreatic beta cells.

13. What are usual dosages of common oral hypoglycemic agents?

The table below contains dosage information for oral hypoglycemia agents.

Dosages for Oral Hypoglycemic Agents

Drug	Usual Daily Dosage
Sulfonylurea — first generation	
Acetohexamide (Dymelor)	500–750 mg once or divided
Chlorpropamide (Diabinese)	250–375 mg once
Tolazamide (Tolinase)	250–500 mg once or divided;
Tolbutamide (Orinase)	1000–2000 mg divided
Sulfonylurea — second generation	
Glimepiride (Amaryl)	1–4 mg once
Glipizide (Glucotrol;	10–20 mg once or divided
Glucotrol XL extended-release tablets)	5–20 mg once
Glyburide (DiaBeta, Micronase;	5–20 mg once or divided;
Glynase, micronized tablets)	3–12 mg once or divided
Alphaglucosidase inhibitors	
Acarbose (Precose)	50–100 mg tid with meals
Miglitol (Glyset)	50–100 mg tid with meals
Thiazolidinediones	
Rosiglitazone (Avandia)	4–8 mg once or divided
Pioglitazone (Actos)	15–45 mg once
Biguanides	
Metformin (Glucophage; Glucophage XR)	1500–2550 mg divided; 1500–2000 mg once
Metformin/glyburide (Glucovance)	500 mg/5 mg bid
Nonsulfonylurea Secretagogues	
Repaglinide (Prandin)	1–4 mg tid before meals
Nateglinide (Starlix)	60–120 mg tid before meals

Adapted from Treatment guidelines Med Lett 1, 2002.

14. Summarize the types of insulin preparations available to treat diabetes mellitus.

The table on the next page characterizes the insulin preparations available.

Characteristics of Insulin Preparations

Insulin Type	Onset of Action	Peak Activity	Duration	Route
Short-acting				
Regular	30–60 min	1–2 hr	5–12 hr	IV, SC, IM
Rapid-acting				
Aspart (NovoLog)	10–30 min	30–60 min	3–5 hr	SC
Lispro (Humalog)	10–30 min	30–60 min	3–5 hr	SC
Intermediate-acting				
NPH/Lente	1–2 hr	4–8 hr	10–20 hr	SC
Long-acting				
Ultralente	2–4 hr	8–20 hr	16–24 hr	SC
Glargine	1–2 hr	No peak	24 hr	SC

IM, intramuscular; IV, intravenous; NPH, neutral protamine Hagedorn; SC, subcutaneous.
Adapted from Treatment Guidelines Med Lett 1, 2002; and
http://diabetes.niddk.nih.gov/dm/pubs/medicines_ez/specific.htm#insulin.

15. **What is the expected decrease in blood glucose levels after the administration of 1 unit of intravenous regular insulin?**

    The blood glucose response to insulin is variable, but a 70-kg adult usually experiences a decrease in blood glucose of 25 to 30 mg/dL after the administration of 1 unit of regular insulin intravenously.

16. **How does insulin glargine differ from other commercially prepared insulins?**

    Insulin glargine is a recombinant DNA analogue of human insulin. It forms microprecipitates in subcutaneous tissue, which delay its absorption and prolong its effects. In contrast to NPH and Ultralente, it exhibits a flat pharmacokinetic profile, with a duration of action of at least 24 hours. It mimics more closely the natural physiological profile of basal endogenous insulin secretion. In the perioperative period, careful attention must be given to its duration of action.

17. **Describe the classic triad of symptoms associated with pheochromocytoma.**

    Pheochromocytoma is an epinephrine and norepinephrine–secreting tumor of chromaffin cells, usually of the adrenal medulla. The classic triad of symptoms associated with pheochromocytoma is (1) headache, (2) palpitations, and (3) sweating. These three symptoms, in association with hypertension, are pathognomonic of the condition. Other manifestations include intermittent facial pallor, anxiety, tremor, hyperglycemia, and ventricular ectopy.

18. Outline the preoperative preparation for a patient with a pheochromocytoma.

Preoperative preparation for patients with pheochromocytomas includes pharmacological measures to control hypertension and arrhythmias and a thorough evaluation for end-organ damage. Preparation should begin at least 2 weeks before surgery. These patients are chronically vasoconstricted as a result of the high levels of circulating catecholamines. Preoperative alpha blockade lowers the blood pressure and allows for normalization of the circulating blood volume.

Phenoxybenzamine is a nonselective alpha adrenergic blocker frequently used to prepare patients for surgery. A starting dose of 10 to 20 mg twice a day is gradually increased to 60 to 250 mg/day in most patients. Side effects include reflex tachycardia, nausea, sedation, gastric irritation, and nasal stuffiness. Prazosin, a specific alpha$_1$ receptor antagonist also may be used preoperatively but is associated with a more profound decrease in blood pressure.

Preoperative beta-adrenergic blockade also may be implemented to control tachycardia and dysrhythmias. It is important that beta adrenergic blocking agents be started only after initiation of alpha-blockade. Blocking beta$_2$-mediated vasodilation, before alpha blockade, can result in unopposed vaso-constriction. A preoperative electrocardiogram and echocardiography help evaluate any cardiac dysfunction.

19. Compare the normal daily cortisol production of the human body with the increased production necessary for major surgery or trauma.

The adrenal cortex normally produces approximately 15 to 20 mg of cortisol daily. During times of stress or trauma, the adrenal cortex produces 100 to 150 mg of cortisol. Increased cortisol secretion may enhance survival by aug-menting the cardiac output, increasing the sensitivity to catecholamines, and mobilizing energy sources.

CONTROVERSY

20. Discuss the current opinion regarding stress-dose steroid administration to surgical patients.

Long-term corticosteroid administration depresses a patient's ability to mount the usual adrenal cortex response to surgical or traumatic stress. The precise dose of corticosteroid or duration of therapy that produces suppression is un-known. Although rare, perioperative vascular collapse can occur in patients with adrenal suppression who do not receive perioperative steroid supplemention.

It is generally accepted that patients who are currently taking physiological doses of corticosteroids or who have taken them for more than 1 month in the past 6 to 12 months are at risk for suppression of the pituitary-adrenal axis. Perioperative steroid supplementation is often implemented for these select individuals. The recommended dose for supplemental corticosteroid administration depends on the degree of surgical stress (see the following table).

Supplemental Corticosteroid Administration

Type of Surgical Stress	Examples of Surgery	Dose of Steroid Supplement
Minor	Inguinal hernia repair	None or minimal (25 mg hydrocortisone equivalent on day of operation only)
Moderate	Open cholecystectomy, lower extremity vascular procedure, total joint replacement, hysterectomy	50–75 mg/day hydrocortisone equivalent for 1–2 days, then resume preoperative dose
Major	Whipple procedure, esophagogastrectomy, total colectomy, cardiopulmonary bypass	100–150 mg/day hydrocortisone equivalent for 2–3 days, then resume preoperative dose

 Key Points

- Excess secretion of growth hormone before puberty produces gigantism, and excess secretion after puberty produces acromegaly.
- The main anesthetic considerations for a patient with acromegaly are difficult airway, hypertension, myocardial hypertrophy, diabetes, and electrolyte abnormalities.
- SIADH is the result of excess ADH. Excess ADH leads to water retention, increased intravascular volume, and dilutional hyponatremia.
- Rapid correction of serum sodium can result in central pontine myelinolysis and permanent neurologic injury.
- Elective surgery should not be performed until a hyperthyroid patient is rendered euthyroid and the resting heart rate is less than 85 to 90 beats/min.
- The patient should be monitored assiduously in the perioperative period for signs and symptoms of thyroid storm (fever, tachycardia, agitation, systolic hypertension, wide pulse pressure).
- Recurrent laryngeal nerve injury is a potential complication of thyroid and parathyroid surgery. Unilateral recurrent laryngeal nerve injury most commonly causes hoarseness, but may be asymptomatic. Bilateral nerve paralysis is evident immediately after extubation. Unopposed adduction of the vocal cords causes stridor, aphonia, or complete airway obstruction.
- A 70-kg adult usually experiences a decrease in blood glucose of 25 to 30 mg/dL after the administration of 1 unit of regular insulin intravenously.

Key Points *continued*

- Insulin glargine is a recombinant DNA analogue of human insulin. It forms microprecipitates in subcutaneous tissue, which delay its absorption and prolong its effects.
- The classic triad of symptoms associated with pheochromocytoma is (1) headache, (2) palpitations, and (3) sweating.
- Phenoxybenzamine is a nonselective alpha-adrenergic blocker frequently used to prepare patients for surgery. Preoperative beta-adrenergic blockade also may be implemented to control tachycardia and dysrhythmias.

 Internet Resources

Endocrine Physiology, Update in Anaesthesia, Issue 14, 2002:
http://www.nda.ox.ac.uk/wfsa/html/u14/u1402_01.htm

Virtual Anaesthesia Textbook:
http://www.virtual-anaesthesia-textbook.com/

Nurse-anesthesia.com:
http://www.nurse-anesthesia.com/

Anaesthetist.com. Thyroid Disease:
http://www.anaesthetist.com/anaes/patient/thyroid.htm

http://www.medstudents.com.br/endoc/endoc8.htm

Bibliography

Dierdorf SF: Anesthesia for patients with diabetes mellitus, *Curr Opin Anaesthesiol* 15:351-357, 2002.

Dougherty TB, Cronau LH Jr: Anesthetic implications for surgical patients with endocrine tumors, *Int Anesthesiol Clin* 36:31-44, 1998.

Farling PA: Thyroid disease, *Br J Anaesth* 85:15-28, 2000.

Jabbour SA: Steroids and the surgical patient, *Med Clin North Am* 85:1311-1317, 2001.

Kaplan NM: Management of hypertension in patients with type 2 diabetes mellitus: guidelines based on current evidence, *Ann Intern Med* 135:1079-1083, 2001.

Lyons FM, Meeran K: The physiology of the endocrine system, *Int Anesthesiol Clin* 35:1-24, 1997.

McAnulty GR, Robertshaw HJ, Hall GM: Anaesthetic management of patients with diabetes mellitus, *Br J Anaesth* 85:80-90, 2000.

O'Riordan JA: Pheochromocytomas and anesthesia, *Int Anesthesiol Clin* 35:99-127, 1997.

Sonksen P, Sonksen J: Insulin: understanding its action in health and disease, *Br J Anaesth* 85:69-79, 2000.

Tasch MD: Corticosteroids and anesthesia, *Curr Opin Anaesthesiol* 15:377-381, 2002.

Surgical Procedures and Anesthetic Management

Genitourinary Surgery

Carl S. Brow, III, and John P. Maye

1. Discuss preoperative considerations specific to patients undergoing genitourinary surgery.

Many patients undergoing genitourinary surgery are elderly and have coexisting diseases. A thorough preoperative examination addressing fluid and electrolyte status, coagulation profiles, and the presence or absence of coronary artery disease is essential to selection of the most appropriate anesthetic for a patient.

A preoperative knowledge of the patient's fluid and electrolyte status is essential. Electrolyte abnormalities and fluid deficits should be corrected before the initiation of the surgical procedure. Urine output is often difficult to measure during genitourinary procedures because of continuous irrigation and simultaneous blood loss from the surgical site. Monitoring renal perfusion and preload in patients with limited cardiac or pulmonary reserve may be done with invasive monitoring and should be anticipated before the start of the surgical procedure.

2. What is first-generation extracorporeal shock wave lithotripsy (ESWL)?

ESWL is a noninvasive means of treating renal and urinary tract stones. The technique was introduced in the early 1980's and revolutionized the treatment of calculus disease. The first-generation lithotripters (Dornier HM-3) required that the patient be immersed in a tub of water. The water served as a coupling agent between the patient and the shock wave energy. Fluoroscopy or ultrasound was used to locate the stone and focus the shock wave energy. Multiple shocks were directed at the stone until the stone eventually disintegrated into particles small enough to pass through the urinary tract.

3. Distinguish second-generation and third-generation ESWL from first-generation ESWL.

Second-generation and third-generation lithotripters do not require immersion in a water bath. A membrane placed over the shock wave generator provides the coupling agent between the patient and the shock wave energy. The second-generation and third-generation lithotripters generate less energy when delivering shock waves. The decrease in energy produces less pain, and these patients usually do not require general or regional anesthesia.

4. Are there contraindications to ESWL?

Absolute contraindications to ESWL include:
- Pregnancy
- Coagulopathies
- Abdominally implanted pacemakers

Relative contraindications include:
- Abdominal aortic aneurysm (may be possible if the aneurysm is <5 cm)
- Severe obesity

In obese patients, accurate focusing of the wave energy on the stone may be technically difficult.

5. What anesthetic techniques are appropriate for second-generation and third-generation ESWL?

Second-generation and third-generation lithotripters generate lower energy shock waves and are usually less stimulating. Intravenous sedation and spinal opioids provide adequate pain relief. Intravenous agents with small volumes of distribution, rapid plasma clearance, and short elimination half-lives seem to be the best choices. Infiltration of local anesthesia at the skin-lithotripter interface site has been used to decrease the cutaneous pain associated with ESWL. At least one investigation found that this method alone seemed to be insufficient in approximately half of patients.

6. State the primary goals of any anesthetic technique for a patient undergoing ESWL.

The primary goals of anesthesia during ESWL are to maintain patient safety and to promote patient comfort. One of the most important components of that goal is to minimize patient movement. Movement during delivery of the shock waves can cause tissue damage to surrounding structures. Diaphragmatic movement during general anesthesia with controlled ventilation may result in significant stone movement. Spontaneous ventilation during general anesthesia is associated with less stone movement. Jet ventilation during general anesthesia also has been used with good results.

7. Describe the anesthetic management of patients undergoing percutaneous nephrolithotomy.

Percutaneous nephrolithotomy is a surgical procedure performed for removal of kidney stones or relief of renal obstruction. A rigid operating scope is inserted into the lower calyx of the kidney under fluoroscopy. Stones are grasped, removed, or pulverized using laser or ultrasound energy. General anesthesia is required for this surgical procedure. Patients usually are positioned prone, although the lateral decubitus position also has been used. Anesthetic concerns related to this surgical procedure are primarily related to positioning and the potential for blood loss.

Continuous irrigation (typically, lactated Ringer's solution or normal saline) through the endoscope is required during this procedure to facilitate visualization and to flush out debris. Large amounts of irrigating fluid may be used depending on the duration of the procedure. Estimating blood loss may be difficult or impossible under these circumstances. Bleeding from the renal structures into the retroperitoneal space may not be detected until a significant amount of blood loss has occurred. Patients who cannot tolerate significant blood loss should have serial hemoglobin determinations. Extravasation of irrigating fluid into the retroperitoneal and abdominal spaces also has been documented. Irrigation output should be closely monitored and compared with the amount used. Circulatory overload may occur if a significant amount of irrigant is absorbed into the vascular compartment.

8. Discuss the most commonly used irrigating solutions for transurethral resection of the prostate (TURP) procedures.

TURP is initiated by inserting a resectoscope into the urethra. Electrocautery is used to resect any hypertrophied prostatic tissue. Continuous irrigation is required to allow visualization, distend the bladder, and flush resected tissue away. Irrigating solutions must be nonionic to prevent dispersal of the electrical current from the electrocautery and clear to allow adequate visualization.

Intravascular absorption of irrigating solutions is a complication of TURP procedures. Irrigating solutions should be nonhemolytic and isotonic. Solutions most commonly used today are mildly hypotonic, which allows for better visualization; these include:
- Glycine 1.5%
- Mannitol 3% to 5%
- Sorbitol 3.5%
- Cytal (a mixture of sorbital 2.7% and mannitol 0.54%)

These solutions are not ideal and may result in adverse effects. Sorbitol may result in hyperglycemia and metabolic acidosis. Mannitol, which increases intravascular volume by drawing extracellular fluid into the vascular space, can lead to circulatory overload and pulmonary edema in susceptible patients. A major metabolite of glycine is ammonia, which in elevated amounts may result in central nervous system depression and coma.

9. Discuss TURP syndrome.

TURP syndrome refers to a collection of symptoms caused by excessive intravascular absorption of irrigating solutions during TURP, leading to hyponatremia, fluid overload, and possibly cerebral edema. TURP syndrome occurs when prostatic venous sinuses are opened during resection of hypertrophied prostatic tissue. Disruption of venous sinuses may lead to uptake of irrigating solutions into the vascular system. Initial symptoms may include central nervous system changes, such as confusion and restlessness. Additional manifestations include nausea, shortness of breath, pulmonary edema, electrocardiogram changes, and hypertension.

The amount of solution absorbed depends on several factors, including (1) the amount of prostate tissue resected, (2) the length of the procedure, and (3) the hydrostatic pressure driving the irrigating solution into the prostatic veins. It has been estimated that the average amount of irrigating solution absorbed is about 20 mL/min of resection time. The vascular uptake of large volumes of irrigating solution leads to increased circulatory volume, hyponatremia, and hypoosmolality. Central nervous system symptoms are due to hyponatremia and acute hypoosmolality, causing free water to move intracellularly and leading to cerebral edema. Central nervous system symptoms, usually confusion and restlessness due to hyponatremia, begin when the serum sodium reaches 120 mEq/L. More severe symptoms, such as coma, seizures, and ventricular dysrhythmias, appear when the serum sodium decreases to less than 115 mEq/L.

10. How is TURP syndrome treated?

Communication with the surgical team is essential. Termination of the surgical procedure is always an alternative. All patients with TURP syndrome should be given oxygen and observed for exacerbation of symptoms. Laboratory tests, including electrolytes, complete blood count, and arterial blood gas analysis, should be performed as soon as possible. Invasive monitoring may be indicated if the patient is hemodynamically unstable.

Treatment is generally symptomatic and guided by the degree of severity. *Mild symptoms* associated with serum sodium concentrations greater than 120 mEq/L can be treated with a loop-type diuretic, fluid restriction, and serial electrolytes. *Moderate-to-severe symptoms* must be treated with ventilatory and circulatory support while the hyponatremia and hypoosmolality is corrected. Hypertonic saline (3%) can be used to treat hyponatremia. Hypertonic saline must be administered slowly ($\leq$100 mL/hr). Hypertonic saline administration and rapid correction of hyponatremia has been associated with central pontine demyelination, caused by rapid osmotic dysequilibrium; this can lead to permanent brain damage.

Problems related to the specific type of irrigating solution should also be corrected, such as hyperglycemia from sorbitol solutions or elevated blood ammonia levels from glycine solutions. Central nervous system symptoms from these causes are often indistinguishable from hyponatremia and hypoosmolality and should be included in the differential diagnosis.

11. What other complications are associated with TURP procedures?

Bleeding, bladder perforation, coagulopathies, and hypothermia are other possible complications associated with TURP. Blood loss frequently occurs from open venous sinuses and arterial sources. The high volume of irrigating solutions makes accurate estimation of blood loss during this procedure virtually impossible.

There are two proposed methods for estimating blood loss during TURP. The first method includes an estimation of 2 to 5 mL of blood loss per minute of resection time. The second method is an estimation of 20 to 50 mL of blood loss per gram of prostate tissue resected. Vital signs and serial hemoglobin determinations should be used to assist in estimating blood loss. Hemodynamic parameters may not be a sensitive indicator of blood loss because the absorption of irrigating solution may mask changes in vital signs.

Bladder perforation may occur from direct injury to the bladder wall by the resectoscope or from overdistention of the bladder. Extraperitoneal perforation causes umbilical, inguinal, or suprapubic pain, which may be difficult to detect regardless of whether general or regional anesthesia is used. Intraperitoneal perforation produces abdominal tenderness and may produce pain in the shoulders from diaphragmatic irritation. Nausea, vomiting, diaphoresis, abdominal rigidity, and hypotension are symptoms that may occur but are usually less specific. If the return of irrigating solution abruptly decreases, bladder perforation should be considered.

Associated coagulopathies may result from the release of plasminogen activator by prostatic tissue. Plasminogen activator is an enzyme that converts plasminogen into plasmin, which breaks down fibrin clots. This can trigger disseminated intravascular coagulation and hemorrhage if high concentrations of plasmin are formed.

12. Describe anesthetic techniques for TURP.

Regional or general anesthesia is required for patients undergoing TURP. *Regional anesthesia* is used in approximately 70% of cases and has been regarded as the superior anesthetic technique. Regional anesthesia allows for earlier detection of complications because the anesthesia provider can assess mental status throughout the procedure. Regional anesthesia provides postoperative pain relief and may be associated with decreased blood loss. Spinal anesthesia is the most frequently employed technique. Sensory block to T10 is the minimal dermatomal level required for adequate anesthesia. A block above T9 should be avoided if possible because pain with bladder perforation is likely to be masked by the high sensory block. Patients who cannot tolerate sudden decreases in blood pressure may benefit from epidural anesthesia or continuous spinal anesthesia carefully titrated to achieve the minimal sensory block needed in a slow controlled manner. General anesthesia is an alternative for patients who have a contraindication to regional anesthesia.

13. Discuss special anesthetic problems that should be considered for patients undergoing open radical genitourinary surgery.

Open radical genitourinary procedures include prostatectomy, nephrectomy, cystectomy, and pelvic lymph node dissection. Prostatectomy with or without pelvic lymph node dissection is the most commonly performed procedure. Although each procedure has its own inherent problems, they all share two major concerns: the potential for significant hemorrhage and positioning.

HEMORRHAGE
The prostate gland and the kidney are both highly vascular organs. Failure to control surgical bleeding or inadvertent damage to nearby major vessels can lead to rapid blood loss. Volume status must be carefully monitored and managed during surgery, and direct arterial blood pressure measurement is usually indicated. Adequate intravenous access is crucial. A second 16-gauge or 14-gauge peripheral line helps facilitate rapid administration of fluids.

POSITIONING
Positioning for prostatectomy and cystectomy may involve the Trendelenburg position for a prolonged time. A decrease in pulmonary reserve and an increase in peak inspiratory pressure may occur as a result of abdominal contents resting against the diaphragm. Prolonged head-down position also can cause venous pooling in the head and neck, possibly leading to airway edema. Positioning for nephrectomy depends on the surgical approach. A flank approach requires placing the patient in a lateral decubitus position with the table flexed and the kidney rest elevated to facilitate surgical exposure. Not only does this position compromise pulmonary function, but also it carries an increased risk for nerve injury.

A dorsal lumbotomy approach requires prone positioning with the table flexed. This position is associated with pulmonary compromise, increased risk of nerve injury, and risk of retinal ischemia.

14. Describe intraoperative measures to decrease blood loss during radical prostatectomy.

Use of intraoperative *blood salvaging* systems has become more common and is a generally accepted practice during prostatectomies. Autologous donation is another strategy that can be used for patients who meet criteria and can schedule the surgery far enough in advance to allow donation.

The use of modest or *controlled hypotension* helps reduce blood loss. In patients in whom there is limited or no concern of hemodynamic compromise, mean arterial pressures of 55 to 65 mm Hg can be tolerated. Regional anesthesia either alone or in combination with general anesthesia is associated with less blood loss.

15. During a radical nephrectomy, the anesthetist notices a rapid increase in peak airway pressures, an increase in end-tidal carbon dioxide concentrations, and a decrease in oxygen saturation. What has most likely occurred?

The surgeons may have inadvertently entered the chest during removal of the kidney. The patient has developed a pneumothorax. The surgeon should be notified immediately, and the patient should be placed on 100% oxygen. An intraoperative chest x-ray confirms the diagnosis, and placement of a chest tube should be considered.

16. Is there a benefit to epidural anesthesia and analgesia for patients undergoing radical genitourinary procedures?

Patients undergoing radical genitourinary procedures can benefit from the pain relief provided by epidural analgesia. One prospective study from 1998 examined the use of epidural anesthesia for patients undergoing radical genitourinary procedures. The findings of this investigation support the use of epidural anesthesia intraoperatively and postoperatively. Patients who received preemptive epidural analgesia or had epidural analgesia continued into the postoperative period were more likely to have lower overall pain scores than the control group. In addition, the preemptive epidural group was more likely to be pain-free 9.5 weeks into the postoperative period.

 Key Points

- Absolute contraindications to ESWL include pregnancy, coagulopathies, and abdominally implanted pacemakers. Relative contraindications include an abdominal aortic aneurysm (may be possible if the aneurysm is <5 cm) and severe obesity.
- Percutaneous nephrolithotomy is a surgical procedure performed for removal of kidney stones or relief of renal obstruction.
- Anesthetic concerns related to percutaneous nephrolithotomy are primarily related to positioning and the potential for blood loss.
- TURP irrigating solutions should be nonhemolytic and isotonic. These include:
  - Glycine 1.5%
  - Mannitol 3% to 5%
  - Sorbitol 3.5%
  - Cytal (a mixture of sorbitol 2.7% and mannitol 0.54%)
- Bleeding, bladder perforation, coagulopathies, and hypothermia are other possible complications associated with TURP.
- TURP syndrome refers to a collection of symptoms caused by excessive intravascular absorption of irrigating solutions during TURP, leading to hyponatremia, fluid overload, and possibly cerebral edema.
- All open radical genitourinary procedures share two major concerns: the potential for significant hemorrhage and positioning.

Internet Resources

Medreviews.com: Advances in Genitourinary Surgery: Highlights From the 114th Meeting of the American Association of Genitourinary Surgeons, April 5-8, 2000, San Antonio, Tex, [Rev Urol. 2000;2(4):203-205, 210]:
http://www.medreviews.com/pdfs/articles/RIU_24_203.pdf

Stonelith V.5: Extracorporeal shockwave lithotripsy system:
http://www.pckmed.com/documents/STONELITH-V5.pdf

History of Anesthesia:
http://www.arss.org/book/anestezi.htm

Bibliography

Gottschalk A, et al: Preemptive epidural analgesia and recovery from radical prostatectomy: a randomized controlled trial, *JAMA* 279:1076-1082, 1998.

Gravenstein D: Anesthesia and renal considerations: extracorporeal shock wave lithotripsy and percutaneous neprolithotomy, *Anesth Clin North Am* 18:953-971, 2000.

Haythornewaite JA, et al: Pain and quality of life following radical retropubic prostatectomy, *J Urol* 160:1761-1764, 1998.

Malhotra V: Anesthesia and renal considerations: transurethral resection of the prostate, *Anesth Clin North Am* 18:883-897, 2000.

Malhotra V, Diwan S: Anesthesia and the renal and genitourinary systems. In Miller R, editor: *Anesthesia,* ed 5, New York, 2000, Churchill Livingstone, pp 1934-1959.

Malhotra V, et al: Intercostal blocks with local infiltration anesthesia for extracorporeal shock wave lithotripsy, *Anesth Analg* 66:85-88, 1987.

Monk TG, Weldon BC: The renal system and anesthesia for urologic surgery. In Barash PG, Cullen BF, Stoelting RK, editors: *Clinical anesthesia,* ed 3, Philadelphia, 1997, Lippincott, pp 945-974.

Ophthalmic Surgery

Meredith L. Muncy

1. Which cranial nerves are involved in the function of the eye?

The following table shows the cranial nerves involved in the function of the eye.

Cranial Nerves Involved in Function of the Eye

Cranial Nerve	Function	Sensory/Motor
II Optic	Provides visual information from the retina	Sensory
III Oculomotor	Innervation of the extraocular muscles Innervation of the pupil and ciliary muscles	Motor
IV Trochlear	Innervation of the superior oblique muscles	Motor
V Trigeminal 1. Ophthalmic		Motor/sensory
a. Lacrimal branch	Innervation of the lacrimal glands	
b. Frontal branch	Innervation of the forehead and the medial upper eyelids	
c. Nasociliary branch	Innervation of the ciliary muscles, iris, and corneas	
2. Maxillary	Innervation of the upper lip, nasal mucosa, and scalp	
3. Mandibular	Innervation of the lower jaw	
VI Abducens	Innervation of the lateral rectus muscles	Motor
VII Facial	Innervation of the muscles of facial expression	Motor/sensory
X Vagus	Parasympathetic innervation associated with the oculocardiac reflex	Motor/sensory

2. What is normal intraocular pressure (IOP), and what affects IOP?

The eye is a rigid globe in which aqueous humor is produced by the ciliary body and removed via the canal of Schlemm. The resulting IOP reflects a balance between these two processes. Normal IOP is 12 to 20 mm Hg. Numerous factors influence IOP; even normal blinking increases the IOP by 5 to 15 mm Hg. Increases in IOP (35 to 50 mm Hg) are seen during coughing, laryngoscopy, and vomiting or similar acute periods of increased venous pressure. Glaucoma causes chronic increases in IOP due to an outflow obstruction of the aqueous humor. Direct pressure on the eye, such as that caused by improper prone positioning, can cause an increase in IOP by changing the shape and size of the eye globe without changing the volume within the eye. Hypercarbia and hypoxia also cause an increase in IOP.

3. What is the oculocardiac reflex?

The "five and dime" reflex, so called because the 5th (trigeminal) and 10th (vagus) cranial nerves are primarily involved, can result from almost any manipulation of the ocular structures. Pressure on the globe or traction on the extraocular muscles can cause many cardiac dysrhythmias. The most common dysrhythmia seen is sinus bradycardia, but others, including asystole, may result. The reflex is seen most commonly in children undergoing extraocular muscle surgery, such as for strabismus, but it can occur in any age group undergoing various ocular procedures. In addition to cardiac dysrhythmias, the awake patient may experience nausea and vomiting and increased sleepiness when the oculocardiac reflex is elicited.

4. Describe appropriate treatment interventions for the oculocardiac reflex.

Usually, asking the surgeon to release pressure or traction on the ocular structures is adequate treatment. If bradycardia persists and causes hemodynamic instability, atropine (10 mcg/kg) should be administered. Surgery should not resume until the heart rate increases. The oculocardiac reflex tends to fatigue, and subsequent stimulation elicits a diminished response. It is controversial whether to administer prophylactic atropine to patients undergoing ocular procedures. The risk of the atropine inducing cardiac dysrhythmias and increasing cardiac demand in the elderly must be weighed against the risk of eliciting the reflex. Many anesthetists routinely administer prophylactic atropine to children undergoing strabismus surgery because increased vagal reflexes are present in this patient group.

5. What considerations must be addressed when preparing a child for ophthalmic surgery?

The most common ophthalmic surgical procedure in children is for strabismus. Although most of these children are healthy, the incidence of strabismus is increased in children with neuromuscular abnormalities, such as muscular dystrophies, cerebral palsy, or myelomeningocele. A thorough health history must be obtained. Strabismus or ptosis can be the only marker for unappreciated neuromuscular disease in an otherwise healthy-appearing child. All children undergoing general anesthesia for ophthalmic surgery should be screened for a family history of malignant hyperthermia (MH) and for previous anesthesia complications associated with MH (masseter muscle spasm, increased temperature). Succinylcholine and other MH-triggering drugs should be avoided if there is any question as to the MH status of a child. Patients with known neuromuscular disease should have a recent cardiac evaluation, including electrocardiogram (ECG) and echocardiogram, if indicated. Children have an increased incidence of the oculocardiac reflex and postoperative nausea and vomiting, probably due to manipulation of the ocular muscles. Treatment of both should be considered.

6. **Summarize common ophthalmic medications that cause concern for the anesthetist.**

Ophthalmic medications are summarized in the following table.

Ophthalmic Medications That Affect Anesthesia

Medication	Description	Systemic Effect
Timolol	Nonselective beta-adrenergic antagonist used in the treatment of glaucoma by decreasing the production of aqueous humor	Systemic absorption associated with bradycardia, bronchospasm, congestive heart failure, and hypotension
Echothiophate	Long-acting anticholinesterase used in the treatment of glaucoma by causing miosis	Systemic absorption associated with reduced plasma cholinesterase activity and resulting prolonged response to succinylcholine and mivacurium
Phenylephrine	Alpha-adrenergic agonist used to produce mydriasis during ocular procedures	Systemic absorption associated with hypertension and dysrhythmias, although rare
Atropine	Anticholinergic used to produce mydriasis during ocular procedures	Systemic absorption associated with central anticholinergic syndrome (agitation, hallucinations, unconsciousness)
Epinephrine	Sympathetic agonist used to produce mydriasis during ocular procedures	Systemic absorption associated with cardiac dysrhythmias and hypertension
Cyclopentolate	Anticholinergic used to produce mydriasis during ocular procedures	Systemic absorption associated with disorientation and psychotic reactions
Acetazolamide	Carbonic anhydrase inhibitor used to decrease IOP	Systemic absorption associated with diuresis and metabolic acidosis

IOP, intraocular pressure.

7. What considerations must be addressed when preparing an elderly patient for ophthalmic surgery under regional anesthesia?

The elderly comprise a large percentage of ophthalmic surgery patients. Elderly patients present with a variety of coexisting diseases, lengthy medical histories, and complicated medication regimens. Before surgery under regional anesthesia, an elderly patient needs to be evaluated for his or her ability to cooperate and lie still and for whether he or she has a history of claustrophobia or acute anxiety attacks. Medication lists must be reviewed for possible drug interactions and to determine which medications should be taken or omitted before surgery. An example of a medication that may be omitted the day of surgery is a diuretic. The patient must lie still for extended periods, which may be nearly impossible with a full bladder. A baseline ECG should be reviewed on every elderly patient and be readily available for comparison in the event of change. Although laboratory tests are not routinely done, appropriate laboratory results should be obtained if the patient is taking antiplatelet drugs or anticoagulants or as medically necessary.

8. When is general anesthesia indicated for ophthalmic surgery?

Any patient who is unwilling or unable to lie still must receive a general anesthetic for ophthalmic surgery. Although many ophthalmic procedures can be performed under local anesthesia, young children and occasionally the elderly are not good candidates for local anesthesia techniques because of their inability to cooperate with the surgeons and lie still for long periods. Heavy sedation must be avoided because when the patient is draped, the airway is not easily managed. Another factor that influences the need for general anesthesia is the type of procedure. Open globe procedures, either due to trauma or planned surgical incision, require general anesthesia to decrease the likelihood of the patient moving or coughing, increasing IOP and extruding ocular contents.

9. How do anesthesia medications affect IOP?

The following table lists anesthesia medications and their effect on IOP.

Anesthesia Medications: Effect on Intraocular Pressure	
Anesthesia Medication	**Effect on Intraocular Pressure**
Succinylcholine	Increase
Nondepolarizing muscle relaxants	None
Inhalational anesthetics (nitrous oxide, volatile agents)	Decrease
Intravenous anesthetics	
Propofol, etomidate, thiopental	Decrease
Ketamine	Variable
Opioids	Decrease

10. Why should nitrous oxide be avoided when sulfur hexafluoride (SF6) is used?

SF6 is used during retinal detachment repairs to form a bubble in the posterior chamber of the eye that flattens the retina and promotes correct healing. This bubble, composed of SF6 and air, expands if nitrous oxide is introduced because nitrous oxide diffuses into the bubble more rapidly than nitrogen can leave the bubble. (Nitrous oxide is 35 times more soluble than nitrogen.) The resulting increased bubble volume increases IOP, decreasing retinal blood flow and possibly compromising the retinal repair. SF6 remains in the posterior chamber for 5 or more days until it is slowly absorbed into the bloodstream. Nitrous oxide should be avoided for at least 10 days after a retinal repair with an SF6 bubble.

11. What equipment must be available when administering regional anesthesia under sedation for ophthalmic surgery?

Although many ophthalmic regional blocks are performed outside the operating room, strict guidelines must be followed to ensure the safety of the patient. Patients receiving ophthalmic blocks should have a functioning intravenous line. Monitoring should include an ECG, noninvasive blood pressure, and pulse oximetry. All ophthalmic block areas should be stocked with appropriate equipment and medications to allow for the induction of general anesthesia in the event of intravascular or optic nerve sheath injection of local anesthetic or resuscitation in the event of a respiratory or cardiac arrest. The following items should be present in every block area:
- Suction
- Oxygen—bag/valve/mask
- Airway equipment—oral airways, laryngoscopes with blades, endotracheal tubes, laryngeal mask airways
- Monitors—ECG, blood pressure monitoring equipment, pulse oximeter, end-tidal carbon dioxide monitor
- Anesthesia medications—induction agents, paralytics, analgesics, amnestics
- Advanced cardiac life support resuscitation medications and equipment

12. List three differences between retrobulbar and peribulbar block techniques.

- With a retrobulbar block, the needle punctures the bulbar fascia and enters the orbital muscle cone. With a peribulbar block, the needle is directed parallel and lateral to the bulbar fascia rather than passing through it. Needle passage through the bulbar fascia often results in a "pop."
- The volume of local anesthetic used in a retrobulbar block is 2 to 4 mL. A peribulbar block requires higher volumes, 4 to 12 mL. The choice of local anesthetic varies, but most anesthetists use a combination of lidocaine and bupivacaine.
- The effectiveness of a retrobulbar block can be evaluated in 2 minutes. A peribulbar block may take 10 to 20 minutes to provide adequate anesthesia and akinesia.

13. What are the primary advantages and limitations to retrobulbar and peribulbar blocks?

Both blocks are effective for various ophthalmic procedures, including cataract extraction, corneal transplant, trabeculectomy, and eyelid reconstruction. The following table lists factors that may influence the choice of regional technique.

Retrobulbar Block Versus Peribulbar Block		
	Retrobulbar Block	**Peribulbar Block**
Advantage	Quick onset of block	Reduced risk of injury to optic nerve, globe perforation, and subdural injection
Limitation	Often requires supplemental cranial nerve VII (facial) block to prevent movement of the eyelid	Causes swelling of the conjunctiva, which may disrupt the surgical field

14. What are the most common injuries associated with anesthesia for ophthalmic surgery?

Most complications related to anesthesia for ophthalmic surgery are sustained during the placement of ocular blocks. The most common injuries are listed in the following table.

Injuries Associated with Anesthesia for Ophthalmic Surgery	
Retrobulbar hemorrhage	Caused by direct needle trauma to orbital vessels; may result in increased IOP
Intravascular Injection	Caused by injection of local anesthetic into local vessels with flow to the cerebral circulation; may result in seizures
Optic nerve sheath injection	Caused by injection of local anesthetic into the nerve sheath surrounding cranial nerve II, which communicates with the midbrain via the optic chiasma; may result in respiratory arrest
Globe rupture	Caused by direct needle trauma to the globe; may result in increased IOP, decreased function, intraocular hemorrhage, and pain
Prolonged nerve/muscle palsy	Caused by direct injection of local anesthetic into muscle or nerve; may result in prolonged ptosis, diplopia, and pain

IOP, intraocular pressure.

15. Discuss considerations in a patient with an open globe injury.

Patients with an open globe injury should be considered as having a "full stomach" if the injury occurs within 8 hours of the patient's last meal. Associated anxiety and pain may delay gastric emptying, placing these patients at risk for aspiration. Extrusion of eye contents and blindness may occur with patient coughing, crying, or bucking on the endotracheal tube. The danger of aspiration coupled with the catastrophic effects of increasing IOP makes the induction of general anesthesia a challenge in these patients. Although no one anesthetic induction is preferred for a patient with an open globe, the goal is a smooth, rapid-sequence induction, with minimal changes in IOP. Succinylcholine and ketamine are generally avoided because of their potential for increasing IOP.

Key Points

- The cranial nerves involved in the function of the eye are as follows: optic, oculomotor, trochlear, trigeminal, abducens, facial, and vagus.
- IOP reflects a balance between the production and removal of aqueous humor in the eye. Normal IOP is 12 to 20 mm Hg.
- IOP can be affected by coughing, laryngoscopy, vomiting, glaucoma, direct pressure on the eye, hypercarbia, and hypoxia.
- With manipulation of ocular structures, the trigeminal and vagus nerves can be stimulated and result in cardiac dysrhythmias, primarily bradycardia. This is called the *oculocardiac reflex*.
- Asking the surgeon to release pressure or traction on the ocular structures is adequate treatment for oculocardiac reflex. If bradycardia persists and causes hemodynamic instability, atropine (10 mcg/kg) should be administered.
- Any patient who is unwilling or unable to lie still must receive a general anesthetic for ophthalmic surgery.
- Most anesthetic drugs, with the exception of succinylcholine and ketamine, have no effect or decrease IOP.
- SF6 is used during retinal detachment repairs to form a bubble in the posterior chamber of the eye that flattens the retina and promotes correct healing. This bubble, comprising SF6 and air, expands if nitrous oxide is introduced because nitrous oxide diffuses into the bubble more rapidly than nitrogen can leave the bubble.
- All equipment necessary for the induction of general anesthesia should be present and ready for use when regional anesthesia or intravenous sedation is used for ophthalmic procedures.
- Succinylcholine and ketamine generally are avoided because of their potential for increasing IOP.

Internet Resources

GASNet: Survey of Anesthesiology—October 2001:
http://www.gasnet.org/sa/2001/05/

Local Anaesthesia for Eye Surgery, Update in Anaesthesia, Issue 12, 2000:
http://www.nda.ox.ac.uk/wfsa/html/u12/u1205_01.htm

Virtual Anaesthesia Textbook:
http://www.virtual-anaesthesia-textbook.com/

The Deep Blue Book: History of Anesthesia:
http://www.arss.org/book/anestezi.htm

Nurse-Anesthesia.com:
http://www.nurse-anesthesia.com/

Ophthalmic Anesthesia Society: EyeAnesthesia.org:
http://www.eyeanesthesia.org/

Bibliography

Brown DL: *Atlas of regional anesthesia*, ed 2, Philadelphia, 1999, WB Saunders, pp 171-178.

Byrd SR, Egbert PR, Gaynon MW, et al: Ophthalmic surgery. In Jaffe RA, Samuels SI, editors: *Anesthesiologist's manual of surgical procedures*, ed 2, Philadelphia, 1999, Lippincott Williams & Wilkins, pp 92-116.

Harvey RR: Anesthesia for ophthalmic procedures. In Nagelhout JJ, Zaglaniczny KL, editors: *Nurse anesthesia*, ed 2, Philadelphia, 2001, WB Saunders, pp 892-921.

Morgan GE, Mikhail MS, Murray MJ, et al: Anesthesia for ophthalmic surgery. In: *Clinical anesthesiology*, ed 3, New York, 2002, Lange Medical Books/McGraw-Hill, pp 761-770.

Stoelting RK, Miller RD: Ophthalmology and otolaryngology. In: *Basics of anesthesia*, ed 4, New York, 2000, Churchill Livingstone, pp 331-335.

Troll GF: Regional ophthalmic anesthesia: safe techniques and avoidance of complications, *J Clin Anesth* 7:163-172, 1995.

Orthopedic Surgery

Lisa J. Thiemann

1. What is the difference between osteoarthritis (OA) and rheumatoid arthritis (RA)?

OA is a degenerative disease resulting from repetitive trauma to the articular joint surface. OA is often limited to the hip and knee joints. RA is a chronic inflammatory autoimmune disease that produces a symmetrical polyarthropathy at synovial joints throughout the body. Complex cell interactions brought about by the inflammatory response destroy synovial tissue and supporting structures. The result is joints that are inflamed, painful, unstable, and with limited range of motion.

2. Describe the systemic involvement of RA.

RA produces significant systemic organ involvement, including the heart, lungs, and kidneys. The immune response associated with RA may result in pericardial thickening, pericarditis, cardiac tamponade, conduction defects, and cardiac valve fibrosis. Patients with RA generally have limited joint movement, and assessment of exercise tolerance can be difficult. Echocardiogram and electrocardiogram (ECG) are useful in preparation for surgery. Patients may also have pulmonary fibrosis and pleural effusion. Hematological disorders associated with the disease include anemia, platelet dysfunction, and thrombocytopenia.

3. Discuss the potential airway management difficulties for patients with RA.

Patients with severe symptoms of RA may have involvement at three areas that are especially relevant to the nurse anesthetist: (1) the cervical spine, (2) the temporomandibular joints, and (3) the cricoarytenoid joints.

Involvement of the *cervical spine* may lead to limited range of motion, atlantoaxial subluxation, or migration of the odontoid process into the foramen magnum. Subluxation can impair vertebral blood flow and compress the spinal cord. Head or neck movement in these settings can have catastrophic results. Radiographs of the cervical spine in flexion and extension are recommended for RA patients with neurological symptoms or symptoms severe enough to require steroid or methotrexate therapy. An awake fiberoptic intubation with neck stabilization should be performed in patients showing neurological symptoms or showing greater than 5 mm atlantoaxial instability.

Patients with *temporomandibular joint* involvement may have limited ability to open the mouth. A nasal approach to intubation may be necessary in these patients.

Patients with *cricoarytenoid* arthritis may present with hoarseness or inspiratory stridor due to narrowing of the glottic opening. A narrowed glottic opening and associated friable, edematous tissue dictates a careful intubation with a smaller endotracheal tube.

4. Discuss the influence of hip fracture location on blood loss.

The anatomical location of the hip fracture has a significant influence on the degree of occult blood loss. Fractures located intracapsularly generally have less blood loss than extracapsular fractures because the capsule tends to act like a tourniquet and contain the blood loss. Examples of intracapsular fractures are subcapital and transcervical fractures. Examples of extracapsular fractures include intertrochanteric, at the base of the femoral neck, and subtrochanteric.

5. Define and describe the fat embolism syndrome (FES).

FES is the embolization of fat into the systemic and pulmonary circulations. It is most commonly seen in patients with fractures of the long bones or pelvis or patients having surgical procedures that increase intramedullary pressure (e.g., reaming the femur). Emboli, in the form of fat or marrow, typically enter the venous circulation. The material may lodge and obstruct the pulmonary microcirculation, increasing pulmonary vascular resistance and right ventricular stroke work. The acute phase of FES can last several hours, and the signs can be delayed for 1 to 3 days. Pulmonary dysfunction is manifested as hypoxemia, dyspnea, and tachypnea. Signs of right ventricular failure may be present. Additional findings may include a petechial rash over the torso and conjunctiva, fever, thrombocytopenia, disseminated intravascular coagulation, and anemia.

6. Identify patient populations at risk for developing FES.

Patients most at risk for developing FES are young adults, owing to a higher incidence of multiple trauma in this group. The elderly constitute the second largest group, owing to the incidence of hip fractures and total joint replacements. The third largest group at risk for developing FES are patients with preexisting diseases, such as pulmonary hypertension, right ventricular dysfunction, and metastatic disease.

7. Discuss the management of patients with FES.

When FES occurs in the operating room under anesthesia, the patient may exhibit sudden bradycardia, hypotension, hypoxemia, jugular venous distention, upper body plethora, rapid decrease in end-tidal carbon dioxide concentration, ischemic changes on the ECG, dysrhythmias, and cardiovascular collapse. The diagnosis may be assisted by finding fat macroglobulinemia in systemic or pulmonary blood and bronchoalveolar lavage showing an increased fat cell content in washings. Pulmonary artery catheter measurements show increased pulmonary artery pressure and decreased cardiac output. Transesophageal echocardiography depicts right ventricular dysfunction and the presence of emboli.

Management of a surgical patient with suspected FES centers on improving right ventricular function, correcting systemic hypotension, and maintaining sufficient oxygenation of tissues. Delivery of 100% oxygen with mechanical ventilation via an endotracheal tube is an important component of care. Hemodynamic support in the form of ephedrine, phenylephrine, epinephrine, or dobutamine may be needed. A central venous or a pulmonary artery catheter helps guide fluid administration and hemodynamic therapy.

8. Identify methods to reduce the degree of fat intravasation.

Rapid stabilization and surgical fixation of long bone and pelvis fractures within 24 hours of injury helps to reduce the incidence of fat intravasation and FES.

9. What is Virchow's triad?

More than 150 years ago, the pathologist Virchow described three main factors that contribute to the formation of thrombi:
- Decreased blood flow
- Vessel injury or inflammation at the site
- Changes in the intrinsic property of the blood (hypercoagulability)

10. Identify patient and surgical risk factors for developing lower extremity thromboembolic complications.

Risk factors for developing deep vein thromboses (DVT) include the following:
- Low cardiac output states
- Prolonged immobilization
- Obesity
- Prior DVT or pulmonary embolism
- Advanced age
- Malignancy

Risk factors specific to the surgical patient include the following:
- Surgery lasting longer than 70 minutes
- Hypothermia
- Intraoperative hypotension or low cardiac output
- Improper positioning
- Dehydration

11. Discuss methods of thromboembolic prevention.

The development of thromboembolism during orthopedic procedures is largely due to *venous stasis* and *hypercoagulability*. DVT prevention is aimed at these two components. Patients should be kept warm and well hydrated. Various pharmacological agents may be used to combat hypercoagulability. Aspirin, low-dose warfarin, and low-molecular-weight heparin have been used. The most appropriate method and duration of pharmacological prophylaxis is still debated. The application of intermittent pneumatic compression boots or graded elastic compression stockings is of proven value. Without prophylaxis, venous thromboembolism may develop in 40% to 80% of patients undergoing orthopedic procedures.

12. Describe the potential complications arising from tourniquet use on an extremity.

Tourniquet use on an extremity may produce pressure-related side effects and systemic effects due to tourniquet inflation. Injury may occur to the underlying skin, nerve, muscle, or blood vessels when the tourniquet is inflated. The extent of injury to these tissues depends on the inflation pressure and duration of inflation. In general, a single tourniquet inflation time greater than 2 hours is not recommended.

Alterations in hemodynamic parameters can occur with inflation and deflation of the tourniquet. These changes are normally well tolerated by healthy individuals, but in patients with preexisting decreased cardiac function, hemodynamic instability may occur. Sudden increases in systemic vascular resistance associated with cuff inflation may lead to congestive heart failure in a susceptible patient. Tourniquet deflation releases vasoactive metabolic by-products into the circulation and decreases systemic vascular resistance. These rapid changes may precipitate myocardial depression, vasodilation, and cardiovascular collapse.

13. Describe the posttourniquet syndrome.

Immediately after tourniquet inflation, ischemic changes begin to develop in tissues distal to the tourniquet. Lactic acidosis, carbon dioxide, extracellular potassium, and inflammatory mediators accumulate in the ischemic limb. With cuff deflation, capillary vessel integrity may be broken, allowing fluid to move into the extravascular spaces. The resulting edema is associated with *posttourniquet syndrome*. This condition can have a significant impact on postoperative healing and develop into a compartment syndrome that may threaten limb viability.

14. Discuss the physiological changes that can occur with methyl methacrylate use.

Mixing methyl methacrylate powder with liquid methyl methacrylate monomer produces an exothermic reaction. The extreme heat from this reaction can produce reflex bradycardia and cardiac arrest. The heat also is capable of expanding intramedullary gases and raising intramedullary pressure such that fat, air, and marrow may be forced into the venous circulation. For this reason, nitrous oxide should be discontinued before insertion of methyl methacrylate.

Systemic absorption of residual methyl methacrylate monomer is capable of producing vasodilation and myocardial depression. In addition to the direct vasoactive effects of methyl methacrylate, reaming of the femur can release tissue thromboplastin, which may result in platelet aggregation, microthrombus formation in the lungs, and cardiovascular instability.

15. Discuss the clinical manifestations of bone cement implantation syndrome (BCIS).

Patients undergoing total hip arthroplasty are at risk for developing BCIS from the introduction of methyl methacrylate used to fixate the prosthesis. Clinical signs of BCIS are similar to FES and include hypoxia, hypotension, dysrhythmias, pulmonary hypertension, and decreased cardiac output. Treatment is aimed at supporting the cardiovascular system and maintaining oxygenation.

Key Points

- The airway involvement of a patient with RA could include limited mobility in the cervical spine, temporomandibular joints, and cricoarytenoid joints.
- Hip fractures located intracapsularly generally have less blood loss than extracapsular fractures because the capsule tends to act like a tourniquet and contain the blood loss.
- Patients at highest risk for FES are young adults; elderly; and patients with preexisting pulmonary disease, right ventricular dysfunction, or metastatic disease.
- Risk factors for developing DVT include low cardiac output states, prolonged immobilization, obesity, prior DVT or pulmonary embolism, advanced age, and malignancy.
- DVT prevention is aimed at prevention of venous stasis and hypercoagulability.
- Posttourniquet syndrome occurs when deflation occurs, and lactic acid, carbon dioxide, extracellular potassium, and other inflammatory mediators are released systemically from the ischemic limb. Fluid moves into the extravascular spaces and edema occurs, which affect postoperative healing.
- Mixing methyl methacrylate powder with liquid methyl methacrylate monomer produces an exothermic reaction. The extreme heat from this reaction can produce reflex bradycardia and cardiac arrest.

Internet Resources

GASnet Search: Orthopedic Surgery:
http://www.gasnet.org/about/search.php?p1=Orthopedic+surgery

Virtual Anaesthesia Textbook:
http://www.virtual-anaesthesia-textbook.com/

Continued

Internet Resources *continued*

British Journal of Anaesthesia Search: Orthopedic Surgery:
http://bja.oupjournals.org/search.dtl

Nurse Anesthesia.com:
http://www.nurse-anesthesia.com/

Anesthesiaweb.com:
http://www.anesthesiaweb.com/

PDA Anesthesia.com: Orthopedic Anesthesia:
http://www.unc.edu/~rvp/RP_Anesthesia/Ortho.html

Orthopedics.com:
http://www.orthobluejournal.com/logon/logon.asp

Bibliography

Fallon KM, et al: Fat embolization and fatal cardiac arrest during hip arthroplasty with methylmethacrylate, *Can J Anaesth* 48:626-629, 2001.

Morgan GE, Mikhail MS, Murray MJ: *Clinical anesthesiology,* ed 3, New York, 2002, Lange Medical Books/McGraw-Hill.

Neal JM: Thromboembolic complications. In Atlee JL, editor: *Complications in anesthesia,* Philadelphia, 1999, WB Saunders, pp 893-895.

Nielsen C: Methylmethacrylate. In Atlee JL, editor: *Complications in anesthesia,* Philadelphia, 1999, WB Saunders, pp 896-897.

Prentice CR: Thromboprophylaxis—which treatment for which patient? *J Bone Joint Surg Br* 82:483-485, 2000.

Propst JW, et al: Segmental wall motion abnormalities in patients undergoing total hip replacement: correlations with intraoperative events, *Anesth Analg* 77:743-749, 1993.

Rodgers A, et al: Reduction of postoperative mortality and morbidity with epidural or spinal anesthesia, *BMJ* 321:1493-1497, 2000.

Weldon BC: Fat embolism syndrome. In Atlee JL, editor: *Complications in anesthesia,* Philadelphia, 1999, WB Saunders, pp 889-892.

Weldon BC, Nielsen C: Extremity tourniquets. In Atlee JL, editor: *Complications in anesthesia,* Philadelphia, 1999, WB Saunders, pp 898-901.

Vascular Surgery

Anthony James Chipas

1. Why is peripheral vascular disease a perioperative concern?

Vascular disease is a common cause of disability and death in Western society. Atherosclerosis of the lower extremities causes symptoms in approximately 3% of persons older than age 50. Greater than 25% of persons older than age 70 have evidence of peripheral arterial disease by noninvasive testing.

2. Define intermittent claudication.

Intermittent claudication is a complex of symptoms caused by ischemia that occurs when metabolic demands in an extremity exceed oxygen supply. The ischemia leads to what patients describe as cramping, tiredness, pain, tension, or weakness in the limb. The symptoms disappear with rest. Over time, as oxygen supply to the limb diminishes, pain develops with minimal exertion and eventually develops at rest. Physical examination of the extremity may show diminished pulses, ulceration, temperature differential, and bruits caused by stenotic lesions.

3. Why should the anesthetist be concerned if an elderly patient with leg pain is having surgery on the hand?

Patients with a history of peripheral vascular disease undergoing either regional or general anesthesia are at risk for developing ischemia in various tissues. Peripheral vascular disease is accompanied by a high incidence of multiple fixed lesions throughout the body, including renal, coronary, and cerebral vessels. These lesions limit the supply of oxygen distal to the obstruction, affecting autoregulation and necessitating higher systemic blood pressures to provide adequate tissue perfusion. Blood supply may be diminished further by hypovolemia and hypotension. Maintaining normal mean arterial blood pressures is important in a patient with a history of peripheral vascular disease, but indiscriminate use of vasoconstrictors, such as phenylephrine, to increase blood pressure during anesthesia should be avoided. In the presence of coronary vessel disease, phenylephrine may increase the incidence of intraoperative myocardial segmental wall abnormalities and increase myocardial oxygen consumption, placing the heart at risk for ischemia.

4. What is Raynaud's phenomenon?

Raynaud's phenomenon is episodic, bilateral, and symmetrical vasospasm of the fingers, which results in cyanosis, pallor, and pain. In some cases, the hands and the feet may be affected, and rarely the disease may involve the nose, chin, or cheeks. Patients may complain that their hands become blue and tingly when cold or when they are emotionally stressed. This phenomenon occurs in 8% of men and 18% of women. Attacks are precipitated by cold or emotional upset and relieved by warmth or relief of stress. Because the cutaneous vessels of the fingers and toes are supplied only by sympathetic vasoconstrictor fibers, increased sympathetic activity may cause profound vasospasm in persons pre-disposed to Raynaud's phenomenon. Vasospasm produced by exposure to cold may cause an extremity to become ischemic even at rest. Vasodilating drugs sometimes are useful in preventing attacks if they are taken before exposure to cold, but they are not successful in all cases and act primarily to provide only temporary relief of symptoms. Arterial catheters should be placed with extreme caution in patients with Raynaud's phenomenon.

5. Summarize the major anesthetic considerations for a patient undergoing carotid endarterectomy.

- Carotid surgery may be performed under general or regional anesthesia. Regional anesthesia is performed with superficial and deep cervical plexus blocks. An advantage of regional anesthesia is the ability to monitor the patient's neurologic function intraoperatively.
- A major goal of anesthetic management for carotid surgery is preserving cerebral blood flow. Blood pressure should be maintained at or slightly above the patient's normal level.
- Isoflurane increases cerebral blood flow and decreases cerebral metabolic rate—favorable properties for a patient undergoing carotid endarterectomy under general anesthesia.
- Surgical manipulation of the carotid sinus can cause pronounced bradycardia. Atropine should be readily available.
- A normal arterial PCO_2 should be maintained with general anesthesia. Vasodilation associated with hypercapnia can cause cerebral steal, and vasoconstriction produced by hypocapnia can decrease cerebral blood flow.
- Hyperglycemia should be avoided.
- Intravenous heparin, 5000 to 10,000 units, is administered immediately before carotid clamping. Intravenous protamine, 50 to 75 mg, usually is administered to reverse residual heparin activity.

6. How can the nurse anesthetist monitor neurological integrity during a carotid endarterectomy?

Several methods currently are used to determine the adequacy of cerebral blood flow. *Stump pressure* determination is based on measurement of arterial blood flow through the circle of Willis from the nonclamped carotid artery. After the operative carotid artery is clamped, a needle is inserted distal to the clamp, and measurements are taken to determine if a pulsatile flow is present and if the mean blood pressure is greater than 60 mm Hg.

Evoked potential monitoring, whether auditory, visual, or somatosensory, is increasingly used. The disadvantage to evoked potential monitoring during surgery is that it restricts anesthesia choice. The recommended anesthetic technique for somatosensory evoked potential monitoring is narcotic based with not more than 0.5 minimal alveolar concentration of inhalational agent. This technique limits the use of inhalational agents, which are effective in controlling blood pressure and decreasing cerebral metabolic requirements.

Outside of the operating room, the *electroencephalogram (EEG)* is a widely used monitor for assessing neurological function. According to Youngberg et al, there are four major disadvantages to conventional EEG analysis during surgery: (1) EEG changes do not appear until severe cerebral ischemia has occurred, (2) EEG changes may not identify small focal changes, (3) the depth of anesthesia and level of ventilation must be kept stable for proper interpretation, and (4) there is a high incidence of false-positive results leading to increased use of shunting.

Transcutaneous Doppler monitoring measures regional cerebral blood flow and detects cerebral emboli that may accompany clamping and unclamping of the carotid artery. Clinical use of transcutaneous Doppler has been promising, but continued research is needed to establish correlations between EEG, transcutaneous Doppler, and regional blood flow. Each of these methods can identify reductions in cerebral perfusion, but none of them is completely reliable during carotid surgery.

7. Discuss the serious risks associated with carotid endarterectomy.

In addition to the intraoperative risks of cerebral ischemia associated with surgery and anesthesia, ischemic injury can occur after the reestablishment of carotid blood flow. Too much oxygen associated with increased blood flow can cause this injury. Ischemic metabolism of substrates, followed by normal metabolism with increased oxygen, leads to the production of oxygen free radicals (oxygen molecules with an uneven number of electrons). These molecules can damage normal cell membranes and cause vasospasm and red blood cell sludging. Treatment includes the use of antioxidants, such as vitamin E or C.

Hypertension and poorly controlled blood pressure are additional concerns in the post–carotid endarterectomy period. Although rare, reperfusion injury after removal of a carotid lesion can lead to cerebral hemorrhage or edema. When the carotid stenosis is eliminated, perfusion pressure distal to the former site of the stenosis is markedly increased. Because autoregulation is disrupted in this area, cerebral blood flow increases with increasing perfusion pressure. Patients at highest risk for reperfusion injury are those who had the greatest degree of presurgical stenosis and the greatest pressure decrease across the carotid lesion. Maintaining control of the blood pressure in the postoperative period can lessen the incidence of this complication.

Airway complications after carotid endarterectomy include hematoma, laryngeal edema, recurrent laryngeal nerve damage, and lymphatic and venous obstruction. The incidence of surgical hematoma after carotid endarterectomy is approximately 1.9%. Post–carotid endarterectomy patients may return to the operating room for surgical control of bleeding or emergency airway management.

Carotid plaque removal may be associated with deterioration of the ipsilateral carotid baroreflex and may contribute to blood pressure instability in the postoperative period. Intravenous vasodilators and adrenergic beta receptor blockers should be available to treat postoperative hypertension and tachycardia.

Other problems that may be present in the postoperative period include residual coagulopathy, hypothermia, dysrhythmias, stroke, and myocardial infarction. Data from the Aspirin and Carotid Endarterectomy Trial suggest that reduced perioperative stroke and death rates occur in carotid endarterectomy patients who receive low-dose aspirin (<325 mg).

Key Points

- Raynaud's phenomenon is episodic, bilateral, and symmetrical vasospasm of the fingers, resulting in cyanosis, pallor, and pain. The hands become blue and tingly when cold or when the person is emotionally stressed.
- Arterial catheters should be placed with extreme caution in patients with Raynaud's phenomenon.
- Anesthetic considerations for carotid endarterectomy include the following:
  - An advantage of regional anesthesia is the ability to monitor the patient's neurologic function intraoperatively.
  - A major goal of anesthetic management for carotid surgery is preserving cerebral blood flow.
  - Surgical manipulation of the carotid sinus can cause pronounced bradycardia.
  - A normal arterial P_{CO_2} should be maintained with general anesthesia.
  - Hyperglycemia should be avoided.
- Several methods are currently used to determine the adequacy of cerebral blood flow, including stump pressure, regional arterial oxygenation, somatosensory evoked potential, and EEG.

Internet Resources

Anesthesia for Carotid Endarterectomy:
http://daccx.bsd.uchicago.edu/manuals/vtmanual/carotids.html

Anesthesia.org: Cervical Plexus Block for Carotid Endarterectomy:
http://www.anesthesia.org/professional/hm/hm_cea_1.html

Internet Resources   *continued*

Anesthesia for Carotid Surgery: Questions and Answers:
http://www.fmsq.org/aaq/membres/documents/resumecongres/DrArchercarotide.pdf

Society of Neurosurgical Anesthesia and Critical Care: Carotid Artery Disease:
http://www.snacc.org/ed/bib/CarotidArteryDisease.html

Virtual Anaesthesia Textbook:
http://www.virtual-anaesthesia-textbook.com/

Bibliography

Cottrell J, Smith D: *Anesthesia and neurosurgery*, ed 4, Philadelphia, 2001, Mosby.

Sigaudo-Roussel D, Evans DH, Naylor AR, et al: Deterioration in carotid baroreflex during carotid endarterectomy, *J Vasc Surg* 36:793-798, 2002.

Smith JS, Roizen MF, Cahalan MK, et al: Does anesthetic technique make a difference? Augmentation of systolic blood pressure during carotid endarterectomy: effects of phenylephrine versus light anesthesia and of isoflurane versus halothane on the incidence of myocardial ischemia, *Anesthesiology* 69:846, 1988.

Taylor DW, Barnett HJ, Haynes, RB, et al: Low-dose and high-dose acetylsalicylic acid for patients undergoing carotid endarterectomy: a randomized controlled trial. ASA and Carotid Endarterectomy Trial Collaborators, *Lancet* 353:2179-2184, 1999.

Weitz JI, Byrne J, Clagett GP, et al: Diagnosis and treatment of chronic arterial insufficiency of the lower extremities: a critical review, *Circulation* 94:3026-3049, 1996.

Youngberg J, et al: *Cardiac, vascular, and thoracic anesthesia*, New York, 2000, Churchill Livingstone.

Cardiac Surgery

Sharon Hawks

1. List the factors that normally affect myocardial oxygen supply.

The following factors affect myocardial oxygen supply:
- Coronary blood flow
- Heart rate (duration of diastole)
- Preload
- Coronary perfusion pressure
- Hemoglobin concentration
- Arterial oxygen content

2. Describe important information obtained from the cardiac catheterization report.

- Despite the increasing use of noninvasive techniques, such as echocardiography, cardiac catheterization is still the gold standard for diagnosing and detailing the *extent of cardiac disease* before cardiac surgery. Stenotic lesions that reduce the vessel diameter greater than 50% are considered significant. Left anterior descending occlusion greater than 90% is the most serious lesion because significant left ventricular decompensation can occur with ischemia.
- *Global and regional evaluation of ventricular function* is possible. Cardiac output, cardiac index, left ventricular ejection fraction, and left ventricular end-diastolic pressure estimate myocardial contractile force and myocardial reserve (see the following table).

Hemodynamic Values Obtained from Cardiac Catheterization Report	
Measurement	**Normal Value**
Right atrial pressure	1–5 mm Hg
Pulmonary artery pressure	$\leq$30/15 mm Hg
	$\leq$22 mm Hg (mean)
Pulmonary capillary wedge pressure	$\leq$12 mm Hg
Cardiac index	2.4–4.2 $L \cdot min^{-1} \cdot m^{-2}$
Ejection fraction	> 60%
Systemic vascular resistance	700–1600 $dyne \cdot sec \cdot cm^{-5}$
Pulmonary vascular resistance	120–160 $dyne \cdot sec \cdot cm^{-5}$

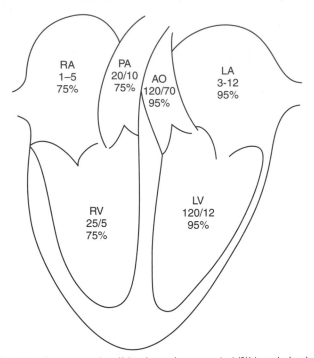

Normal cardiac pressures (mm Hg) and normal oxygen content (%) in each chamber.

- Cardiac catheterization assesses *valvular function.*
- *Baseline pulmonary artery pressures* are provided by cardiac catheterization (see the figure above).

3. **What are key anesthetic goals during induction of the cardiac patient for coronary artery bypass graft (CABG) procedures?**

- Monitor the electrocardiogram closely, especially leads II and V for dysrhythmias and indications of ischemia.
- Preoxygenate well.
- Induce intravenous anesthesia slowly and smoothly with the goal of avoiding tachycardia and hypertension. Anesthetic agent dosing is usually inversely related to ventricular function.
- Avoid using nitrous oxide. Nitrous oxide is seldom used because of its tendency to expand intravascular air bubbles that may form during cardiopulmonary bypass (CPB).
- Intubate quickly to minimize stimulation and associated hemodynamic changes.
- Maintain coronary perfusion pressure by avoiding hypotension, especially decreases in diastolic blood pressure. Small doses of phenylephrine, 50 mcg intravenously, or ephedrine, 5 to 10 mg intravenously, may be necessary if the blood pressure decreases more than 20% from baseline.

4. What cardiovascular medications should be set up and ready for use for cardiac surgery?

A good rule is to have at least one inotrope (epinephrine, dobutamine, dopamine), one vasodilator (nitroglycerin, nitroprusside, nicardipine), and one vasoconstrictor (phenylephrine, norepinephrine) available and ready for use as an intravenous infusion and in syringes for intravenous bolus administration. In addition, atropine, ephedrine, and calcium chloride should be drawn up and ready for administration.

5. How does the ejection fraction guide anesthetic management?

The ejection fraction is equal to the volume of blood ejected with each stroke volume (SV), divided by the end-diastolic volume (EDV). In a healthy heart, the ejection fraction is approximately 0.6 or greater. The ejection fraction is often expressed as a percentage:

$$80 \text{ mL (SV)} \div 120 \text{ mL (EDV)} = 0.66 \text{ or } 66\%$$

Knowing the patient's preoperative ejection fraction is especially instructive in guiding anesthesia maintenance. An ejection fraction less than 40% indicates suboptimal left ventricular performance. In these patients, anesthesia maintenance with a potent inhalational agent may depress left ventricular performance to unacceptable levels. Patients with poor ventricular function may benefit more from a narcotic-based anesthetic, which would support left ventricular function.

6. What are the anesthesia implications of sternotomy?

Two key interventions are required before sternotomy and sternal spread:
- Deepen the anesthesia in anticipation of profound surgical stimulation.
- Turn off the ventilator and hand ventilate the patient to prevent inflation and accidental injury to the lungs during sternotomy. The lungs should be observed for equal and full inflation after the chest is open.

7. Why is cardioplegia used in cardiac surgery?

Cardioplegic solutions are potassium-based solutions used to provide cardiac quiescence—a flaccid, noncontracting heart. Cardioplegia, mild-to-moderate hypothermia, and topical cooling of the heart with ice slush reduce myocardial oxygen consumption dramatically and preserve myocardial viability during periods of ischemia.

8. Why should a pulmonary artery catheter be used instead of a central venous pressure catheter to monitor cardiac function during cardiac surgery?

Benefits of a pulmonary artery catheter include the ability to:
- Assess right and left ventricle volume status separately
- Evaluate right and left ventricular function separately
- Evaluate pulmonary vascular dynamics
- Assess valvular function

For patients with different right and left ventricular function, volume status may be difficult to determine with the use of a central venous pressure catheter alone. For select patients with adequate left ventricular function, some institutions are foregoing the use of the pulmonary artery catheter and relying on information provided by the central venous pressure catheter. In this population of patients, the function of the right heart is assumed to mirror function on the left.

9. **Is the radial artery a reliable measure of blood pressure for a patient undergoing cardiac surgery?**

The radial artery is the most common site for invasive blood pressure monitoring. In many patients ($\leq 70\%$), the radial artery pressure is significantly lower than the aortic pressure at the completion of CPB. Typically, as the patient warms completely, this discrepancy ceases.

10. **Discuss important considerations during CPB.**

- The lungs are not ventilated during CPB, and resultant atelectasis may occur.
- On the start of bypass, a decrease in mean arterial blood pressure (MAP) often occurs secondary to hemodilution. Until the aorta is cross-clamped and the heart is cooled and in full asystole, cardiac ischemia is a risk. MAP of 55 to 65 mm Hg should be maintained to ensure adequate flow to all organ systems, most notably the brain and the kidneys. Blood pressure may be adjusted by varying pump flow rates, administering vasopressors (phenylephrine, methoxamine [Vasoxyl]) or vasodilators (sodium nitroprusside, phentolamine [Regitine]), or titrating anesthetic agents.
- Anesthetic depth should be sufficient to prevent awareness, to suppress sympathoadrenal response to surgical stimulation, and to prevent spontaneous movement.
- Temperature should be measured at two sites—one core site (bladder, nasopharyngeal, tympatic membrane, pulmonary artery catheter) and one shell (i.e., outer body) site (rectal, skin).
- Hypothermia, the duration of surgery, and decreases in perfusion pressure during CPB can cause peripheral neuropathy and ischemic injury to soft tissue. Extra attention should be directed to positioning the patient correctly and to padding pressure points well.
- Measures to optimize renal function should be considered for patients with preexisting renal dysfunction (serum creatinine > 1.5 mg/dL), especially diabetic and hypertensive patients. These measures include the use of mannitol, dopamine, or furosemide during CPB.

11. **What is the proper dose of heparin for CPB?**

Intravenous heparin should be administered into a central venous line approximately 3 minutes before initiation of CPB to prevent acute disseminated intravascular coagulation. Heparin dosing is recorded in USP units. The initial dose for CPB is 300 to 400 USP units/kg. The calculated dose for a 70-kg patient is 21,000 to 28,000 units. The most common commercial preparation of heparin is 100 units/mg (1,000 units/mL), but concentrations vary.

After administration through a central line, heparin peaks in about 1 minute. With small doses (100 to 150 USP units/kg), the elimination half-time of heparin is about 1 hour. With larger doses of heparin (300 to 400 USP units/kg), the elimination half-time is 2 hours or more. Hypothermia and CPB prolong the duration of heparin. Significant anticoagulation can last 4 to 6 hours during CPB. Additional heparin usually is administered in 5000- to 10,000-unit increments.

12. How is heparin activity measured during cardiac surgery?

The activated coagulation time (ACT) is the most widely used method to assess the anticoagulant response of heparin during CPB. The ACT should be checked 2 to 5 minutes after the initial heparin dose, after initiating CPB, after each supplemental dose of heparin, and every 30 to 60 minutes during the procedure to confirm adequate anticoagulation. Centers differ, but generally during CPB, the ACT is maintained at values longer than 400-480 seconds.

13. Discuss considerations with regard to aortic and venous cannulation.

The aortic cannula usually is placed in the ascending aorta, and hypotension can occur with aortic cannulation consequent to sudden blood loss. A systolic blood pressure of 100 mm Hg or less decreases the incidence of blood loss and aortic dissection with cannulation. When the aortic cannula is correctly placed, volume can be administered by the perfusionist to correct hypotension. Venous cannulation in the right atrial appendage is a potential source of atrial arrhythmias. The surgeon should be notified if arrhythmias persist.

14. Why is hypothermia initiated for CPB surgery, and what are the physiologic consequences?

Intentional systemic hypothermia is induced for CPB to decrease cellular metabolism and total body oxygen consumption. Core temperature usually is reduced to 30°C to 32°C after initiation of CPB. Physiologic consequences of hypothermia include reversible coagulopathy, platelet dysfunction, myocardial depression, and impaired metabolism of citrate and drugs.

15. What goals must be achieved before CPB is terminated?

- The patient should be warmed to a core temperature greater than 36°C and a shell temperature greater than 33°C before terminating CPB. Sweating during rewarming is common and should not be mistaken for "light" anesthesia.
- The lungs should be reexpanded fully, removing all areas of atelectasis.
- Pacing, if indicated, is initiated.
- A heart rate of 80 to 100 beats/min is generally necessary to maintain a satisfactory cardiac output because patients may have reduced ability to increase

their stroke volume. Sinus tachycardia greater than 120 beats/min should be treated before CPB termination.

16. List factors that predict an increased risk for difficulty weaning from CPB.

The following factors predict an increased risk for difficulty:
- Preoperative ejection fraction less than 45%
- Elderly patient
- Prolonged CPB (>2 to 3 hours)
- Angiotensin-converting enzyme use (excessive vasodilation)
- Pre-CPB period ischemia

17. What pharmacologic agents may be used to assist with weaning from CPB?

Low systemic vascular resistance is common at the completion of CPB, and alpha adrenergic receptor agonists, such as phenylephrine, may be used to improve systemic blood pressure. If the blood pressure does not respond and volume replacement is adequate, inotropes (dopamine, dobutamine, epinephrine) may be needed. Milrinone may be used if systemic vascular resistance is high and cardiac output is low. If inotropes do not increase the blood pressure and cardiac output, an intraaortic balloon pump may be indicated. Calcium has been used to increase blood pressure when weaning from CPB, but its use is usually reserved for reversing hypotension from hypocalcemia, calcium channel blockers, and cardiac toxicity from hyperkalemia. Calcium should be administered only after the heart has been reperfused (at least 15 minutes after aortic cross-clamp release) because intracellular hypercalcemia can worsen reperfusion injury.

18. When is protamine administered?

Protamine is administered intravenously when the patient is off CPB and stable hemodynamically. Protamine is an alkaline cationic protein derived from salmon sperm. It binds to the anionic heparin molecule and neutralizes its effect. Protamine neutralizes heparin in a ratio 1 mg:100 U.

Protamine dosing at the end of the procedure usually is calculated based on the total dose of heparin administered at the initiation of CPB. Generally, 0.5 to 1 mg of protamine is administered for each 100 U of heparin administered. For example, 30,000 U (300 mg) of heparin may be reversed by 150 to 300 mg of protamine.

Protamine should always be administered slowly (30 to 50 mg/min). Rapid administration is associated with decreased systemic and pulmonary pressures and decreased venous return. This response may be blunted by volume loading and slow administration. Patients with prior exposure to NPH insulin or who are allergic to fish are at a higher risk for allergy to protamine.

19. What is an acceptable hematocrit for a post-CPB patient?

The "acceptable" hematocrit has long been, and continues to be, a controversial subject. Most institutions accept a safe lower limit hematocrit level in a stable patient with good left ventricular function of 23% to 25%.

20. Why is a cardiac surgery patient at risk for intraoperative and postoperative thrombocytopenia?

Patients presenting for cardiac surgery may be receiving one of many types of antiplatelet drugs (aspirin, indomethacin, nonsteroidal antiinflammatory drugs, glycoprotein IIb/IIIa inhibitors). These agents are associated with qualitative defects of platelet function. During CPB, circulating platelets may be damaged or destroyed, creating a potential quantitative platelet defect. The bleeding patient with a platelet count less than 100,000/mm^3 may require platelet transfusions.

21. What percentage of patients undergoing cardiac surgery experience immediate postoperative cognitive decline?

Of patients undergoing cardiac surgery, 50% to 80% experience immediate postoperative cognitive decline.

22. List risk factors for cognitive decline after cardiac surgery.

- Older age
- Severity of cardiac disease
- Presence or history of cerebrovascular disease
- Diabetes mellitus and hyperglycemia
- Duration of CPB
- Duration of aortic cross-clamping

 Key Points

- Factors that affect myocardial oxygen supply are coronary blood flow, heart rate, preload, coronary perfusion pressure, hemoglobin concentration, and arterial oxygen content.
- Key anesthetic goals during induction for CABG procedures are monitor electrocardiogram closely for signs of ischemia; preoxygenate well; institute slow, smooth induction; do not use nitrous oxide; intubate quickly; and maintain coronary perfusion pressure.
- Cardioplegic solutions are potassium-based solutions used to provide cardiac quiescence— a flaccid, noncontracting heart. Cardioplegia, mild-to-moderate hypothermia, and topical cooling of the heart with ice slush reduce myocardial oxygen consumption dramatically and preserve myocardial viability during periods of ischemia.
- The ACT is the most widely used method to assess heparin's anticoagulant response during CPB.

Continued

Key Points *continued*

- Considerations during aortic and venous cannulation are sudden blood loss and cardiac arrhythmias.
- Before CPB is terminated, the following must be done:
  - Warm to core temperature greater than 36°C
  - Reexpand lungs
  - Use cardiac pacing if indicated
  - Establish heart rate of 80 to 100 beats/min
- Factors predicting difficult weaning from CPB include:
  - Preoperative ejection fraction less than 45%
  - Elderly patient
  - CPB longer than 2 to 3 hours
  - Use of angiotensin-converting enzyme inhibitors
  - Pre-CPB period ischemia
- Pharmacological agents that may assist with weaning from CPB are adrenergic receptor agonists, inotropes, and calcium.
- Protamine always should be administered slowly (≤30 to 50 mg/min).
- A safe lower limit hematocrit level in the stable patient (post CBP) with good left ventricular function is 23% to 25%.
- Risk factors for cognitive decline after cardiac surgery are older age, severity of cardiac disease, presence or history of cerebrovascular disease, diabetes, duration of CPB, and duration of aortic cross-clamping.

Internet Resources

The Perfusion Home Page:
http://www.perfusion.com/

CardiacEngineering.com: Anesthesia for Minimally Invasive Cardiac Surgery: Made Ridiculously Simple:
http://www.cardiacengineering.com/Midcabg.htm

The Virtual Anaesthesia Textbook: Anaesthesia for Cardiothoracic Surgery:
http://www.virtual-anaesthesia-textbook.com/vat/cardiac.html

Central neuraxial analgesia in cardiac surgery, The Mount Sinai Journal of Medicine:
http://www.mssm.edu/msjournal/69/v69_1&2_045_050.pdf

GASNet Search: Cardiac Anesthesia:
http://www.gasnet.org/about/search.php?p1=cardiac+anesthesia

Nurse-Anesthesia.com:
http://www.nurse-anesthesia.com/

Bibliography

Bojar R, Warner K: *Manual of perioperative care in cardiac surgery*, ed 3, Malden, MA, 1999, Blackwell Science.

Hensley FA, Martin, DE, Gravlee GP: *A practical approach to cardiac anesthesia*, ed 3, Philadelphia, 2003, Lippincott Williams & Wilkins.

Newman M, Kirchner JL, Phillips-Bute B, et al: Longitudinal assessment of neurocognitive function after cardiac surgery: postoperative decline predicts long-term (5-year) neurocognitive deterioriation, *N Engl J Med* 344:395-402, 2001.

Stern DH, Gerson JI, Allen FB, et al: Can we trust the direct radial artery pressure immediately following cardiopulmnary bypass? *Anesthesiology* 62:557-561, 1985.

Thomas S, Kramer J: *Manual of cardiac anesthesia*, ed 2, New York, 1993, Churchill Livingstone.

Tuman KJ, McCarthy RJ, Spiess BD, et al: Effect of pulmonary artery catheterization on outcome in patients undergoing coronary artery bypass surgery, *Anesthesiology* 70:199-206, 1989.

Ear, Nose, and Throat Surgery

Kasey P. Bensky

1. List and describe the conditions necessary to support an airway fire.

Conditions that support an airway fire include:
- Spark
- Combustible material
- Oxygen

There is an increased risk of airway fire whenever there is the potential for a spark in the airway, material present that will burn, and oxygen to support the fire. The laser and the bovie are the most common causes of a spark in the airway. The material present in the airway is typically the endotracheal tube (ETT), but also may be sponges or drapes. Any ear, nose, and throat (ENT) procedure in which a laser or bovie is used in the airway should be treated as a situation with an increased risk of an airway fire.

2. List measures the certified registered nurse anesthetist (CRNA) can take to decrease the incidence of an airway fire.

- Use a laser-approved ETT when a laser is in use. A red rubber ETT wrapped with approved laser tape and the Mallinckrodt Laser flex tube are appropriate choices.
- Decrease the fraction of inspired oxygen (FIO_2) to less than or equal to 30%.
- Place moist sponges around the patient's airway.
- Place saline in the ETT cuff.
- Provide a seal with the ETT cuff or moist sponges; this decreases the oxygen leaking into the upper airway.

3. Which gases are appropriate to lower the FIO_2 to decrease the risk of an airway fire, and why?

Air and helium are appropriate to lower the FIO_2. Air is mostly nitrogen. Nitrogen and helium do not support combustion. Oxygen and nitrous oxide (N_2O) support combustion.

4. **Describe the steps in the treatment of an airway fire.**
   - Immediately disconnect the anesthesia circuit and turn off the oxygen.
   - Remove the ETT.
   - Extinguish the ETT fire.
   - Remove any smoldering ETT pieces from the airway.
   - Resume ventilation with air until it is certain that no debris is left burning in the airway, then switch to 100% oxygen.
   - Examine the airway, and treat the patient accordingly.
   - Save all involved materials and devices for later investigation.

5. **Discuss appropriate ETTs for laser airway surgery.**

   RED RUBBER ENDOTRACHEAL TUBE WRAPPED WITH FOIL TAPE
   The ETT should be wrapped with foil tape designed for laser surgery. The purpose of the foil tape is to reflect the laser beam. This wrap keeps the beam from penetrating the ETT and causing a fire. When preparing the tube, it should be wrapped starting at the cuffed end of the tube and wrapped in an overlapping spiral fashion until the pilot balloon is reached. This should be done without gaps, lumps, or bumps in the wrap. Gaps allow an opening for the laser to reach the ETT. Lumps and bumps may cause damage to the airway when the tube is inserted or removed. A red rubber ETT has a higher ignition temperature than a polyvinyl chloride ETT.

   MALLINCKRODT LASER FLEX ENDOTRACHEAL TUBE
   This is a metal tube with two cuffs on the end. The cuff is the only portion of this ETT that is combustible. One difficulty with the tube is that it has thick walls. A tube with an internal diameter of 5 cm has an external diameter similar to that of a regular 7-cm internal diameter ETT. This must be kept in mind when airway space is limited.

6. **When providing anesthesia for laser airway surgery, what should be placed in the ETT cuff and why?**

   Saline or saline with methylene blue should be placed in the ETT cuff to provide fluid to extinguish a fire should the laser come in contact with the cuff. Methylene blue provides a noticeable blue color in the airway if the cuff is ruptured.

7. **When setting up to do a suspension microdirect laryngoscopy, what extra equipment should be available in the operating room?**

   The following equipment is recommended:
   - Venturi ventilator
   - Racemic epinephrine with a nebulizer
   - Appropriate laser ETTs
   - Saline for the ETT cuff
   - Various sizes of regular ETTs

8. **During a suspension microdirect laryngoscopy, the patient develops premature ventricular contractions. List some potential causes of the premature ventricular contractions.**

Potential causes include the following:
- Hypoxemia
- Hypercarbia
- Laryngeal stimulation
- Light anesthesia

9. **Discuss the manifestations and treatment of postoperative airway edema.**

The postoperative patient with airway edema is anxious and restless. The airway obstruction may result in muscle retraction, cyanosis, stridor, tachypnea, and tachycardia. The patient with airway edema should be assisted into the sitting position and administered humidified oxygen. The patient's oxygen saturation should be monitored closely. Nebulized racemic epinephrine can be administered until the heart rate reaches an unacceptable level. If this occurs without a reduction in symptoms, the CRNA may need to secure the airway by either intubation or tracheostomy. Endotracheal intubation requires a smaller ETT than was used during the procedure. Different sizes of ETTs should be readily available. If laryngoscopy and intubation is unsuccessful, the patient may require a tracheostomy performed by the ENT surgeon or other emergency airway intervention by the CRNA.

10. **Describe the treatment of a laryngospasm.**

Laryngospasm is a reflex closure of the vocal cords. A patient with a complete laryngospasm is unable to move air in or out of the lungs, and it is impossible to mask ventilate the patient. The first step to treat a laryngospasm is to administer positive-pressure ventilation with 100% oxygen. If this does not quickly alleviate the spasm, the CRNA needs to administer succinylcholine via an intravenous or intramuscular route. The dose of succinylcholine is 20 to 40 mg in an adult patient and 1 mg/kg in a pediatric patient.

11. **List potential complications related to a tonsillectomy, and describe the treatment or prevention of each complication.**
- Hypovolemia from hemorrhage
  - Administer adequate amounts of fluid to replace the blood loss and deficit resulting from NPO (nothing-per-mouth) status.
  - Check a hematocrit when indicated.
  - Administer blood products as necessary.
- Laryngospasm
  - Suction the airway before extubation.
  - Extubate the patient either awake or under deep general anesthesia.
  - If a laryngospasm occurs, provide positive-pressure ventilation.
  - If this does not break the laryngospasm, administer a small dose of intravenous or intramuscular succinylcholine.

- Airway fire
  - Maintain the FIO_2 at 30% or less to help decrease the likelihood of an airway fire.
  - See Question 4 for the treatment of an airway fire.

12. When is bleeding after a tonsillectomy most likely to occur?

Typically, bleeding after a tonsillectomy occurs within 6 hours after surgery or by postoperative day 6. The incidence of postoperative bleeding is approximately 0.3% to 0.6%.

13. Describe the signs and symptoms of a right main stem intubation.

The signs and symptoms of a right main stem intubation include the following:
- Decrease in the oxygen saturation on the pulse oximeter
- Decreased breath sounds on the left side
- Decreased end-tidal carbon dioxide
- Increased $PaCO_2$
- Wheezing
- ETT moved from where it was originally taped

14. List ENT procedures that may have the potential for a large blood loss.

The following ENT procedures have the potential for a large blood loss:
- Neck dissections
- Tonsillectomy
- Nasal surgery
- Sinus surgery

Nasal and sinus surgical procedures consist of a slow oozing of blood, and the longer the procedure, the greater the blood loss.

15. Describe the CRNA's responsibility when a surgeon has placed a throat pack.

The CRNA should chart when the pack was placed and when it was removed. The CRNA should confirm that the throat pack has been removed before extubating the patient.

16. Describe dysrhythmias that are frequently encountered in ENT surgery.

- *Tachycardia* during ENT surgery is typically the result of a very stimulating procedure.
- *Bradycardia* may be encountered during ENT surgery. It may be the result of carotid artery stimulation during a radical neck procedure or stimulation of the laryngeal area.
- *Premature ventricular contractions* may occur during ENT surgery as the result of inadequate ventilation during the procedure.

17. Describe times in the ENT room when the anesthetist must pay extremely close attention to the patient's airway.

The anesthetist must pay close attention to the patient's airway at the following times:
- When the surgeon is placing the mouth gag
- During Venturi ventilation
- During laser surgery of the airway
- When suspension laryngoscopy begins
- When the surgeon is holding the mask airway of the patient
- During a tracheostomy
- Whenever the surgeon turns the patient's head

18. List four ENT procedures that may be posted on the operating room schedule as either an urgent or an emergency case.

- Epistaxis
- Tonsillectomy for peritonsillar abscess
- Choanal atresia
- Bleeding postoperative tonsillectomy

19. List extraordinary items that may be required for a radical neck dissection.

- Fluid warmer
- Patient warmer
- Two intravenous lines
- Arterial line
- Central line
- Foley catheter
- Extra ETTs and tracheostomy tubes

20. Describe the effect of N_2O on the middle ear.

N_2O rapidly diffuses into air-filled cavities. This occurs 34 times faster than air diffuses out of the cavity. This rapid entrance of N_2O into the middle ear results in an increase in the middle ear pressure. When N_2O is discontinued, it rapidly diffuses out of the middle ear. This may result in negative pressure within the middle ear. This negative pressure within the middle ear may result in serous otitis.

21. What type of ear procedure would not be affected by N_2O?

A myringotomy with or without tube placement would not be affected by N_2O. When a hole is produced in the tympanic membrane, the middle ear no longer is a closed, air-filled space. It ventilates to the atmosphere, alleviating pressure changes within the middle ear.

Key Points

- Measures that decrease the incidence of airway fires are FiO_2 less than or equal to 30%, saline in ETT cuff, moist sponges in the airway, and use of secondary gases that do not support combustion (air and helium).
- The steps in treatment of an airway fire are:
  - Immediately disconnect the anesthesia circuit and turn off the oxygen.
  - Remove the ETT.
  - Extinguish the ETT fire.
  - Remove any smoldering ETT pieces from the airway.
  - Resume ventilation with air until certain that no debris is left burning in the airway, then switch to 100% oxygen.
  - Examine the airway, and treat the patient accordingly.
  - Save all involved materials and devices for later investigation.
- Symptoms of postoperative airway edema include muscle retraction, cyanosis, stridor, tachypnea, and tachycardia.
- Treatment of postoperative airway edema includes the sitting position, humidified oxygen, racemic epinephrine and, as an extreme measure, mechanical or surgical securing of the airway (intubation or tracheostomy).
- The potential complications related to tonsillectomy are hypovolemia from hemorrhage, laryngospasm, and airway fire.
- Bleeding after a tonsillectomy occurs within 6 hours after surgery or the 6th postoperative day.
- The signs of right mainstem intubation are:
  - Decreased oxygen saturation
  - Decreased breath sound of left side
  - Decreased end-tidal carbon dioxide
  - Increased arterial partial pressure of carbon dioxide
  - Wheezing
  - Migration of ETT

 Internet Resources

The Virtual Anaesthesia Textbook: Anaesthesia for ENT, ophthalmic, dental, and facial surgery:
http://www.virtual-anaesthesia-textbook.com/vat/ent.html

GASNet Video Library:
http://www.gasnet.org/videos/index.php

Nurse-Anesthesia.com:
http://www.nurse-anesthesia.com/

Bibliography

Barash PG, Cullen BF, Stoelting RK, editors: *Clinical anesthesia*, ed 4, Philadelphia, 2001, Lippincott Williams & Wilkins.

Groudine SB, Hollinger I, Jones J, et al: New York State guidelines on the topical use of phenylephrine in the operating room, *Anesthesiology* 92:859-864, 2000.

McGoldrick K, editor: *Anesthesia for ophthalmic and otolaryngologic surgery,* Philadelphia, 1992, WB Saunders.

Nagelhout JJ, Zaglaniczny KL, editors: *Nurse anesthesia,* ed 2, Philadelphia, 2001, WB Saunders.

Omoigui S, editor: *The anesthesia drugs handbook,* ed 2, St. Louis, 1995, Mosby.

Professional Nurses Organization: *Patient safety—coping with OR fires: four qualities that you need,* Amityville, NY, 1999, Professional Nurses Purchasing Group.

Sosis MB, Dillon FX: Saline-filled cuffs help prevent laser-induced polyvinylchloride endotracheal tube fires, *Anesth Analg* 72:187-189, 1991.

Stoelting RK: *Pharmacology and physiology in anesthetic practice,* ed 3, Philadelphia, 1998, JB Lippincott.

Chapter 36

Noncardiac Thoracic Anesthesia and One-Lung Ventilation

Craig K. Huard

1. Why is it important to review diagnostic tests, such as arterial blood gases, and pulmonary function tests, before thoracic surgery?

Review of diagnostic tests is crucial to characterize and quantify the risk of surgery and anesthesia to the patient. Preoperative *arterial blood gases* can indicate hypoventilation and carbon dioxide retention. Arterial carbon dioxide tension ($PaCO_2$) greater than 45 mm Hg indicates an increased risk of postoperative complications.

Pulmonary function tests use spirometry, which is inexpensive and effective, as the cornerstone of initial assessment. Forced vital capacity, forced expiratory volume in 1 second, residual volume-to-total lung capacity ratio, and maximal breathing capacity are commonly measured. Pulmonary function test values linked to increased risk of postoperative pulmonary complications are listed in the following table. Other pulmonary function tests may involve split-lung function studies that use ventilation with radioisotopes, in conjunction with perfusion scans, to determine regional viability of lung tissue that would remain after surgery. Simulation of remaining pulmonary vascular compliance can be achieved with selective pulmonary artery occlusion, utilizing a balloon tipped catheter. In general, a mean pulmonary artery pressure greater than 35 to 40 mm Hg, $PaCO_2$ greater than 60 mm Hg, PaO_2 less than 45 mm Hg, or pulmonary vascular resistance greater than 190 dynes·sec·cm^5 suggests a poor risk or inoperable thoracic condition.

Pulmonary Function Tests	
Measurement	**Value Associated with Increased Postoperative Risk**
FVC	<50% of predicted
FEV$_1$	<50% of FVC or <2 L
RV/TLC	<50% of predicted
MBC	<50% of predicted or <50 L/min

FFV$_1$, forced-expiratory volume in 1 second; FVC, forced vital capacity; MBC, maximal breathing capacity; RV/TLC, residual volume-to-total lung capacity ratio.

2. **Many patients undergoing thoracic surgery are chronic smokers. What are the benefits of smoking cessation before thoracic surgery and the time frames involved for accrual of benefits?**

   Smoking increases airway irritability and secretions. Mucociliary transport, forced vital capacity, and forced midexpiratory flow rate ($FEF_{25\%-75\%}$) all decrease with prolonged smoking. Acutely, 48 hours of smoking cessation decrease the patient's carboxyhemoglobin level. Accompanying this decrease is a rightward shift in the oxyhemoglobin dissociation curve, increasing oxygen availability to the tissues. The greatest benefits (improved ciliary function, reduction in sputum production, and increase in $FEF_{25\%-75\%}$) occur 4 to 6 weeks after smoking cessation.

3. **Describe the mechanism of hypoxic pulmonary vasoconstriction (HPV).**

   HPV is a protective autoregulation mechanism that diverts blood flow away from hypoxic lung regions toward better oxygenated regions. The stimulus for HPV is alveolar oxygen tension (PAO_2) and mixed venous oxygen tension (PvO_2). Within limits, a decreased PAO_2 or PvO_2 produces vasoconstriction in local pulmonary blood vessels.

4. **What factors inhibit HPV?**

   The following factors inhibit HPV:
   - High pulmonary artery pressure. At greater than 16 to 18 mm Hg, vessels constricted by hypoxia dilate owing to increased hydrostatic pressure. Conditions such as mitral stenosis, left heart failure, and volume overload may increase pulmonary vascular pressure.
   - Abnormal pH. A normal pH allows a maximal HPV response.
   - Local infection
   - Hypothermia
   - Inhaled anesthetics. Inhalational agents depress HPV in a dose-dependent manner. Intravenous agents do not seem to affect HPV.

5. **List absolute and relative indications for one-lung ventilation (OLV).**

Absolute Indications (to isolate a lung)	Relative Indications (to facilitate surgical exposure)
Bronchopleural fistula	Lobectomy, pneumonectomy
Bullae or bronchial rupture	Thoracic aortic aneurysm repair
Lung infection	Upper esophageal resection
Copious bleeding in one lung	Thoracic spine surgeries via the anterior approach
	Thoracospocy

6. **Identify the possible complications associated with using a double-lumen tube (DLT).**

   Complications associated with use of a DLT include the following:
   - Tracheal or bronchial lacerations
   - Bronchial wall tissue damage due to excessive cuff inflation. To limit pressure on the mucous membranes, the bronchial cuff should be deflated when positioning the tube except when OLV is absolutely indicated.

- Increased incidence of postsurgical infection
- Tracheal rupture

7. Identify the common causes of a malpositioned DLT.

Common causes of a malpositioned DLT are as follows:
- Improper positioning of a DLT in the right main stem bronchus with resulting blockage of right upper lobe ventilation. The distance from the carina to the right upper lobe bronchus is typically about 2.5 cm in men and 2 cm in women.
- Insufficient insertion of the DLT into the bronchus, with the bronchial lumen orifice above the carina (bilateral breath sounds are noted when ventilating through the bronchial lumen)
- Left-sided tube occluding the left upper lobe orifice

8. Describe the method used to insert a DLT.

The concave curvature of the DLT tip should face anterior when first placed in the mouth. When the tip passes the vocal cords, the tube is rotated 90 degrees toward the desired main stem. It is advanced until moderate resistance is met, approximately 29 cm.

9. What methods may be used to verify proper placement of an endobronchial tube?

After placement, the following steps are initiated:
- The tracheal cuff is inflated, and breath sounds are auscultated bilaterally.
- The bronchial cuff is inflated, and bilateral breath sounds are assessed again.
- Each lumen is clamped individually, and OLV is confirmed, using auscultation and inspection of chest wall movement.
- A fiberoptic bronchoscope (FOB) is used to verify placement.

The FOB is considered by most the standard for final confirmation of DLT placement. When viewed from the tracheal lumen of the DLT, the FOB view should show the carina and the dome of the bronchial cuff in the selected main stem bronchus. There should not be herniation of the bronchial cuff over the carina because blockage of the opposite main stem can occur. Passing the FOB through the bronchial lumen of the DLT should result in a view (for a left-sided DLT) of the left upper lobe bifurcation. On the right, the right upper lobe bifurcation must be clear, and the FOB can confirm this with a view through the fenestration that exists in the bronchial cuff. Most practitioners use the left-sided DLT for right and left lung separation because of the difficulty in placing and maintaining placement of the right-sided DLT.

10. Describe the physiological changes associated with the lateral decubitus position.

Four scenarios may be used to contrast the changes observed with the lateral decubitus position versus the supine position.

- *Awake, closed chest, spontaneously breathing:* With this scenario, tidal volume is preferentially delivered to the dependent lung coinciding with increased blood flow to the dependent lung. Ventilation-perfusion ratios are unchanged; shunted blood flow to total blood flow shunt fraction is not greatly altered from the supine position.
- *Awake, open chest, spontaneously breathing:* Rarely seen for extended periods, this scenario produces a mediastinal shift and paradoxical respirations. Lack of negative pleural pressure in the nondependent hemithorax causes a downward mediastinal shift as the dependent hemithorax draws air in. Paradoxical respiration occurs as air flows into the nondependent lung during expiration, causing the collapsed lung to inflate as the dependant lung deflates.
- *Anesthetized, closed chest, paralyzed:* In this scenario, ventilation favors the nondependent lung, whereas blood flow is greatest in the dependent lung. The decreased functional residual capacity observed with anesthesia is accentuated in this scenario due to loss of diaphragmatic contraction, downward mediastinal shift, and abdominal content pressure on the diaphragm. Overall, ventilation-perfusion mismatch is greatly increased.
- *Anesthetized, open chest, paralyzed:* An open chest creates an even larger ventilation-perfusion mismatch than in the previous scenario. The nondependent lung is overventilated further, and the dependent lung is underventilated further. Most of the blood flow is to the dependent lung.

11. Describe the physiological changes observed in an anesthetized patient undergoing OLV in the lateral decubitus position.

Venous admixture or shunt increases with OLV in the lateral decubitus position. The shunt associated with two-lung ventilation in the lateral decubitus position is about 5% of the cardiac output for each lung, or 10% total. During OLV, the total shunt may approach 30%, even with an intact HPV response. Factors contributing to an increased venous admixture include the following:

- Absorption atelectasis in the dependent lung due to dependent lung exposure to a high FIO_2
- Decreased lung volume in the dependent lung due to general anesthesia, paralysis, compression by mediastinal weight, and secretions
- Vasoconstriction in hypoxic segments of the dependent lung, with blood flow directed to the nondependent, nonventilated lung
- Transudation of fluid into the dependent lung, decreasing functional residual capacity and increasing airway closure.

12. What ventilation settings are employed for thoracic anesthesia and OLV?

Tidal volumes of 8 to 12 mL/kg are recommended for the initiation of OLV. Higher tidal volumes can increase shunt fraction by increasing airway pressures and vascular resistance in the ventilated lung, directing blood flow toward the nonventilated lung. Lower tidal volumes can result in atelectasis. Practitioners must pay close attention to intraoperative indicators, such as pulse oximetry, peak airway pressure, returned tidal volume, and arterial blood gases, to choose and adjust the appropriate tidal volume setting. FIO_2 of 0.8 to 1.0 is advised.

13. What can the practitioner do to manage hypoxemia during OLV?

- Confirm tube placement and increase the FIO_2.
- Implement continuous positive airway pressure, 5 to 10 cm H_2O, to the nonventilated lung.
- Apply positive end expiratory pressure, 5 to 10 cm H_2O, to the dependent lung.
- Intermittently inflate and deflate the surgical lung, if possible.
- Ask the surgeon to occlude the pulmonary artery of the nonventilated lung (if a pneumonectomy is planned).

14. Describe the proper use of the Univent tube.

The Univent tube is a standard endotracheal tube containing a special low-pressure/high-volume blocker balloon. The balloon is attached to a movable tube, housed in a small channel in the anterior aspect of the parent tube. Initially placed as a regular endotracheal tube, the Univent tube is rotated 90 degrees toward the desired main stem, and the balloon is pushed forward. The blocker balloon is inflated with 6 to 8 mL of air. Residual air in the lung may be suctioned out via the blocker lumen or gently squeezed out by the surgeon.

Alternatively an FOB may be used as a stylet to advance the Univent tube into the desired main stem. When the blocker is placed, the Univent tube is withdrawn into the trachea.

The table lists benefits and limitations of the Univent tube.

Benefits and Limitations of Univent Tube	
Benefits	**Limitations**
Right or left blockade possible	Single size (7.0 mm)
Selective segment or entire lung blockade possible	Overdistention of blocker balloon may result in balloon herniation over the carina
Less likely to be displaced than DLT	Overdistention of blocker balloon may cause damage to tissue
Suction, lavage, oxygen delivery, or jet ventilation possible through blocker lumen	
Postoperative ventilation does not require ETT change	

DLT, double-lumen tube; ETT, endotracheal tube.

Key Points

- In general, a mean pulmonary artery pressure greater than 35 to 40 mm Hg, $Paco_2$ greater than 60 mm Hg, Pao_2 less than 45 mm Hg, or a pulmonary vascular resistance greater than 190 dyne·sec·cm^5 suggests a poor risk or inoperable thoracic condition.

- Acutely, 48 hours of smoking cessation decreases the patient's carboxyhemoglobin level. Accompanying this is a rightward shift in the oxyhemoglobin dissociation curve, increasing oxygen availability to the tissues. The greatest benefits (improved ciliary function, reduction in sputum production, and increase in $FEF_{25\%-75\%}$) occur 4 to 6 weeks after smoking cessation.

- HPV is a protective autoregulation mechanism that diverts blood flow away from hypoxic lung regions toward better oxygenated regions. The stimulus for HPV is alveolar oxygen tension and mixed venous oxygen tension.

- High pulmonary artery pressure, abnormal pH, local infection, hypothermia, and inhaled anesthetics inhibit HPV.

- Absolute indications for OLV are bronchopleural fistula, bullae or bronchial rupture, lung infection, and copious bleeding in one lung.

- Possible complications associated with using a DLT are tracheal or bronchial lacerations, bronchial wall tissue damage due to excessive cuff inflation, increased incidence of postsurgical infection, and tracheal rupture.

- Tidal volumes of 8 to 12 mL/kg are recommended for the initiation of OLV.

- The practitioner can manage hypoxemia during OLV by:
  - Confirming tube placement and increase the FIo_2
  - Implementing continuous positive airway pressure, 5 to 10 cm H_2O, to the nonventilated lung
  - Applying positive end-expiratory pressure, 5 to 10 cm H_2O, to the dependent lung
  - Intermittently inflating/deflating the surgical lung, if possible
  - Asking the surgeon to occlude the pulmonary artery of the nonventilated lung

- The Univent tube is a standard endotracheal tube containing a special low-pressure/high-volume blocker balloon.

Internet Resources

The Virtual Anesthesiologist: Anesthesia for cardiothoracic surgery:
http://www.anesthesiology.de/Links/Cardiothoracic_Anesthesia/
cardiothoracic_anesthesia.htm

University of Rochester Medical Center Department of Anesthesiology: Thoracic anesthesia II (CA-3) rotation:
http://web.anes.rochester.edu/resident/GandO/ThoracicCA3.doc

Internet Resources   *continued*

Case Western Reserve University: MetroHealth Medical Center Department of Anesthesiology: Anesthetic considerations for thoracic aortic surgery: http://www.metrohealthanesthesia.com/edu/card/TAorta02.htm

University of Chicago: Anesthesia and critical care. vascular thoracic anesthesia manual: http://daccx.bsd.uchicago.edu/manuals/vtmanual/vtmanual.html

Campos JH, Massa FC, Kernstine KH: The incidence of right upper-lobe collapse when comparing a right-sided double-lumen tube versus a modified left double-lumen tube for left-sided thoracic surgery, Anesth Analg 90:535-540, 2000; http://www.anesth.uiowa.edu/readabstract.asp?PMID=10702432

Bibliography

Brodsky JB, Fitzmaurice B: Modern anesthetic techniques for thoracic operations, *World J Surg* 25:162-166, 2001.

Eisenkraft JB, Cohen E, Neustein SM: Anesthesia for thoracic surgery. In Barash P, Cullen B, Stoelting R, editors: *Clinical anesthesia,* ed 4, Philadelphia, 2001, Lippincott Williams & Wilkins, pp 813-851.

Klein U, et al: Role of fiberoptic bronchoscopy in conjunction with the use of double lumen tubes for thoracic anesthesia: a prospective study, *Anesthesiology* 88:346-350, 1998.

Levitzky MG: *Pulmonary physiology,* ed 5, New York, 1999, McGraw-Hill, pp 136-137.

Shah J, Bready LL: Anesthesia for thoracoscopy, *Anesthesiol Clin North Am* 19:156-164, 2001.

Neuroskeletal Surgery

Kathleen A. Cook

1. Review the blood flow to the spinal cord.

The blood flow to the spinal cord commonly is thought of as being supplied by the single anterior and paired posterior spinal arteries (PSAs). These vessels depend on a network of collateral vessels to help them provide an adequate blood supply to the spinal cord. The two PSAs arise from the posterior inferior cerebellar arteries or the vertebral arteries at the level of the foramen magnum. They supply the posterior one third of the spinal cord, traveling down its posterolateral region. The single anterior spinal artery (ASA) also arises from the vertebral arteries. Its origin is more cephalad, just below the vertebrobasilar junction. The ASA supplies the anterior two thirds of the spinal cord as it courses along the median fissure of the spinal cord. Damage or impaired blood flow through the ASA results in a motor deficit and loss of pain and temperature sensation.

The combined flow from the ASA and the PSAs alone is only enough to support the metabolic needs of the cervical cord. Additional flow to the lower spinal cord regions is supplied by the radicular (also known as the segmental) arteries that anastomose with the ASA and PSAs. The radicular arteries originate from the vertebral, deep cervical, intercostal, and lumbar arteries. Their anatomical distributions are highly variable. The cervical and lumbar regions receive twice the amount of blood flow than is delivered to the thoracic cord.

2. What is the significance of the artery of Adamkiewicz?

The artery of Adamkiewicz (also called the *arteria radicularis magna*) is the largest and most consistent radicular artery. This important artery is located in the thoracolumbar region. Its point of entry can be anywhere from T5 to L3, but it enters from T9 to T12 in 60% of individuals. The artery of Adamkiewicz supplies blood to the ASA and is responsible for most of the spinal cord blood flow beneath its point of entry.

3. Define the "watershed" areas of the spinal cord.

The areas of the spinal cord most susceptible to ischemic damage when arterial flow is compromised are mainly in the thoracic region. Relatively long distances between the radicular arteries and sluggish flow through them make these areas most vulnerable. The areas at greatest risk are T4 and L1 anteriorly and T1 to T3 posteriorly.

4. How does spinal cord blood flow compare with cerebral blood flow?

Total blood flow to the spinal cord is roughly 40% of the blood flow to the brain. It is approximately 60 mL/100 g of tissue/min. Flow to the gray matter is about 60 mL/100 g of tissue/min, whereas flow to the white matter is approximately 20 mL/100 g of tissue/min. The differences in flow between tissue types are commensurate with metabolic demand.

5. Do autoregulation and carbon dioxide reactivity play a role in the control of spinal cord blood flow?

Autoregulation of spinal cord blood flow exists, just as it does within the brain. Within the autoregulatory limits, the spinal cord vasculature either dilates or constricts in response to changes in perfusion pressure, maintaining a constant flow. Pressure limits of spinal cord autoregulation are 50 to 150 mm Hg. Outside the limits of autoregulation, spinal cord blood flow becomes pressure dependent.

Spinal cord blood flow responds to changes in carbon dioxide tension similar to the cerebral blood flow. Flow increases when carbon dioxide levels are high and decreases when arterial carbon dioxide is lowered.

Autoregulation and carbon dioxide responsiveness are altered after injury to the spinal cord. Preservation of spinal cord perfusion is a major anesthetic goal in any circumstance in which the spinal cord is at risk for ischemia.

6. Discuss the best method of neurological monitoring to prevent postoperative paralysis.

The traditional "wake-up test," previously thought of as the standard for intraoperative neurological monitoring during many types of spine surgery, has mostly been replaced by evoked potential monitoring. The wake-up test is not a benign procedure, with loss of intravenous lines, endotracheal tubes, and spine fixation devices; air embolism; pain; and recall as potential risks.

A survey published in 1995 suggested that sensory evoked potential monitoring decreased the overall incidence of neurological deficits in spinal surgeries. The greatest accuracy of the sensory evoked potential monitoring was seen when the evoked potentials were stable intraoperatively.

Theoretically, it makes sense that motor evoked potential (MEP) monitoring would be the definitive tool for detection of neurological injury intraoperatively. The incompatibility of MEPs and many anesthetic agents precluded their widespread use in the past. As the MEP techniques undergo refinement, greater success is being achieved with their use with general anesthesia.

7. What are the anesthetic implications when using MEPs?

If myogenic transcranial MEPs are being recorded, the recommendations for anesthetic technique are shown in the following table. Simply stated, total intravenous anesthesia is often the most appropriate technique when using MEPs.

Recommendations for Anesthetic Technique

Compatible Agents	Incompatible Agents
Opioids	Volatile inhalational agents
Etomidate	Neuromuscular blockade with loss of >2 twitches in train of four
Ketamine	Nitrous Oxide > 50%
Low-dose propofol	Induction doses of thiopental or midazolam

8. Which patients may benefit from high-dose methylprednisolone therapy?

High-dose methylprednisolone therapy may be efficacious for patients with acute spinal cord injury and for patients with severe spine disease undergoing major spinal surgery.

9. What is the recommended dose of methylprednisolone for spinal cord–injured patients?

Guidelines recommend a bolus dose of methylprednisolone, 30 mg/kg, administered over 15 minutes, followed 45 minutes later by a 23-hour infusion at 5.4 mg/kg/hr if pharmacological treatment is initiated within 8 hours of injury. Recommendations from the National Acute Spinal Cord Injury Study III published in 1997 state that if therapy is initiated 3 to 8 hours after injury, the total duration of methylprednisolone therapy should be 48 hours.

10. Identify the pitfalls of high-dose steroid therapy.

Immunosuppression and *wound infections* are major risks associated with perioperative steroid therapy. Gastrointestinal bleeding in a patient population already predisposed to stress ulcers, myopathy, hyperglycemia, and decubitus ulcers also is associated with high-dose corticosteroid therapy.

11. Discuss the indications for an awake intubation for patients undergoing elective cervical spine surgery.

Limitations to mobility of the cervical spine, whether anatomical or orthotic, may necessitate intubation with the patient awake and spontaneously breathing. Patients with known cervical spine disease who have exacerbation of neurological symptoms during head or neck movement are best intubated with the neck in a neutral position while awake and spontaneously breathing. A high index of suspicion for cervical spine instability should be maintained in patients with: severe lumbar degenerative disease (high correlation with concomitant cervical disease), rheumatoid arthritis, Down syndrome, and Klippel-Feil syndrome.

12. What are the possible complications of surgery on the cervical spine via an anterior approach?

Possible complications applicable to operations in this anatomical region are listed in the following table. Recurrent laryngeal nerve injuries are due to intraoperative retraction or dissection. A left-sided surgical approach decreases the incidence of this complication but is technically more difficult for a right-handed surgeon.

Complications of Surgery via Anterior Approach

Airway	Nerve Injuries	Vascular	Others
Accidental intraoperative extubation due to dislodgment of head-halter traction Airway obstruction Laryngeal edema	Recurrent laryngeal nerve injury External laryngeal nerve injury Phrenic nerve injury Horner's syndrome	Carotid artery injury Vertebral artery injury Superior or inferior thyroid artery injury Wound hematoma	Thoracic duct injury Perforation of the esophagus Dural tear Hoarseness

13. How often do airway complications occur after anterior cervical spine surgery?

The incidence of postoperative airway complications is about 6%, with one third of these patients requiring reintubation.

14. Which patients undergoing anterior cervical spine surgery are most likely to experience postoperative airway complications?

A retrospective review of more than 300 anterior cervical spine cases revealed the following risk factors as predictive of airway compromise:
• Operative time greater than 5 hours
• Multilevel operations that exposed more than three vertebrae including C2, C3, or C4
• Blood loss greater than 300 mL

15. What areas of the spine are most susceptible to trauma?

Traumatic spinal cord injuries are most common in the middle to lower cervical spine, C5-7, and the thoracolumbar junction, T12-L1. These are the least protected and most mobile areas of the spinal column.

Approximately 40% of all spinal cord injuries are due to motor vehicle accidents. The most commonly injured levels of the spine in motor vehicle accidents are C5 and C6. Approximately half of all spine injuries are cervical, whereas thoracic, lumbar, and sacral injuries constitute the other 50%.

16. What areas of the spine are most susceptible to disease?

Spinal stenosis occurs more often in the lumbar spine than in the cervical region. The lumbar levels most commonly involved are the L3-4 and the L4-5 interspaces. It is common for multiple levels to be involved.

Degenerative disc disease (spondylosis) occurs in the lumbar spine six times more frequently than in the cervical spine. The spinal levels most commonly compromised are L4-5 and L5-S1.

17. Identify the major anesthetic implications of the anterolateral surgical approach to the thoracolumbar spine.

Anesthetic implications of the anterolateral surgical approach to the thoracolumbar spine include the following:
* Lateral decubitus positioning and associated implications
* Possible thoracotomy and request for one-lung ventilation for operations above T10
* Prolonged lung retraction. Pulmonary reserve should be assessed preoperatively; postoperative mechanical ventilation may be required.
* Large blood loss. Coagulation status should be assessed preoperatively.

18. What is scoliosis?

Scoliosis is a disorder causing abnormal curves from side to side, front to back, or top to bottom of the spinal column. The curves create lateral and rotational deformities of the ribs and the vertebral column.

19. What causes scoliosis?

Idiopathic scoliosis accounts for about 80% of cases. Medical conditions that may cause scoliotic changes include congenital abnormalities (e.g., spina bifida), neuromuscular disorders (e.g., cerebral palsy, muscular dystrophies), and various syndromes (e.g., Marfan syndrome, neurofibromatosis, osteogenesis imperfecta). Traumatic insults to the spinal column can also lead to scoliotic deformities.

20. Why is the Cobb angle important?

The Cobb angle is a method of measuring the degree of curvature of the spinal column. A curve of 10 degrees or greater indicates scoliosis. Clinical experience has shown that the greater the angle of curvature, the greater the progression of the deformity and severity of complications. The Cobb angle correlates with systemic manifestations.

21. Describe the most significant medical complications associated with scoliosis.

As the degree of curvature increases, the thoracic cage narrows, causing derangements of cardiovascular and pulmonary function. Evidence of restrictive lung disease (decreased inspiratory capacity and vital capacity) appears with curves greater than 65 degrees. Significant respiratory compromise occurs with angles of 90 degrees and greater, with dyspnea on exertion evident at 100-degree curvatures. As the angle of curvature progresses beyond 120 degrees, pulmonary vascular hypertension, right ventricular hypertrophy, cor pulmonale, and alveolar hypoventilation occur.

22. How is scoliosis corrected?

In most cases, the spinal column curvature remains small enough so that surgical intervention is not required. Curvatures of 25 to 40 degrees are managed with orthotic bracing and radiographic evaluation every 4 to 6 months. If the angle of curvature exceeds 40 to 50 degrees, surgery is indicated. When operative treatment is necessary, the surgical procedure performed depends on the type of scoliosis being corrected. For idiopathic adolescent scoliosis, the most common operation is posterior spinal fusion with instrumentation and bone grafting. With neuromuscular scoliosis, more complex combined anterior and posterior techniques (staged or same-day surgeries) are common.

23. What are the most important anesthetic implications of surgical repair of scoliosis?

Anesthetic preoperative evaluation should focus on the severity of the scoliosis, the presence of confounding medical comorbidities, and the type of surgical intervention planned. Cardiopulmonary instability and major blood loss are the two most critical intraoperative complications for the anesthetist to anticipate.

 Key Points

- The artery of Adamkiewicz (also known as the arteria radicularis magna) is the largest and most consistent radicular artery. This important artery is located in the thoracolumbar region. This artery supplies blood to the ASA and is responsible for most of the spinal cord blood flow beneath its point of entry.
- Total blood flow to the spinal cord is roughly 40% of the blood flow to the brain. It is approximately 60 mL/100 g of tissue/min.
- Pressure limits of spinal cord autoregulation are 50 to 150 mm Hg. Outside the limits of autoregulation, spinal cord blood flow becomes pressure dependent.
- Spinal cord blood flow responds to changes in carbon dioxide tension similar to the cerebral blood flow. Flow increases when carbon dioxide levels are high and decreases when arterial carbon dioxide is lowered.

Key Points   *continued*

- High-dose methylprednisolone therapy may be efficacious for patients with acute spinal cord injury and for patients with severe spine disease undergoing major spinal surgery.
- Recurrent laryngeal nerve injuries can result from surgery on the cervical spine via an anterior approach.
- Traumatic spinal cord injuries are most common in the middle to lower cervical spine, C5-7, and the thoracolumbar junction, T12-L1.
- Spinal stenosis occurs more often in the lumbar spine than in the cervical region. The lumbar levels most commonly involved are the L3-4 and the L4-5 interspaces.
- Scoliosis is a disorder causing abnormal curves from side to side, front to back or top to bottom of the spinal column. The curves create lateral and rotational deformities of the ribs and the vertebral column.
- The Cobb angle is a method of measuring the degree of curvature of the spinal column. The Cobb angle correlates with systemic manifestations.
- The significant medical complications associated with scoliosis are derangements of cardiovascular and pulmonary function.
- Cardiopulmonary instability and major blood loss are the two most critical intraoperative complications for the anesthetist to anticipate.

Internet Resources

Anesthesia for Spine Surgery:
http://www.anesthesia.org.cn/asa2002/rcl_source/236_Black.pdf

Clinical monitoring of the brain and spinal cord:
http://www.anesthesia.org.cn/asa2002/rcl_source/532_Sloan.pdf

Society of Neurosurgical Anesthesia and Critical Care Education Material:
http://www.snacc.org/Ed.html

Virtual Anesthesia Textbook:
http://www.virtual-anaesthesia-textbook.com/

Nurse-Anesthesia.com:
http://www.nurse-anesthesia.com/

Bibliography

Bracken MB: Methylprednisolone and acute spinal cord injury: an update of the randomized evidence, *Spine* 26:S47-S54, 2001.

Geller EB, Najm IM: Intraoperative neurophysiologic monitoring of the spinal cord. In Herkowitz HN, Garfin SR, Balderston RA, et al, editors: *Rothman-Simeone, the spine*, Philadelphia, 1999, WB Saunders, pp 1662-1667.

Johnson RM, et al: Surgical approaches to the spine. In Herkowitz HN, Garfin SR, Balderston RA, et al, editors: *Rothman-Simeone, the spine,* Philadelphia, 1999, WB Saunders, pp 1502-1569.

Kawaguchi M, et al: Low dose propofol as a supplement to ketamine-based anesthesia during intraoperative monitoring of motor-evoked potentials, *Spine* 25:974-979, 2000.

Mahla ME: Cervical spine in anesthesia. In Cucchiara RF, Black S, Michenfelder JD, editors: *Clinical neuroanesthesia,* ed 2, New York, 1998, Churchill Livingstone, pp 396-400.

Mahla ME, Horlocker TT: Vertebral column and spinal cord surgery. In Cucchiara RF, Black S, Michenfelder JD, editors: *Clinical neuroanesthesia,* ed 2, New York, 1998, Churchill Livingstone, pp 403-436.

Nesathurai S: Steroids and spinal cord injury: revisiting the NASCIS 2 and NASCIS 3 trials, *J Trauma* 45:1088-1093, 1998.

Parsa AT, Miller JI: Neurosurgical diseases of the spine and spinal cord: surgical considerations. In Cottrell JE, Smith DS, editors: *Anesthesia and neurosurgery,* ed 4, St. Louis, 2001, Mosby, pp 539-553.

Sagi HC, et al: Airway complications associated with surgery on the anterior cervical spine, *Spine* 27:949-953, 2002.

Scheufler KM, Zentner J: Total intravenous anesthesia for intraoperative monitoring of the motor pathways: an integral view combining clinical and experimental data, *J Neurosurg* 96:571-579, 2002.

Scoliosis Research Society (SRS): In depth review of scoliosis, 2000, available online: URL http://www.srs.org/htm/library/review/review00.htm.

Stambough JL, Simeone FA: Neurologic complications in spine surgery. In Herkowitz HN, Garfin SR, Balderston RA, et al, editors: *Rothman-Simeone, the spine,* Philadelphia, 1999, WB Saunders, pp 1725-1726.

Stier GR, et al: Spinal cord: injury and procedures. In Newfield P, Cottrell JE, editors: *Handbook of neuroanesthesia,* ed 3, Philadelphia, 1999, Lippincott Williams & Wilkins, pp 234-235.

Stier GR, et al: Spinal cord injury. In Cottrell JE, Smith DS, editors: *Anesthesia and neurosurgery,* ed 4, St. Louis, 2001, Mosby, pp 715-730.

Tencer AF: Biomechanics of spinal trauma. In Cotler JM, Simpson JM, An HS, et al, editors: *Surgery of spinal trauma,* Philadelphia, 2000, Lippincott Williams & Wilkins, pp 61-112.

Zuckerberg AL, Yaster M: Anesthesia for orthopedic surgery. In Motoyama EK, Davis PJ, editors: *Smith's anesthesia for infants and children,* St. Louis, 1996, Mosby, pp 605-619.

Neurosurgical Principles

Steve L. Alves

1. Discuss the physiological elements of intracranial pressure (ICP).

Brain (80%), blood (12%), and cerebrospinal fluid (CSF) (8%) are enclosed within a rigid bone structure, the cranium. An increase in the volume of one of these three components is balanced by an equal decrease in another, to prevent a rise in ICP. ICP is the pressure measurement transduced from the lateral ventricles or over the cerebral cortex. Normal values range from 10 to 20 mm Hg. Potential causes of increased ICP are listed in the following box.

Potential Causes of Increased Intracranial Pressure

- Communicating or obstructive hydrocephalus
- Intracranial masses
- Head trauma
- Bleeding cerebral aneurysm
- Arteriovenous malformations
- Cerebrovascular accident with edema

Intracranial compliance measures the change in ICP in response to a change in intracranial volume. A small increase in volume does not normally increase ICP. If the volume continues to increase, a point is reached where further addition of volume produces a marked rise in ICP. The body minimizes increases in ICP by the following mechanisms:
- Displacing CSF from the cranial to the spinal compartments
- Increasing the absorption and decreasing production of CSF
- Decreasing the cerebral blood volume

2. Describe possible consequences of increased ICP.

Signs and symptoms associated with increased ICP include headache, vomiting, papilledema, pupillary changes, alterations in consciousness, and behavioral changes. The classic *Cushing's triad*—hypertension, bradycardia, and changes in respiration—is probably due to brainstem ischemia and indicates a severe increase in ICP. Severe elevations in ICP can cause decreased cerebral perfusion pressure and catastrophic herniation of the brain.

3. **Describe the process of anesthesia induction for patients with increased ICP.**

Preventing further increases in ICP is an important goal for anesthetic induction of a patient with an elevated ICP. Hyperventilation in a conscious and co-operative patient during the preintubation phase helps reduce $Paco_2$ and ultimately decreases cerebral blood volume and ICP. Commonly used intravenous agents, such as barbiturates, propofol, and etomidate, lower cerebral blood flow (CBF) either by reducing the cerebral metabolic rate of oxygen consumption ($CMRO_2$) or by cerebral vasoconstriction. In addition, to minimize the risk of hypertension during induction, intravenous lidocaine and beta adrenergic receptor antagonists such as esmolol and labetalol are recommended. Narcotics, although less useful in reducing CBF, are commonly used to blunt the sympathetic response to laryngoscopy and tracheal intubation.

4. **What are the key features of cerebral metabolism?**

The brain accounts for about 20% of the total body oxygen consumption. Approximately 60% of cerebral oxygen consumption is used to support nerve cell energy requirements. The $CMRO_2$ averages 3 to 3.5 mL/100 g tissue/min, which is approximately seven times greater than the average metabolic rate of the body. Because the $CMRO_2$ is so high, cerebral blood flow obstruction can result in rapid loss of consciousness. Perfusion must be reestablished within minutes to avoid irreversible cellular damage.

Brain cells use glucose as their chief energy source, at a rate of approximately 5 mg/100 g tissue/min. Acute sustained hypoglycemia produces neuronal injury and death. Hyperglycemia has been shown to accelerate cellular brain injury in the presence of cerebral hypoxia.

5. **Describe the fundamental components of cerebral CBF.**

CBF is coupled with $CMRO_2$. Increases in $CMRO_2$ lead to increases in CBF. Normal CBF is approximately 50 mL/100 g tissue/min. Total CBF in adults averages 750 mL/min, or approximately 15% to 20% of the cardiac output. CBF values less than 20 to 25 mL/100 g tissue/min are associated with cerebral ischemic changes, as evidenced by slowing of electroencephalogram waveforms. Rates less than 10 mL/100 g tissue/min may produce irreversible brain damage.

CBF is directly proportional to $Paco_2$ between the values of 20 and 80 mm Hg. For every 1 mm Hg change in $Paco_2$, CBF changes by approximately 1 to 2 mL/100 g/min (see the figure on page 339). The effects of $Paco_2$ on CBF are rapid and are the result of changes in the pH of CSF and cerebral tissue. Elevated blood oxygen tensions have minimal or no effect on CBF, but Pao_2 levels less than 50 mm Hg greatly increase CBF.

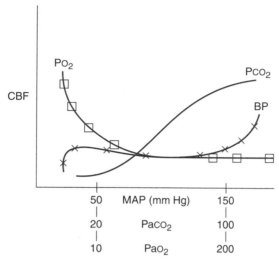

Regulation of cerebral blood flow. *(From Duke J: Anesthesia secrets, Philadelphia, 2000, Hanley & Belfus, p 250.)*

Hypothermia decreases $CMRO_2$ and CBF. For every 1°C decrease in body temperature, the $CMRO_2$ and CBF decrease by 7%. *Hyperthermia* has the opposite effect. Increased temperatures increase $CMRO_2$ and CBF.

6. Is CBF autoregulated?

Within limits, changes in mean arterial blood pressure (MAP) have little effect on CBF. The autoregulatory limits are MAP values between 60 and 160 mm Hg. These values may be shifted to the right with chronic hypertension. If the blood pressure fluctuates beyond these autoregulatory limits, CBF becomes pressure dependent. Stroke or cerebral edema can result from MAP greater than 160 mm Hg.

7. What are the determinants of cerebral perfusion pressure (CPP)?

$$CPP = MAP - ICP$$

If the cerebral venous pressure, estimated by the central venous pressure (CVP), is greater than the ICP, the following equation applies:

$$CPP = MAP - CVP$$

A normal CPP is 70 to 110 mm Hg. Increases in ICP greater than 30 mm Hg can compromise CPP (and CBF) despite a normal MAP. Patients with CPP values less than 50 mm Hg may show a slowing of electroencephalogram waveforms, and perfusion pressures less than 25 mm Hg may produce brain damage.

8. Identify the effects of anesthetic agents on cerebral dynamics.

The table below highlights common inhalational and intravenous anesthetic agents and their influence on cerebral physiology. Decreased neuronal metabolic demand in combination with increased CBF is associated with volatile anesthetics. These effects, called *luxury perfusion,* may be advantageous during surgical cases that increase the risk of global ischemia.

The effects of volatile agents may be less advantageous with focal ischemia. Under these conditions, vasodilation in healthy brain areas may draw blood flow away from maximally dilated ischemic areas, a process called *cerebral steal.* Hypercarbia, nitroglycerin, and nitroprusside have similar effects.

Barbiturates and hyperventilation cause vasoconstriction in normal or healthy areas of the brain. These interventions shunt blood flow to diseased areas of the brain, a process called the *Robin Hood effect* or *reverse steal.*

Effects of Anesthetic Agents on Cerebral Dynamics

Agent	CMRO$_2$	CBF	CSF Production	CSF Absorption	CBV	ICP
Intravenous Agents						
Barbiturates	↓↓↓↓	↓↓↓	±	↑	↓↓	↓↓↓
Benzodiazepines	↓↓	?	±	↑	↓	↓
Etomidate	↓↓↓	↓↓	±	↑	↓↓	↓↓
Ketamine	±	↑↑	±	↓	↑↑	↑↑
Lidocaine	↓↓	↓↓	?	?	↓↓	↓↓
Opioids	±	±	±	↑	±	±
Propofol	↓↓↓	↓↓↓	?	?	↓↓	↓↓
Inhalational Agents						
Desflurane	↓↓↓	↑	↑	↓	?	↑↑
Enflurane	↓↓	↑↑	↑	↓	↑↑	↑↑
Halothane	↓↓	↑↑↑	↓	↓	↑↑	↑↑
Isoflurane	↓↓↓	↑	±	↑	↑↑	↑
Nitrous oxide	↓	↑	±	±	±	↑
Sevoflurane	↓↓↓	↑	?	?	?	↑↑

↑ = increase; ↓ = decrease; ± = little or no change; ? = unknown.
CBF, cerebral blood flow; CBV, cerebral blood volume; CMRO$_2$, cerebral metabolic rate of oxygen consumption; CSF, cerebro spinal fluid; ICP, intracranial pressure.
From Alves SL, Yermal SJ: Assessment of the neurosurgical patient. In Waugaman WR, Foster SD, Rigor BM, editors: Principles and practice of nurse anesthesia, ed 3, Stamford, CT, 1999, Appleton & Lange.

9. **Summarize fluid management guidelines for patients undergoing neurosurgical procedures.**
   - Glucose-containing solutions should be avoided, unless specifically indicated (e.g., hypoglycemia).
   - Preoperative fluid deficits and intraoperative blood and fluid losses should be replaced with isotonic crystalloids or colloids.
   - Generally, patients with space-occupying lesions are kept "dry." A relative hypovolemic state limits cerebral edema, facilitates surgical exposure, and helps keep the ICP from increasing.

10. **Discuss the anesthetic goals for managing patients with elevated ICP or intracranial lesions or both.**

    Patients with increased ICP should be premedicated cautiously, if at all. Respiratory depression may increase the $PaCO_2$ and ICP. The anesthetic induction should be tailored to avoid further increases in ICP. The stimulus associated with intubation may be effectively blunted with thiopental, opiates, and lidocaine. Nondepolarizing muscle relaxants are often preferred for intubation because succinylcholine produces a mild and transient increase in ICP.

    Intraoperatively, fluid administration and diuretics are tailored to limit further increases in ICP. Blood pressure should be monitored continually with the aim of maintaining adequate CPP. Ventilation management is an important adjunct to any neuroanesthetic technique. Most centers aim for a $PaCO_2$ level of 25 to 30 mm Hg. The following box and the box on page 342 provide an overview of the goals of anesthesia care for patients with elevated ICP and intracranial lesions.

Methods to Decrease Intracranial Pressure

- Positioning (avoid head-down position)
- Hyperventilation (maintain $PaCO_2$ 25 to 30 mm Hg)
- Cerebrospinal fluid drainage
- Diuretics (furosemide, 0.5 to 1 mg/kg intravenously, mannitol, 0.25 to 1 g/kg intravenously)
- Corticosteroid (relieve localized cerebral edema that may develop around an intracranial tumor)
- Barbiturates

---

11. **Why does the sitting position place the neurosurgical patient at risk for venous air embolism (VAE)?**

    When pressure within an open vein or sinus is subatmospheric, air may be entrained into the venous circulation and lodge in the pulmonary circulation. If the patient has a patent foramen ovale (10% to 25% incidence), the entrained air may pass into the arterial circulation, a *paradoxical air embolism*. The presence of air in the arterial circulation potentially can result in cerebral ischemia or coronary occlusion.

> ## Maintenance of Anesthesia for Intracranial Lesion
>
> - Treatment of hypertension with a direct vasodilator (nitroglycerin or nitroprusside) may increase cerebral blood flow and intracranial pressure despite a simultaneous reduction in systemic pressure
> - Skeletal muscle paralysis is often maintained during intracranial surgery because unexpected movement may lead to increased intracranial pressure or bulging of the brain
> - Central venous pressure monitoring helps guide fluid management
> - Brainstem manipulation may exacerbate dysrhythmias
> - Urine output should be maintained at a minimal rate of 0.5 to 1 mL/kg/hr
> - Doppler transducer (placed between the second and third intercostal spaces, just to the right of the sternum) is used for detection of venous air embolism in patients at risk (e.g., sitting position, any procedure in which the operative site is above the level of the heart)
> - Initiate measures to avoid reaction to the tracheal tube during awakening

12. List the main determinants of morbidity and mortality associated with VAE.

The following are determinants of morbidity and mortality associated with VAE:
- Amount of air entrained
- Rate of air entry
- Whether the patient has a patent foramen ovale
- Preexisting cardiopulmonary function and reserve

13. List important measures to prevent intraoperative VAE.

- Employ positive-pressure ventilation.
- Ensure adequate hydration.
- Minimize head elevation.
- Employ careful surgical technique.
- Avoid nitrous oxide for procedures requiring the sitting position or in patients with known intracardiac defects.
- Avoid drugs that increase venous capacitance (e.g., nitroglycerin).
- Position central venous catheter high in the right atrium, with preparation for aspiration of entrained air.

14. Name the physiological consequences associated with VAE in the neurosurgical patient.

Cardiovascular	Respiratory	Central Nervous System
Dysrhythmias	Hypercarbia	Neurological deficits
Hypotension/hypertension	Hypoxemia	Coma
Change in heart sounds	Pulmonary hypertension	Stroke
Murmurs	Pulmonary edema	
Electrocardiogram evidence of ischemia		
Acute right ventricular failure		
Cardiac arrest		

15. What are the most sensitive monitors for detecting intraoperative VAE?

Precordial Doppler positioned over the right heart (a "roaring" sound indicates air embolism) and *two-dimensional transesophageal echocardiography* are the most sensitive monitors. Decreased end-tidal carbon dioxide (valid only if cardiac output and blood pressure remain stable) and increased pulmonary artery pressures are other important manifestations.

16. Summarize important treatment measures when VAE is detected.

- Ask the surgeon to flood the operative field with fluids, pack the wound, and apply bone wax to skull edges.
- Stop nitrous oxide, and administer 100% oxygen.
- Provide jugular vein compression to increase cerebral venous pressure temporarily and slow air entrainment.
- Aspirate the right atrial catheter in an attempt to retrieve the entrained air.
- Administer intravenous fluid vigorously to increase central venous pressure.
- Provide cardiovascular support.
- Change patient position to a left lateral position to dislodge possible cardiac air entrapment.

 Key Points

- The three physiological components of ICP are brain, blood, and CSF. Normal values range from 10 to 20 mm Hg.
- Symptoms of increased ICP include headache, vomiting, papilledema, pupillary changes, alterations in consciousness, and behavioral changes.
- The classic Cushing's triad—hypertension, bradycardia, and changes in respiration—is probably due to brainstem ischemia and indicates a severe increase in ICP.
- Severe elevations in ICP can cause decreased cerebral perfusion pressure and catastrophic herniation of the brain.
- Preventing further increases in ICP is an important goal for anesthetic induction of a patient with an elevated ICP. Hyperventilation in a conscious and cooperative patient during the preintubation phase helps reduce $Paco_2$ and ultimately decreases cerebral blood volume and ICP.
- $CMRO_2$ averages 3 to 3.5 mL/100 g tissue/min, which is approximately seven times greater than the average metabolic rate of the body.
- Normal CBF is approximately 50 mL/100 g tissue/min. Total CBF in adults averages 750 mL/min, or approximately 15% to 20% of the cardiac output.
- CBF is autoregulated between MAP values of 60 to 160 mm Hg.
- The formula for determination of CPP is:
  - CPP = MAP – ICP

Continued

Key Points   *continued*

- If the cerebral venous pressure, estimated by the CVP, is greater than the ICP, the following equation applies:
  - CPP = MAP – CVP
- With the exception of ketamine, intravenous agents decrease cerebral blood volume and ICP.
- When pressure within an open vein or sinus is subatmospheric, air may be entrained into the venous circulation and lodge in the pulmonary circulation.
- Important measures to prevent intraoperative venous air embolism are:
  - Employ positive-pressure ventilation.
  - Ensure adequate hydration.
  - Minimize head elevation.
  - Employ careful surgical technique.
  - Avoid nitrous oxide for procedures requiring the sitting position or in patients with known intracardiac defects.
  - Avoid drugs that increase venous capacitance (e.g., nitroglycerin).
  - Position central venous catheter high in the right atrium, with preparation for aspiration of entrained air.

Internet Resources

GASNet: Management of the Patient with Intracranial Hypertension:
http://www.gasnet.org/lectures/ruskin.icp/icp_files/frame.htm

Virtual-Anaesthesia Textbook:
http://www.virtual-anaesthesia-textbook.com/

Update in Anaesthesia: Neuropharmacology – Intracranial Pressure and Cerebral Blood Flow:
http://www.nda.ox.ac.uk/wfsa/html/u09/u09_019.htm

Nurse-Anesthesia.com:
http://www.nurse-anesthesia.com/

Bibliography

Aker J: Neuroanatomy, physiology, and neuroanesthesia. In Nagelhout JJ, Zaglaniczny KL, editors: *Nurse anesthesia*, ed 2, Philadelphia, 2001, WB Saunders.

Albin M: *Textbook of neuroanesthesia with neurosurgical and neuroscience perspectives,* New York, 1997, McGraw-Hill.

Alves SL, Yermal SJ: Assessment of the neurologic system in the adult. In Waugaman WR, Foster SD, Rigor BM, editors: *Principles and practice of nurse anesthesia,* ed 3, Stamford, CT, 1999, Appleton & Lange.

Cottrell JE, Smith DS: *Anesthesia and neurosurgery,* ed 3, St. Louis, 1994, Mosby-Year Book.

Cucchiara RF, Black S, Michenfelder JD: *Clinical neuroanesthesia,* ed 2, New York, 1998, Churchill Livingstone.

Morgan GE, Mikhail MS, Murray MJ: *Clinical anesthesiology,* ed 3, New York, 2002, Lange Medical Books/McGraw-Hill.

Newfield P, Cottrell JE: Handbook of neuroanesthesia, ed 3, Philadelphia, 1999, Lippincott Williams & Wilkins.

Laparoscopic Surgery

Kirstin Michelle Lawler

1. What are major benefits of laparoscopic surgery versus an open laparotomy technique?

Advantages of the laparoscopic technique include smaller abdominal incision, reduced pain, less diaphragmatic dysfunction, better postoperative pulmonary function, decreased incidence of ileus, early ambulation, shorter hospital stay, and early return to normal activities.

2. List some commonly performed laparoscopic procedures.

Some of the more commonly performed laparoscopic procedures include:
- Cholecystectomy
- Inguinal and hiatal hernia repair
- Appendectomy
- Nephrectomy
- Colectomy
- Tubal ligation
- Uterine procedures
- Thoracoscopy
- Adrenalectomy
- Vagotomy
- Diagnostic procedures

3. Name absolute and relative contraindications for laparoscopy.

Laparoscopy is *contraindicated* if a patient has a bowel obstruction, ileus, peritonitis, diaphragmatic hernia, intraperitoneal hemorrhage, or severe cardio-respiratory disease. *Relative contraindications* include advanced pregnancy (after 23 weeks' gestation), morbid obesity, inflammatory bowel disease, large abdominal mass, increased intracranial pressure, hypovolemia, ventricular shunt, and peritoneojugular shunt.

4. What pressure level is the peritoneal cavity insufflated to with laparoscopy?

Usually an intraabdominal pressure of 12 to 15 mm Hg is used to provide the desired degree of distention. Pressure should not exceed 19 mm Hg.

5. Which characteristics would make the ideal insufflating gas?

Ideally an insufflating gas would not support combustion. It would be without color or odor. It would be physiologically inactive and soluble in plasma. Nitrous oxide and oxygen have been used; however, both support combustion. Nitrogen, argon, and helium have been studied; however, because of their low blood gas solubility, venous gas embolism would be a more serious risk with these agents. Carbon dioxide (CO_2) is the most widely used insufflating gas.

6. What sudden hemodynamic change might the nurse anesthetist observe with trocar insertion, peritoneal stretching, or organ manipulation, and why?

Bradycardia or complete sinus arrest or both may occur as a result of vagal stimulation. This is usually resolved by removing the stimulus, although treatment with a vagolytic drug may be necessary.

7. How does pulmonary function change during pneumoperitoneum?

CO_2 insufflation into the peritoneal cavity causes an increase in $Paco_2$ due to the absorption of CO_2 from the peritoneal cavity. Increased $Paco_2$ reaches a plateau 10 to 30 minutes after the beginning of CO_2 insufflation in most cases. If there is an unexpected increase in $Paco_2$ after this plateau, other causes should be investigated. Decreased thoracic and lung compliance caused by general anesthesia and the supine position is exacerbated by intraperitoneal CO_2. This may lead to a decrease in functional residual capacity relative to the closing volume, and ventilation-perfusion mismatch. Peak inspiratory pressures and intrathoracic pressures increase. Impaired respiratory compliance associated with pneumoperitoneum does not seem to be clinically relevant in patients without preexisting lung disease. It is recommended that insufflation pressure be minimized in patients with pulmonary disease to help prevent postoperative complications.

8. Is end-tidal CO_2 ($ETCO_2$) an adequate monitor for predicting $Paco_2$ during laparoscopy?

In most young, healthy patients, $ETCO_2$ is a reliable monitor to predict $Paco_2$. CO_2 insufflation should not alter the $Paco_2$-$ETCO_2$ gradients significantly. It has been shown, however, that in patients with comorbidities (American Society of Anesthesiologists II-IV), $Paco_2$ does not consistently correlate with $ETCO_2$. Direct measurement of $Paco_2$ via an arterial blood sample would be more appropriate in these patients, if the CO_2 tension is in question.

9. Describe four main respiratory complications associated with intraperitoneal CO_2 insufflation.

- *Extraperitoneal insufflation of CO_2* has been described as one of the most common complications of laparoscopy (0.4% to 2%). An increase in $ETCO_2$ after plateau may suggest CO_2 subcutaneous emphysema. This increase in

$ETCO_2$ may be difficult to control by adjusting ventilation, and may require a temporary halt to surgery until CO_2 is eliminated. This complication quickly resolves after insufflation ceases and does not usually interfere with tracheal extubation after surgery.

- *Endobronchial intubation* can occur as a result of the diaphragm and carina being displaced cephalad during pneumoperitoneum. Signs of this complication include increased airway pressure and decreased oxygen saturation.
- *Gas embolism* is a rare but potentially deadly complication of laparoscopic surgery. An embolus may occur because of trocar placement into a vessel or gas insufflation into an abdominal organ. Signs of an embolus include tachycardia, arrhythmias, hypotension, increased central venous pressure, altered heart tones (millwheel murmur), cyanosis, electrocardiogram changes reflecting right heart strain, pulmonary edema, and cardiovascular collapse. If an embolus is suspected, insufflation should be stopped and the pneumoperitoneum released. The patient should be placed in the head-down, left lateral decubitus position to attenuate gas moving to the pulmonary circulation. Ventilation with 100% oxygen should be initiated. If present, central venous or pulmonary artery catheters should be aspirated for gas.
- *Pneumothorax* is another rare but life-threatening complication. This injury may be a result of diaphragmatic or pleural tears that occur during the surgery. Gas also may enter the pleural space through embryonic remnants of channels, which communicate between the peritoneal cavity and the pleural and pericardial sacs. Weaknesses in the aortic and esophageal hiatus and the diaphragm also may be entry points. Signs of a pneumothorax include increased airway pressure, hemodynamic instability, oxygen desaturation, unexpected hypoxemia, and hypercarbia. If there is no associated pulmonary trauma, the pneumothorax caused by nitrous oxide or CO_2 may resolve spontaneously in 30 to 60 minutes after exsufflation. If this is the case, thoracentesis may be avoided. If injury is a result of pulmonary trauma, or if cardiopulmonary compromise is present, immediate thoracentesis is necessary.

10. Name the main hemodynamic changes that occur with pneumoperitoneum.

Mean arterial pressure (MAP), systemic vascular resistance, left ventricular end-diastolic wall stress, central venous pressure, and pulmonary artery occlusion pressure all are increased. Cardiac index is decreased. Heart rate remains unchanged or is slightly increased.

11. Describe how pneumoperitoneum can lead to an increase in MAP.

Increased intraabdominal pressure causes an increase in intrathoracic pressure, which, along with mechanical stimulation of peritoneal receptors, causes an increased release of vasopressin. Increased vasopressin combined with direct compression of abdominal arteries leads to an increase in systemic vascular resistance and an increase in MAP.

12. How is preload affected by pneumoperitoneum?

Preload is decreased because of compression on the vena cava, pooling of blood in the legs, and increased venous resistance.

13. Are patients with cardiac disease affected adversely by a pneumoperitoneum?

The degree of cardiovascular change is similar to that occurring in patients without cardiovascular disease; however, the results of these changes can be more detrimental in patients with cardiovascular disease. Changes that may be well tolerated in a healthy adult are not as well tolerated in patients with cardiac disease.

14. Compare the effects of Trendelenburg and reverse Trendelenburg positions on cardiorespiratory function.

Trendelenburg position is often used to improve visualization by shifting abdominal contents out of the surgical field. This displacement causes the diaphragm to move cephalad, impairing pulmonary function, which may result in atelectasis and hypoxemia. Functional residual capacity, total lung volume, and diaphragmatic excursion are decreased, whereas intrathoracic pressure is increased. Cardiovascular changes include improved venous return and increase in central blood volume. The baroreceptor response to the increase in pressure may produce vasodilation and bradycardia.

Reverse Trendelenburg position is usually more favorable to pulmonary status and may attenuate the adverse ventilatory effects of the pneumoperitoneum. Cardiovascular effects are more pronounced in the head-up position. Venous return, cardiac output, and MAP decrease beyond the decreases caused by the insufflated abdomen. Venous stasis in the lower extremities also is worsened in this position.

15. How is respiratory function affected after laparoscopy?

Oxygen demand is increased, although to a lesser degree than after an open procedure. Forced expiratory volume, forced expiratory flow, and forced vital capacity are decreased by about 25% for 24 hours or more after laparoscopic cholecystectomy. Pulmonary dysfunction is less pronounced than what patients experience after an open procedure.

16. Does laparoscopic surgery place patients at a higher risk for postoperative nausea and vomiting?

Abdominal insufflation and manipulation of peritoneal contents places patients at a high risk for postoperative nausea and vomiting. Women undergoing gynecological surgery are at a particularly high risk. Prophylactic antiemetics may attenuate postoperative nausea and vomiting. Prophylactic decompression of the stomach with an oral or nasogastric tube has become common clinical practice.

17. Describe some unique aspects of postoperative pain in these patients.

Overall, postoperative pain is reduced compared with an open surgical technique. Pain associated with laparoscopy often is described as visceral, whereas pain after an open laparotomy is described as parietal. Shoulder pain is a common result of diaphragmatic irritation. Eighty percent of patients report neck and shoulder pain 24 hours after laparoscopy. Local anesthetics and nonsteroidal anti-inflammatory drugs are important adjuncts in postoperative pain management after laparoscopy.

18. List some important anesthesia considerations in caring for a pregnant patient undergoing emergency laparoscopy.

The surgery ideally should be performed before the 23rd week of pregnancy, during the second trimester for optimal surgical conditions and to minimize the risk of preterm labor. Anesthetic goals should include the following:
- Maintain fetal blood flow.
- Position the patient in a left uterine tilt.
- Avoid extreme positioning changes.
- Limit insufflation pressures to 12 mm Hg or less.
- Use continuous fetal heart rate monitoring.
- Tocolytics may be used prophylactically to stop preterm labor (use is *controversial*).
- Maintain physiological maternal alkalosis; arterial blood gas analysis may be warranted.

CONTROVERSY

19. Should nitrous oxide be omitted from anesthetics for patients undergoing laparoscopy?

The use of nitrous oxide during laparoscopic surgery is controversial. The concerns are mainly related to the potential for increased postoperative nausea and vomiting and bowel distention during surgery, which may reduce surgical access. Some studies have shown no clinical differences when the anesthetic included air or nitrous oxide. Other studies contend that bowel distention and postoperative nausea are significant when nitrous oxide is used. An additional concern is related to the use of electrocautery and laser during a laparoscopic procedure in which the concentrations of nitrous oxide in the peritoneal cavity are high enough to support combustion of bowel gases, if the bowel is perforated. A prudent approach would be to eliminate nitrous oxide from the anesthetic for these procedures if possible.

Key Points

- An intraabdominal pressure between 12 and 15 mm Hg is used to provide the desired degree of distention. Pressure should not exceed 19 mm Hg.
- Bradycardia or complete sinus arrest may occur as a result of vagal stimulation with placement of the trocar, peritoneal stretching, or organ manipulation.
- CO_2 insufflation into the peritoneal cavity causes an increase in $Paco_2$ due to the absorption of CO_2 from the peritoneal cavity.
- In most young, healthy patients $ETCO_2$ is a reliable monitor to predict $Paco_2$. CO_2 insufflation should not significantly alter the $Paco_2$-$ETCO_2$ gradients.
- Extraperitoneal insufflation of CO_2 has been described as one of the most common complications of laparoscopy (0.4% to 2%).
- Abdominal insufflation and manipulation of peritoneal contents places these patients at a high risk for postoperative nausea and vomiting. Women undergoing gynecologic surgery are at a particularly high risk.
- Shoulder pain is a common result of diaphragmatic irritation; 80% of patients report neck and shoulder pain 24 hours postlaparoscopy. Local anesthetics and nonsteroidal antiinflammatory drugs are important adjuncts in postoperative pain management after laparoscopy.

Internet Resources

GASNet: Remifentanil compared with alfentanil for ambulatory surgery using total intravenous anesthesia, Survey of Anesthesiology, October 1997:
http://www.gasnet.org/sa/1997/05/01.php

Anesthesiaweb:
www.anesthesiaweb.com

Capnography: A Comprehensive Educational Website: capnography and laparoscopy:
http://www.capnography.com/lapscopy/lapscopy.htm

Bibliography

Cunningham AJ, Mcaleese JAM: Anesthesia for laparoscopic surgery. In Barash PG, Cullen BF, Stoelting RK, editors: *Clinical anesthesia*, ed 3, Philadelphia, 1997, Lippincott Williams & Wilkins, pp 991-999.

Gainer VG, Wong HV: Anesthesia for laparoscopic surgery. In Nagelhout JJ, Zaglaniczny KL, editors: *Nurse anesthesia*, ed 2, Philadelphia, 2001, WB Saunders, pp 705-714.

Joris JL: Anesthesia for laparoscopic surgery. In Miller RD, editor: *Anesthesia*, vol 2, ed 5, Philadelphia, 2000, Churchill Livingstone, pp 2003-2023.

Joshi GP: Complications related to abdominal surgery with an emphasis on laparoscopy. In Benumof JL, Saidman LJ, editors: *Anesthesia and perioperative complications,* ed 2, St. Louis, 1999, Mosby, pp 665-684.

Morgan GE, Mikhail MS, Murray MJ: Anesthesia for patients with respiratory disease. In: *Clinical anesthesiology,* ed 3, Stamford, CT, 2002, Appleton & Lange, pp 511-524.

Rauh R, et al: Influence of pneumoperitoneum and patient positioning on respiratory system compliance, *J Clin Anesth* 13:361-365, 2001.

Anesthetic Considerations for Select Patient Groups

Obstetrics and Anesthesia

Donna Jean Funke

1. What causes anemia in pregnancy?

An increase in maternal intravascular fluid volume begins in the first trimester and results in an average expansion of about 1000 to1500 mL at term. The plasma volume increases 45% to 50%, whereas the red blood cell volume increases by only 15% to 20%. This disproportionate increase in plasma volume accounts for the relative dilutional anemia of pregnancy. It takes about 8 weeks after delivery for the blood volume to return to normal. A hemoglobin level less than 11 g/dL or hematocrit less than 33% usually represents anemia secondary to iron deficiency.

2. What is the average blood loss with delivery?

The increased vascular volume offsets the 400- to 600-mL blood loss that accompanies vaginal delivery and the average 1000 mL blood loss that accompanies cesarean section. Normally, blood loss at delivery is well tolerated.

3. What would a high hemoglobin level in pregnancy indicate?

A hemoglobin level greater than 14 g/dL may indicate a low-volume state caused by preeclampsia, hypertension, or inappropriate diuretics.

4. How does cardiac output change in the parturient?

Cardiac output increases, the result of increased stroke volume. By 28 to 32 weeks' gestation, the heart rate also increases 10 to 15 beats per minute.

5. During labor, when does the largest increase in cardiac output occur?

The largest increase in cardiac output occurs immediately after delivery (see the table on page 358). Typically, cardiac output, heart rate, and stroke volume return to nonpregnant levels within 2 weeks after delivery.

6. Why is maternal hypotension a concern?

Maternal systolic blood pressure less than 90 to 95 mm Hg is a concern because it may be associated with a decrease in uterine blood flow. Even in the presence of a healthy uteroplacental unit, decreases in maternal systolic blood pressure to

Cardiac Output During Labor	
Labor Stage	**Cardiac Output Changes**
Latent phase	Increases 15%
Active phase	Increases 30%
Second stage	Increases 45%
Postpartum	Increases 80%

less than than 100 mm Hg for longer than 10 to 15 minutes may be associated with progressive fetal acidosis and bradycardia.

7. Define supine hypotension syndrome.

When the parturient assumes the supine position, compression of the inferior vena cava by the gravid uterus decreases venous return, resulting in decreased cardiac output and hypotension. Nausea, vomiting, diaphoresis, and changes in cerebration may accompany this syndrome. The gravid uterus also may compress the lower abdominal aorta, leading to arterial hypotension in the lower extremities and decreases in uteroplacental perfusion. This arterial hypotension may occur despite a "normal" blood pressure measured in the arm.

8. Describe the treatment for supine hypotension syndrome and aortocaval compression.

Prevention is preferred to treatment. The gravida at term should be encouraged to assume a lateral position. Alternatively, left uterine displacement in the supine position is effective by moving the gravid uterus off the inferior vena cava or aorta. Displacement of the uterus to the left can be accomplished manually or by elevation of the right hip 10 to 15 cm, with a blanket or foam rubber wedge. Alternatively, tipping the operating or delivery table 15 degrees to the left is effective. Drugs causing vasodilation or techniques causing sympathetic blockade further decrease venous return to the heart in the presence of vena caval obstruction.

9. Discuss typical upper airway findings in the parturient.

Capillary engorgement of the mucosa causes swelling of the nasal and oral pharynx, larynx, and trachea. As a result, the parturient may have nasal congestion and voice changes. Manipulation of the upper airway requires special care. Aggressive suctioning or placement of airways and careless laryngoscopy may result in trauma and bleeding. The nasal airway is especially prone to causing epistaxis. When endotracheal intubation is performed, a smaller sized, 6.5-to-7.0 mm, cuffed, oral tube is required because swelling of the false vocal cords often decreases the glottic opening.

10. How is the patient's minute ventilation affected by pregnancy?

Minute ventilation is increased by 50% above nonpregnant levels at term, primarily the result of increased tidal volume. Progesterone sensitizes the respiratory center to carbon dioxide. Ventilatory augmentation produces a respiratory alkalosis with compensatory renal excretion of bicarbonate and partial pH correction.

11. What happens to the functional residual capacity (FRC) during pregnancy?

With enlargement of the uterus, the diaphragm is forced cephalad, decreasing the FRC. FRC is decreased further with supine, lithotomy, and Trendelenburg positions and with obesity. The reduced FRC, in conjunction with the increased oxygen consumption associated with pregnancy, can lead to a precipitous decline in Pao_2, especially during periods of apnea. Supplemental oxygen during labor and an increased fraction of inspired oxygen during general anesthesia are prudent.

12. Is inhalational agent uptake affected by pregnancy?

The combination of increased minute ventilation and decreased FRC increases the rate at which changes in alveolar concentrations of inhaled anesthetics can be achieved. Induction, emergence, and changes in depth of anesthesia are faster in parturients.

13. Can one type of anesthetic decrease oxygen consumption by the parturient more than another?

Oxygen consumption increases by about 20% during pregnancy, in response to demand by the growing conceptus and maternal tissues. During labor, oxygen consumption can increase by an additional 100% because of increased cardiorespiratory work. Regional analgesia during the first and second stages of labor eliminates this additional increase in oxygen consumption.

14. What happens to the oxyhemoglobin dissociation curve during pregnancy?

The oxyhemoglobin dissociation curve shifts to the right, with P50 values increasing from 26 to 30 mm Hg by term; this facilitates oxygen unloading to the fetus.

15. Why are parturients at risk for aspiration?

The enlarging uterus changes the angle of the gastroesophageal junction, leading to relative incompetence of the physiological sphincter mechanism. Progesterone also decreases gastrointestinal motility.

Parturients are vulnerable to regurgitation of gastric contents (Mendelson's syndrome). Maternal "bearing down" efforts and the lithotomy position during the second stage of labor and delivery make silent regurgitation a threat. Opioids, diazepam (Valium), and atropine all decrease lower esophageal sphincter tone and prolong gastric emptying time.

16. Discuss what can be done to prevent pulmonary aspiration.

Pregnant patients should always be considered to have a "full stomach" regardless of the time of their last meal. Use of the nonparticulate antacid, sodium citrate (30 mL, 0.3 Mol/L) is recommended. Metoclopramide (10 mg) or an H_2 receptor blocker is often administered before regional or general anesthesia. A rapid-sequence induction technique is required for general anesthesia. The mechanical effects of a gravid uterus on the stomach are resolved in a few days postpartum; the other gastrointestinal changes revert back to nonpregnant states within 6 weeks postpartum.

17. Why is the parturient at risk for deep venous thrombosis?

The blood of the parturient is "hypercoagulable." Plasma levels of platelets; the clotting factors, VII, VIII, IX, and X; and thrombin are increased. This "hypercoagulable state" is beneficial in limiting blood loss at delivery, but it places the parturient at risk for thromboembolic complications.

18. Does the decrease in plasma cholinesterase (pseudocholinesterase) activity affect anesthesia care?

Plasma cholinestererase levels decrease from the 10th week of gestation to 6 weeks postpartum. There may be prolongation of the neuromuscular blocking effects of succinylcholine or mivacurium in postpartum, but not term, pregnant patients. This prolongation may be related to the larger volume available for drug distribution in pregnancy, which may offset decreased hydrolysis of the drug. Practitioners are advised to use a peripheral nerve stimulator to guide neuromuscular blockade.

19. How does progesterone affect the central nervous system?

Progesterone has a sedative effect on the mother. There is an increase in the parturient's sensitivity to inhalational anesthetic agents. Anesthesia requirements for inhalational agents in the postpartum period return to normal in 3 to 5 days.

20. Are the required doses of local anesthetic agents for spinal and epidural anesthesia different in the parturient?

A wider dermatomal spread of sensory anesthesia is observed in parturients after epidural anesthesia. This may be explained by the following:
- Swelling of the epidural veins, which decreases the volume of cerebrospinal fluid in the vertebral column
- Labor-induced increases in cerebrospinal fluid pressure
- Increased neurosensitivity to local anesthetics

The anesthetist should reduce doses of local anesthetics in the pregnant patient by 30% to 50%. There may be increased sensitivity to local anesthetics for epidural or spinal anesthesia 36 hours postpartum.

21. Name a common neurological dysfunction in the postpartum period.

Backache is a frequent complaint in parturients; the incidence is not altered by regional anesthesia.

22. On what does the integrity of the uteroplacental circulation depend?

Uterine blood flow $=$ [uterine arterial pressure − uterine venous pressure] ÷ uterine vascular resistance

The integrity of the uteroplacental circulation depends on adequate uterine blood flow and normal placental function. At term, uterine blood flow represents 10% of the cardiac output, or 700 mL/min (compared with 50 mL/min in the nonpregnant uterus). At least 80% of the uterine blood flow normally supplies the placenta, and the remainder goes to the myometrium.

23. What are major factors that decrease uterine blood flow during pregnancy?

Pregnancy maximally dilates uterine vessels, so autoregulation is absent. Any condition that decreases mean maternal arterial pressure or increases uterine vascular resistance decreases uterine blood flow. Hypotension, vasoconstriction, and uterine contractions are the major factors that decrease uterine blood flow (see the following table).

Factors That Decrease Uterine Blood Flow		
Decrease Uterine Arterial Pressure	**Increase Uterine Arterial Resistance**	**Increase Uterine Venous Pressure**
Hypovolemia/hemorrhage	Catecholamines (stress)	Uterine contractions; drug-induced hypertonus (oxytocin)
Hypotension induced by drugs or sympathetic blockade	Vasopressors (phenylephrine)	Skeletal muscle hypertonus (seizures)
Aortocaval compression	Severe hypocapnea ($Paco_2$ <20 mm Hg)	Vena caval compression

24. What is an appropriate drug to treat sustained hypotension in a parturient patient?

Ephedrine is the vasopressor of choice for hypotension during pregnancy because it increases the blood pressure by inotropic and chronotropic effects on the heart, without decreasing uterine blood flow. The uterine muscle has alpha and beta receptors. Alpha$_1$ receptor stimulation causes uterine contraction. Beta$_2$ receptor stimulation produces relaxation. Maternal release of catecholamines or administration of an alpha-adrenergic agonist drug (mephentermine, metaraminol, methoxamine) increases blood pressure, but may paradoxically reduce uterine blood flow because of the associated uterine contraction. Low-dose phenylephrine (40 mcg intravenous boluses) may be an acceptable alternative to ephedrine if tachycardia is contraindicated.

25. Define the determinants of diffusion across the placenta.

Although the placenta acts as a barrier to the passage of drugs, nonionized, fat-soluble, low-molecular-weight drugs may be transferred rapidly from the mother to the fetus. Minimizing the maternal blood concentration of a drug is the most important method of limiting the amount that ultimately reaches the fetus. Transfer to the fetus can be decreased by intravenous injection of a drug during uterine contraction because maternal blood flow to the placenta is markedly decreased at this time.

26. Define ion-trapping.

Fetal uptake of a substance that crosses the placenta may be facilitated by the lower pH of fetal compared with maternal blood. The lower fetal pH means that weakly basic drugs (local anesthetics, opioids) that cross the placenta in the nonionized form become ionized in the fetal circulation. Because an ionized drug cannot readily cross the placenta back to the maternal circulation, this drug accumulates in the fetal blood.

27. Describe fetal oxygen balance.

Fetal oxygen transfer depends on the oxygen affinity and the oxygen-carrying capacity of maternal and fetal blood. To aid oxygen transfer, the fetal hemoglobin dissociation curve shifts to the left, producing a greater fetal hemoglobin affinity for oxygen compared with maternal hemoglobin. Additionally, fetal hemoglobin concentration is usually 15 g/dL compared with 12 g/dL in the mother. The higher oxygen affinity and the higher oxygen-carrying capacity of fetal blood benefits the fetus.

28. Summarize mechanisms that can produce fetal acidosis during maternal hyperventilation.

The figure on page 363 summarizes the mechanisms that can produce fetal acidosis.

29. What is the most serious fetal risk associated with maternal surgery during pregnancy?

Intrauterine asphyxia is the most serious fetal risk. Potential causes of fetal oxygen deprivation include maternal hypotension, maternal hypoxemia, umbilical cord compression, umbilical cord prolapse, and placental abruption.

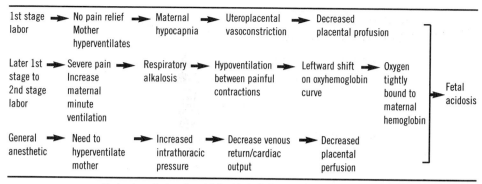

Mechanisms that produce fetal acidosis during maternal hyperventilation.

30. Describe the effects of inhalational agents on the fetus.

The volatile halogenated anesthetic agents can directly depress the *fetal cardio-vascular system and central nervous system.* Volatile agents may indirectly affect the fetus by producing maternal hypotension, which may decrease uterine blood flow and lead to fetal asphyxia.

Nitrous oxide specifically may have adverse effects on DNA synthesis. This proposed effect is controversial, but as a precaution, many practitioners avoid nitrous oxide administration to mothers during the first two trimesters of pregnancy.

31. Why are beta-receptor agonists used to treat premature labor?

Stimulation of beta$_2$-adrenergic receptors causes relaxation of uterine smooth muscle, arresting premature labor (tocolysis). Side effects of beta-adrenergic agonists include hypokalemia and hyperglycemia. Potassium is redistributed from the extracellular to the intracellular compartments. Beta-adrenergic stimulation increases blood glucose and insulin levels. Beta$_1$-adrenergic stimulation causes an increase in myocardial oxygen demand, contractility, and heart rate. Premature ventricular contractions and palpitations are common with use of these agents. The administration of beta agonists results in down-regulation of beta receptors over time, resulting in decreased tocolytic effect during long-term therapy. Ritodrine (Yutopar) is approved by the U.S. Food and Drug Administration for inhibition of preterm labor.

Ritodrine, a selective beta$_2$ agonist, has the following properties:
- Ritodrine increases maternal heart rate by about 40 beats/min.
- Systolic blood pressure increases, and diastolic blood pressure decreases.
- The manufacturer recommends no more than 2 L of fluid over 24 hours because of the potential for pulmonary edema.

32. What are the effects of magnesium sulfate?

Magnesium causes relaxation of vascular, bronchial, and uterine smooth muscle by altering calcium transport and availability. Motor end-plate sensitivity and muscle membrane excitability also are depressed. Magnesium sulfate is used to treat *preterm labor* and *preeclampsia* (pregnancy-induced hypertension).

Intravenous dosaging for preeclampsia or preterm labor is as follows:
- Loading dose is 4 to 8 g over 20 minutes followed by 1 to 2 g/hr.
- Serum levels of 4 to 8 mEq/L are required for tocolytic effects.

Levels need to be monitored to avoid toxic doses, which are dose dependent. Hypermagnesemia is associated with skeletal muscle weakness, hyporeflexia, central nervous system depression, and vasodilation (see the following table). Treatment involves discontinuation of magnesium, administration of calcium (calcium gluconate 10%, 1 to 10 mL intravenously, infused slowly), diuresis, and cardiovascular and airway support.

Effects of Hypermagnesemia

9 mEq/L	10 mEq/L	15 mEq/L	>25 mEq/L
Increased P-R interval Widened QRS	Lose deep tendon reflexes	Respiratory depression/ paralysis, Atrioventricular block	Cardiac arrest

33. Discuss common uterotonic agents.

Oxytocin (Pitocin) is a synthetic preparation that selectively acts on the smooth muscle cells of the uterus to increase uterine muscle tone and the frequency of contractions. It is commonly used to induce or augment labor and to prevent postpartum hemorrhage. To avoid hypotension, a dilute intravenous mixture (2 units per 100 mL of solution) is recommended. In large doses, pitocin has been shown to exhibit an antidiuretic effect.

Ergot alkaloids are considered the drug of choice when oxytocin fails to produce adequate uterine contraction. Uterine tone is increased through direct alpha adrenergic stimulation. Ergonovine maleate (Ergotrate) and methylergonovine maleate (Methergine) may precipitate maternal hypertension by causing direct peripheral vasoconstriction. Administer intramuscularly or very slowly intravenously.

Prostaglandins (prostaglandin $F_{2\alpha}$) are used if uterine contraction is not effective after oxytocin or ergot alkaloids. Smooth muscle constriction may produce hypertension, bronchoconstriction, and pulmonary vasoconstriction. A common choice is carboprost tromethamine (Hemabate), 250 mcg intramuscularly.

34. Provide a brief overview of fetal heart rate (FHR) patterns.

- FHR patterns are examined at baseline between contractions and in association with uterine contractions.

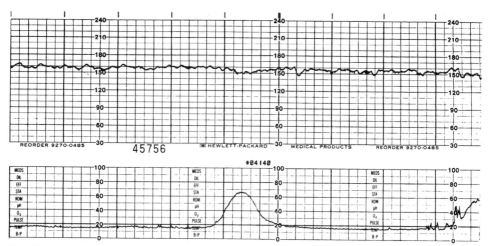

Normal beat-to-beat and long-term variability with a fetal heart rate (FHR) of 150 to 160 beats/min. The distance between the heavy vertical lines represents 60 seconds. The lighter vertical lines are 10 seconds apart. The top graph is the FHR tracing; the bottom is intrauterine pressure. The rise in the bottom graph under the time stamp *04:40 is a uterine contraction. FHR and uterine pressure are measured directly.

- Normal FHR is 110 to 160 beats/min between contractions. FHR greater than 160 beats/min in a term fetus is tachycardia.
- FHR less than 110 beats/min in a term fetus is bradycardia.
- FHR variability is one of the most important parameters for the recognition of intrauterine fetal well-being, an intact central nervous system regulatory mechanism, and good fetal reserve. Beat-to-beat FHR variability refers to the small changes in rate from one beat to the next. Long-term variability is the short-lived acceleration of FHR in response to fetal movement or other uterine stimuli. A normal FHR varies 5 to 20 beats/min at baseline. The figure above shows normal beat-to-beat and long-term variability in heart rate (irregular graph pattern).

Causes of FHR patterns are as follows:

Fetal Tachycardia	Fetal Bradycardia	Fetal Heart Rate Acceleration or Deceleration
Prematurity (decreased parasympathetic nervous system activity near term)	Fetal heart block	Post paracervical block
	Fetal asphyxia	Maternal administered drugs (beta blockers)
	Postterm pregnancy	
Mild fetal hypoxia	Decreased maternal oxygen	Hypothermia
Fetal anemia	Umbilical cord compression	Acute maternal hypotension
Maternal fever		Decreased uterine blood flow (hypertonus)
Maternal administered drugs (terbutaline, ephedrine)		Decreased umbilical blood flow (cord compression, cord prolapse)

35. Describe early, late, and variable FHR decelerations.

EARLY DECELERATIONS

Early decelerations (see the figure below) begin when the contraction begins, and they return to baseline when the contraction ends—a mirror image. Maximal FHR slowing occurs at the peak intensity of the contraction. Heart rate change is usually no more than 20 beats/min. Early decelerations usually do not signal fetal distress. Causes include vagal stimulation, fetal head compression with increased intracranial pressure (parturient pushing too early against an insufficiently dilated cervix), and increased volume of blood entering the fetal circulation during contractions triggering the baroreceptor reflex. Treatment is with atropine if necessary.

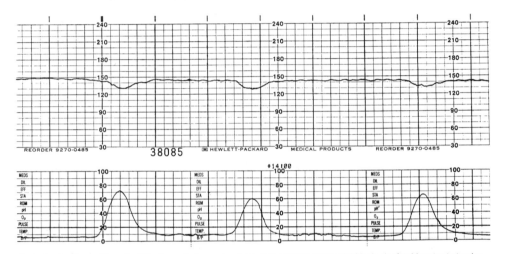

Early decelerations with each of the three uterine contractions. Note also the poor variability in the fetal heart rate tracing.

LATE DECELERATIONS

Late decelerations (see the figure on page 367) are characterized by a delay (10 to 30 sec) between the onset of the uterine contraction and the beginning of FHR slowing. The peak of FHR deceleration occurs after uterine contraction. The onset and return are gradual and smooth. Late decelerations signal fetal compromise. They are classified as *severe* if the FHR decreases by more than 45 beats/min. Causes include maternal hypotension (reduced uterine blood flow), fetal hypoxia, and fetal acidosis. Treatment involves improving maternal and fetal placental blood flows and instituting maternal hyperoxia. Immediate delivery may be needed.

VARIABLE DECELERATIONS

Variable decelerations (see the figure on page 367) are the most common of all FHR patterns. They are variable in appearance, duration, depth, and shape. Generally, they are abrupt in onset and recovery. This pattern is often benign, indicating that the fetus is responding to stress. Variable decelerations are classified as *severe* and associated with fetal asphyxia if the FHR decreases by

60 beats/min or if they last 60 seconds or longer. Causes include umbilical cord compression, first stage of labor, and substantial head compression during maternal voluntary expulsive efforts late in the second stage of labor.

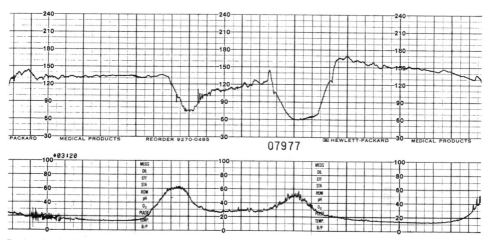

Two late decelerations in a woman with a placental abruption. The first deceleration is significant even though it is only 10 beats/min. Any late deceleration is a poor sign. Note the poor variability indicating that the fetus is already decompensated.

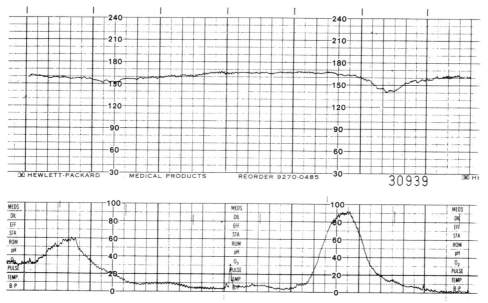

Two variable decelerations on a baseline of poor long-term variability. The first deceleration recovers slowly, probably indicating fetal decompensation. Before recovery is complete, a second uterine contraction occurs, prompting another variable decleration. This second deceleration meets any criteria for severity. The FHR drops more than 60 beats/min, the FHR decreases to a rate of 60 beats/min, and the deceleration persists for greater than 60 seconds. The first uterine contraction did not relax to baseline before the second one began. The irregularity of the uterine pressure graft is artifact.

36. Describe the stages of labor.

Progress of labor refers to increasing cervical dilation, effacement, and descent of the fetal presenting part through the vagina with time.

FIRST STAGE
The first stage begins with the onset of regular contractions and concludes when the cervix is fully dilated. This stage is subdivided into the *latent* and *active* phases, lasting 7 to 13 hours in the primigravida and 4 to 5 hours in the multigravida. The latent phase is a preparatory phase of labor, during which, despite regular contractions, there is little cervical dilation. The contractions cause softening and thinning (or effacement) of the cervix. The active phase is characterized by rapid changes in cervical dilation.

SECOND STAGE
The second stage begins with complete dilation of the cervix until delivery of the fetus. This stage usually lasts less than 2 hours.

THIRD STAGE
The third stage extends from delivery of the infant until the placenta is expelled, typically taking 15 to 30 minutes.

37. Differentiate between visceral and somatic pain; how does pain change during labor?

Childbirth is associated with two distinct kinds of pain, visceral and somatic. *Visceral pain* is caused by uterine contractions and dilation of the cervix. *Somatic pain* is due to stretching of the vagina and perineum by descent of the fetus.
- *First stage:* Afferent visceral pain impulses from the uterus and cervix travel in nerves that enter the spinal cord at T10-L1 (see the figure on page 369).
- *Late first stage and second stage:* Somatic pain impulses from stretching of the vagina and the distention and tearing of the perineum travel via the pudendal nerves to the spinal cord at S2-4.

38. List the advantages of regional analgesia in the parturient.

Advantages of regional analgesia include the following:
- Ability to achieve segmental bands of analgesia during labor, reducing levels of catecholamines in the maternal circulation
- Unlikely to produce drug-induced depression in the fetus or mother
- Avoids the risks of general anesthesia (aspiration, failed intubation); maternal airway reflexes remain intact
- Means to provide surgical anesthesia if necessary
- Mother remains awake and can react to her newborn early in the postpartum period

39. What are the advantages of a caudal block?

A caudal block is produced by injection of local anesthetic solution into the lowest part of the epidural space that lies in the sacral canal. Compared with

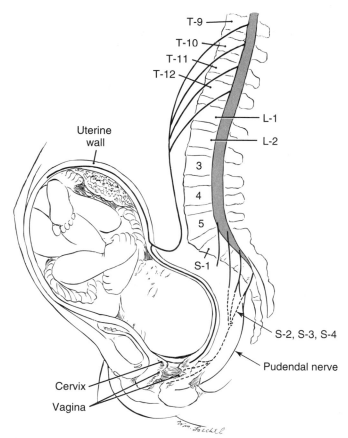

Lower thoracic, lumbar, and sacral regions of the spine showing spinal cord, nerve roots, and sensory innervation to the uterus, cervix, and vagina.

continuous lumbar epidural analgesia, there is a lower incidence of inadvertent dural puncture, and perineal analgesia is profound.

40. What are the disadvantages of a caudal block?

Difficulties associated with the caudal technique include identifying the sacral hiatus and keeping the sacral area clean. The technique nearly always blocks the sacral spinal cord, which may inhibit rotation of the fetal head and delay the second stage of labor. The biggest concern is accidental injection of local anesthetic solution into the fetal head.

41. What are the advantages of a paracervical block?

A paracervical block is performed by the obstetrician. It involves injection of a local anesthetic, usually via the transvaginal approach, into the mucosa of the cervicouterine junction. Fibers of the T10, T11, and L1 nerves are blocked, providing pain relief for the first stage of labor. A paracervical block eliminates visceral pain by anesthetizing the sensory fibers from the uterus, cervix, and upper vagina. Somatic pain and the urge to bear down are not affected. Maternal sympathetic nervous system blockade does not occur.

42. What are the disadvantages of a paracervical block?

Anesthesia from the paracervical block is not effective during the second stage of labor because sensory fibers from the perineum are not blocked. Additionally, there is a high incidence of fetal bradycardia that develops 2 to 10 minutes after injection of the local anesthetic, lasting 3 to 30 minutes. Bradycardia produced by paracervical block is often associated with decreased fetal oxygenation and fetal acidosis.

43. Describe anesthesia obtained from a pudendal nerve block.

A pudendal block may be performed by the obstetrician during the second stage of labor or just before delivery. In combination with perineal infiltration of local anesthetic, this block provides anesthesia to the perineum. It can be performed by either the perineal or the transvaginal route with the patient placed in the lithotomy position.

44. What is the most common regional block for labor analgesia?

A *lumbar epidural regional technique* most commonly is performed for labor analgesia. A lumbar epidural catheter usually is placed when the patient is in established labor. If augmentation with oxytocin is anticipated, the block can be started earlier. Dilute local anesthetic or opioid solutions or both are used to provide adequate analgesia, while minimizing marked motor blockade, which can contribute to malposition and inadequate expulsive efforts. Low doses of local anesthetics or opioids are often sufficient during the first part of labor to provide an effective T10-L1 segmental block. As labor progresses, anesthetic doses may be increased to cover the increased pain of the late first and second stages of labor and the distribution of the pudendal nerve (S2-4). The first stage of labor usually is not prolonged by the administration of epidural anesthesia. The second stage of labor may be prolonged by 20 to 40 minutes.

45. Review obstetrical epidural local anesthetics.

The table on page 371 summarizes obstetrical epidural local anesthetics.

46. Discuss important considerations for regional anesthesia for cesarean section.

- Regional anesthetic (lumbar epidural or spinal) is often chosen for elective cesarean section, particularly when maternal awareness is desirable. A regional anesthetic minimizes newborn depression, and avoids the risks of general anesthesia (aspiration, failed intubation).

Obstetrical Epidural Local Anesthetics

Anesthetic	Description	Concern
Bupivacaine	Commonly used local anesthetic for labor analgesia because of high-quality analgesia with minimal motor blockade; relatively long duration of action and lack of tachyphylaxis; highly protein bound and placental passage low	Cardiotoxicity; bupivacaine toxicity from accidental intravascular injection has been associated with cardiac arrest resulting in difficult resuscitation or death.
Lidocaine (Xylocaine)	Commonly used for cesarean delivery because of its quick onset (5 min) and shorter duration (60 min/plain; 75 min/epidural)	Higher placental transfer; possible neurotoxic damage to the mother (cauda equina syndrome)
Chloroprocaine	Short plasma half-life (rapid breakdown by plasma pseudocholinesterase) with little drug crossing the placenta. Quick onset (4-6 min), short duration (30-60 min); may require repetitive dosing	Antagonism of injected epidural opioids and bupivacaine; the rapid onset of the block may be associated with a higher incidence of hypotension; earlier preparations contained preservatives that prevented decomposition, but led to neurotoxicity and complaints of back pain
Ropivacaine (Naropin)	Amide local anesthetic; less potent than bupivacaine with cardiotoxicity intermediate between lidocaine and bupivacaine; may get a selective nonmotor block during labor and delivery	
Levobupivacaine (Chirocaine)	Reduced cardiotoxicity compared with ropivacaine; slow onset of action, prolonged duration of anesthesia and inferior sensory blockade compared with bupivacaine	

- A sensory level of T4 is desirable for a cesarean section, although an awake parturient may experience some discomfort with exteriorization of the uterus and traction on the abdominal viscera at this level.
- Epidural anesthesia for cesarean section requires large doses of local anesthetics, which may cross the placenta and potentially affect the fetus. The anesthesia provider must ensure proper catheter placement with a test dose before administering a full local anesthetic dose.
- Administer a nonparticulate oral antacid (sodium citrate, 15 to 30 mL) within 1 hour of the procedure.

- Administer intravenous dextrose-free balanced salt solution immediately before the regional technique (at least 500 mL for an epidural anesthetic and 1000 to 2000 mL for a spinal anesthetic).
- Administer supplemental oxygen to the mother.
- After regional block placement, position the mother with left uterine displacement.
- Compare maternal blood pressure and FHR with baseline. Prepare to treat hypotension with additional volume expansion and 5 to 10 mg of ephedrine as needed.

47. What should be done if the regional block fails?

If the sensory block is not satisfactory, supplemental analgesia can be achieved safely by incremental administration of low-dose opioids or ketamine (0.1 to 0.25 mg/kg) or inhaled nitrous oxide in oxygen. It is paramount that maternal laryngeal reflexes remain intact. General anesthesia and endotracheal intubation may be required.

48. Summarize important considerations for general anesthesia for cesarean section.

- Evaluate the airway in advance. If difficulties are anticipated, consider an awake oral fiberoptic tracheal intubation. Review the algorithm on page 373 for management of the difficult airway.
- Administer a nonparticulate oral antacid (sodium citrate 15 to 30 mL) within 1 hour of induction.
- Place the mother in left uterine displacement.
- Preoxygenate the mother for 3 to 5 minutes or substitute with four or five deep breaths, with a well-fitting mask.
- Administer cricoid pressure and initiate a rapid-sequence induction (e.g., thiopental sodium, 3 to 4 mg/kg intravenously, followed by succinylcholine, 80 to 100 mg intravenously). A defasciculating muscle relaxant drug need not be administered because increased progesterone levels seem to prevent fasciculations. If succinylcholine cannot be used, rocuronium, 0.6 mg/kg, may be substituted.
- Inability to intubate the trachea and provide effective ventilation of the lungs is the leading cause of maternal death related to anesthesia.
- When endotracheal tube placement is confirmed by capnography, the obstetrician may proceed with the skin incision. In the predelivery interval, anesthesia may be maintained with 50% nitrous oxide and 50% oxygen at high flow rates, with 0.5 minimal alveolar concentration of halogenated agent. The small dose of volatile anesthetic decreases the likelihood of maternal awareness and does not increase maternal blood loss. A few minutes before delivery is anticipated, the concentration of volatile anesthetic may be increased to provide uterine relaxation.
- Avoid maternal hyperventilation because it may decrease uterine blood flow.
- After cutting of the cord, a narcotic and an amnestic can be used to deepen the anesthesia.
- Extubate only when the patient is fully awake and able to protect the airway.

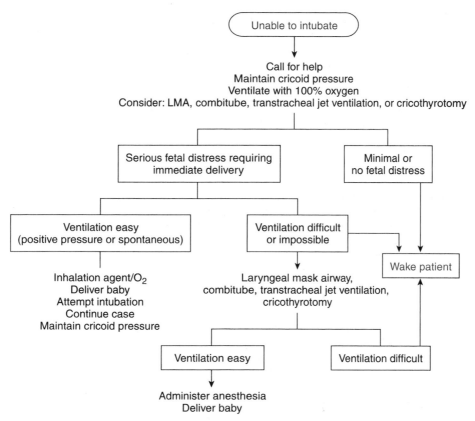

Algorithm for management of the difficult intubation.

Key Points

- A disproportionate increase in plasma volume accounts for the relative dilutional anemia of pregnancy.
- A hemoglobin level less than 11 g/dL or hematocrit less than 33% usually represents anemia secondary to iron deficiency.
- An average of 400 to 600 mL of blood is lost during vaginal delivery, and an average of 1000 mL is lost during a cesarean section.
- A hemoglobin level greater than 14 g/dL may indicate a low-volume state in the parturient caused by preeclampsia, hypertension, or inappropriate diuretics.
- To avoid supine hypotension syndrome and aortocaval compression, left uterine displacement in the supine position is effective by moving the gravid uterus off the inferior vena cava or aorta.
- Capillary engorgement of the mucosa causes swelling of the nasal and oral pharynx, larynx, and trachea, increasing the risk for bleeding when manipulating the airway of the parturient.

Continued

Key Points   *continued*

- With enlargement of the uterus, the diaphragm is forced cephalad, decreasing the FRC. FRC is decreased further with supine, lithotomy, and Trendelenburg positions and obesity.

- The oxyhemoglobin dissociation curve shifts to the right, with P50 values increasing from 26 to 30 mm Hg by term; this facilitates oxygen unloading to the fetus.

- A rapid-sequence induction technique is required for general anesthesia in a pregnant patient.

- The blood of the parturient is "hypercoagulable," placing the parturient at risk for thromboembolic complications.

- Plasma cholinestererase levels decrease from 10 weeks of gestation to 6 weeks postpartum. There may be prolongation of the neuromuscular blocking effects of succinylcholine or mivacurium in postpartum, but not term, pregnant patients.

- Ephedrine is the vasopressor of choice for hypotension during pregnancy because it increases the blood pressure by inotropic and chronotropic effects on the heart, without decreasing uterine blood flow.

- Nonionized, fat-soluble, low-molecular-weight drugs may be transferred rapidly from the mother to the fetus.

- Common uterotonic agents are oxytocin, ergotrate, methergine, and prostaglandins.

- Visceral pain is caused by uterine contractions and dilation of the cervix. Somatic pain is due to stretching of the vagina and perineum by descent of the fetus.

- Fibers of the T10, T11, and L1 nerves are blocked with a paracervical block, providing pain relief for the first stage of labor. A paracervical block eliminates visceral pain by anesthetizing the sensory fibers from the uterus, cervix, and upper vagina.

- A pudendal block provides anesthesia to the perineum.

- A lumbar epidural regional technique is most commonly performed for labor analgesia.

- Important considerations for regional anesthesia for cesarean section are:
  - A regional anesthetic minimizes newborn depression and avoids the risks of general anesthesia (aspiration, failed intubation)
  - A sensory level of T4 is desirable for a cesarean section
  - Epidural anesthesia for cesarean section requires large doses of local anesthetics, which may cross the placenta and potentially affect the fetus
  - Administer intravenous dextrose-free balanced salt solution immediately before the regional technique
  - Administer supplemental oxygen to the mother
  - After regional block placement, position the mother with left uterine displacement

- Important considerations for general anesthesia for cesarean section are:
  - Evaluate the airway in advance
  - Administer a nonparticulate oral antacid within 1 hour of induction
  - Place the mother in left uterine displacement

Key Points *continued*

- Preoxygenate the mother for 3 to 5 minutes or substitute with four or five deep breaths, with a well-fitting mask
- Administer cricoid pressure, and initiate a rapid sequence induction
- Inability to intubate the trachea and provide effective ventilation of the lungs is the leading cause of maternal death related to anesthesia
- When endotracheal tube placement is confirmed by capnography, the obstetrician may proceed with the skin incision
- Avoid maternal hyperventilation because it may decrease uterine blood flow
- After cutting of the cord, a narcotic and an amnestic can be used to deepen the anesthesia
- Extubate only when the patient is fully awake and able to protect her airway

Internet Resources

The Virtual Anesthesiologist: Anesthesia for Obstetrics:
http://www.anesthesiology.de/Links/Anesthesia_for_Obstetrics/anesthesia_for_obstetrics.htm

Hypertextbook of Regional Anaesthesia for Obstetrics:
http://www.manbit.com/oa/oaindex.htm

Nurse-Anesthesia.com:
http://www.nurse-anesthesia.com/

Update in Anesthesia: Cumulative index arranged by issue:
http://www.nda.ox.ac.uk/wfsa/html/pages/up_issu.htm

Anesthesiaweb:
http://www.anesthesiaweb.com/
http://www.csen.com/anesthesia/index5.htm
http://www.vh.org/adult/provider/anesthesia/obanesthesia/
http://www.virtual-anaesthesia-textbook.com/

Bibliography

American Association of Nurse Anesthetists: *Guidelines for the management of the obstetrical patient for the certified registered nurse anesthetist,* Chicago, 1998, American Association of Nurse Anesthetists.

American Society of Anesthesiologists: *Guidelines for regional anesthesia in obstetrics,* 1991, American Society of Anesthesiologists.

Chestnut D: *Obstetric anesthesia principles and practice,* ed 3, Philadelphia, 2004, Mosby.

Crawforth K: The AANA Foundation Closed Malpractice Claims study: obstetric anesthesia, *AANA J* 70:97-104, 2002.

Datta S: *The obstetric anesthesia handbook,* ed 3, Philadelphia, 2000, Hanley & Belfus.

Fiedler M: Obstetric anesthesia. In Nagelhout J, Zaglaniczny K, editors: *Nurse anesthesia,* ed 2, Philadelphia, 2002, WB Saunders, pp 1089-1131.

Hawkins JL, Chang J, Calloghan W, et al: Anesthesia-related maternal mortality in the United States 1991-1996: an update, *Anesthesiology* A1046, 2002.

Hughes S, Levinson G, Rosen M: *Shnider and Levinson's anesthesia for obstetrics,* ed 4, Philadelphia, 2002, Lippincott Williams & Wilkins.

Moore C, Fragneto R: The obstetric patient. In Waugaman W, Foster S, Rigor B, editors: *Principles and practice of nurse anesthesia,* ed 3, Stamford, CT, Appleton & Lange, 1999, pp 3117-3142.

Norris M: Labour analgesia: What are the (new) options? Refresher course outline, *Can J Anaesth* 45:138-143, 1998.

Practice Guidelines for Obstetrical Anesthesia: A report by the American Society of Anesthesiologists Task Force on Obstetrical Anesthesia, *Anesthesiology* 90:600-611, 1999.

Rosen MA: Management of anesthesia for the pregnant surgical patient, *Anesthesiology* 91:1159-1163, 1999.

Stoelting R, Miller R: *Basics of anesthesia,* ed 4, Philadelphia, 2000, Churchill Livingstone, pp 341-363.

High-Risk Obstetrical Anesthesia

Joanne Pearson

1. How often does obesity complicate pregnancy?

Obesity (weight > 300 lb at delivery) is a common complicating factor of pregnancy. More than 25% of parturients are obese. There is a significant increase in the incidence of obstetrical complications and a 2-fold to 12-fold increase in mortality in obese parturients.

2. What are notable physiological changes seen in an obese parturient?

Physiological changes are summarized in the following table. It is especially crucial to monitor an obese parturient when she is placed in the supine or Trendelenburg position. These positions can cause serious deterioration of oxygenation and cardiac compromise.

Physiological Changes in Obese Parturient

System	Increase	Decrease
Pulmonary	Oxygen consumption Carbon dioxide production Ventilation-perfusion mismatch	Pulmonary mechanics Pulmonary reserve Functional residual capacity (FRC) Tidal volume Vital capacity
Cardiovascular	Blood volume Cardiac output, blood pressure Left ventricular hypertrophy Pulmonary hypertension	
Gastrointestinal	Gastric volume* Hiatal hernia Aspiration risk	Gastric pH*
Endocrine	Diabetes mellitus	
Coagulation	Deep vein thrombosis Pulmonary embolism	

*It is controversial whether this effect of obesity is additive to the effects of pregnancy.

3. Is the clinical anesthetic management of an obese parturient different than that of a normal pregnant woman?

An obese parturient is likely to have concomitant medical disorders. Early anesthetic assessment should be an important priority. A simple pulse oximetry reading can provide basic information about oxygenation. Arterial blood gases may be indicated for symptomatic patients. Intravenous access should be established early because this may be difficult in some patients. Appropriately sized equipment must be available. Airway management and intubation also may be difficult. Lumbar epidural anesthesia is a good choice for analgesia and anesthesia in an obese parturient because it reduces oxygen consumption and attenuates the increase in cardiac output with delivery. Epidural placement may be more technically difficult in these patients. Use of the sitting position may help to identify the epidural space. When incidental dural puncture occurs, continuous spinal analgesia is a viable option.

4. Differentiate preeclampsia and eclampsia.

The following table lists criteria for preeclampsia and eclampsia.

Preeclampsia and Eclampsia		
	Preeclampsia	**Eclampsia**
Hypertension	Diastolic BP >90 mm Hg or systolic BP >140 mm Hg or increase above baseline diastolic >15 mm Hg or increase above baseline systolic >30 mm Hg	Diastolic BP >110 mm Hg or systolic BP >160 mm Hg; findings on two occasions
Proteinuria	>300 mg protein/24 hr or >1 g/L in two random specimens	3+ or 4+ on a urine analysis or >5 g in a 24-hr urine collection
Edema	Generalized edema (>1+) after 12 hr of bed rest or weight gain >5 lb in 1 wk	Generalized edema and prone to pulmonary edema
Liver function		Impaired
Neurological		Headache, visual disturbances, seizures
Thrombocytopenia		<150,000 platelet count

Adapted from ACOG Technical Bulletin: Hypertension in pregnancy, Int J Gynecol Obstet 53:175-183, 1996.

5. Define the HELLP syndrome.

HELLP refers to **h**emolysis, **e**levated **l**iver enzymes, and **l**ow **p**latelets. There is significant morbidity and mortality for a mother with HELLP syndrome. Most patients develop the syndrome before 36 weeks of gestation; 30% develop it postpartum. Women suspected of having HELLP syndrome should be monitored carefully intrapartum and postpartum. Treatment includes immediate delivery. If delivery is postponed, the status of the mother and the fetus may deteriorate quickly.

6. Why are some parturients placed on magnesium sulfate?

Magnesium sulfate may be used to treat *pregnancy-induced hypertension (PIH)* and *preterm labor*. Important therapeutic effects include the following:
- Smooth muscle relaxation in the uterus and blood vessels
- Decreased acetylcholine release at the neuromuscular junction, with decreased muscle fiber excitability
- Antiepileptic effect

Magnesium levels should be monitored carefully, especially in patients with renal impairment. Therapeutic levels are 4 to 7 mEq/L. Magnesium toxicity can cause somnolence, muscle weakness, attenuation of deep tendon reflexes, and respiratory arrest. The effects of nondepolarizing muscle relaxants may be more pronounced in a patient receiving magnesium sulfate. Magnesium sulfate is usually continued into the postpartum period until most of the symptoms of PIH have abated.

7. How prevalent is PIH?

PIH complicates 6% to 10% of all pregnancies. PIH may cause significant morbidity and mortality in parturients who were completely healthy before pregnancy. The cause of PIH is poorly understood. Blood pressure usually decreases in pregnancy so that any elevation is considered abnormal.

8. Discuss important anesthetic interventions for a patient with PIH.

The definitive treatment for PIH is delivery of the fetus. An epidural should be placed early if the ultimate goal is delivery. A recent (<6 hours) platelet count should be obtained before catheter placement. Excellent catheter placement is paramount because glottic edema may make airway management and intubation a challenge should regional analgesia fail. Other important anesthetic considerations associated with PIH include the following:
- *Hypertension:* Treatment should be aggressive to maintain a blood pressure less than 140/90 mm Hg. Hydralazine and labetalol are commonly used agents. Careful blood pressure monitoring is crucial.
- *Hydration status:* Fluid management is complex. These patients are vasoconstricted and potentially fluid depleted, yet prone to pulmonary edema. Adequate hydration is important to promote renal blood flow and urine output. In the presence of oliguria and questionable hemodynamic status, central venous pressure monitoring should be considered.
- *Epigastric pain:* A complaint of epigastric pain requires immediate attention. Epigastric discomfort may be an ominous symptom in these patients, signaling

stretching of the liver capsule and impending hepatic rupture. A computed tomography scan can diagnose hepatic enlargement or subcapsular hemorrhage.

• *Seizure activity:* Seizures may be treated with a barbiturate or midazolam. Some of the older benzodiazepines are suspected to be teratogenic and should be avoided. Key interventions include maintaining adequate oxygenation, treating hypertension aggressively, and monitoring magnesium levels closely. Twenty-seven percent of PIH seizures occur in the postpartum period.

9. How common is diabetes during pregnancy?

Diabetes mellitus is the most common complication affecting pregnant women. Pregnancy is sometimes called a *diabetogenic* condition. Increased levels of placental lactogen, prolactin, cortisol, progesterone, and estrogen can elevate blood glucose. Preeclampsia occurs more frequently in pregnant diabetics. Significant fetal abnormalities associated with maternal diabetes include macrosomia, polyhydramnios, intrauterine growth retardation, and retarded fetal pulmonary maturation.

10. List special anesthetic considerations for a pregnant diabetic patient.

• Perform early assessment for possible urgent delivery.
• Complications of obesity (more common in diabetics) may be present.
• Continuous glucose management is needed during labor and delivery (maintain plasma glucose at 90 to 110 mg/dL).
• Glucose requirements decrease abruptly after delivery (obtain hourly finger-stick tests for blood glucose determination until stable).
• Fetus is likely to experience hypoglycemia after birth.
• Epidural anesthesia decreases circulating catecholamines, improves placental blood flow, and facilitates instrumental or emergent delivery.
• Infuse non–glucose-containing intravenous solutions for fluid replacement.
• Ensure that a neonatologist is available for delivery.

11. What problems arise with fetal macrosomia?

Macrosomia may precipitate the need for *instrumented* or *cesarean delivery. Emergent delivery* also may be necessary owing to a low tolerance for stress and poor placental blood flow in these fetuses.

12. Name the most common obstetrical complications influencing anesthetic management.

The following complications commonly influence management:
• Prematurity
• Preterm labor
• Multiple gestations
• Abnormal presentation

13. How does preterm labor affect anesthetic management?

Pharmacological intervention for preterm labor can have significant effects on anesthetic management. Treatment for preterm labor may include magnesium sulfate, beta$_2$ adrenergic receptor agonists, calcium channel blockers, and prostaglandin inhibitors. Pharmacological interactions with anesthetic agents and muscle relaxants should be considered. Uterine relaxation provided by these drugs does not end with delivery. The patient may have significant uterine atony after delivery, precipitating possible postpartum hemorrhage.

14. Do multiple gestations change the basic physiology of pregnancy?

A multiple gestation pregnancy changes the physiology of pregnancy proportional to the number of gestations. Increased cardiac output, relative anemia, compromised pulmonary function, and the increased size of the uterus all place the mother at greater risk. The expansively stretched uterine tissue and pharmacological intervention for preterm labor aggravate uterine atony.

15. Identify some high-risk scenarios for the multiple gestation parturient.

High-risk scenarios are presented in the following table.

High-Risk Scenarios

Scenario	Anesthetic Intervention
Increased blood loss with delivery	Place a large-bore intravenous catheter; type and crossmatch for blood
Large uterus	Aspiration prophylaxis; extreme left uterine displacement
Instrumental or emergent delivery; subsequent gestation cord prolapse or abruption	Place optimal functioning epidural early; use carbonated 3% chloroprocaine for rapid block onset; convert to general anesthesia if necessary
Internal fetal manipulation or subsequent gestation entrapment	Nitroglycerin, 50–100 mcg IV, for uterine relaxation; high concentrations of volatile agent under general anesthesia
Uterine atony	Aggressive treatment with oxytocin (Pitocin), methylergonovine (Methergine), or prostaglandin F$_{2\alpha}$ (Hemabate)

16. How does abnormal fetal presentation affect anesthetic care of the parturient?

- *Breech presentation* is the most common abnormal presentation. External cephalic version (manual turning of the fetus) can be attempted to change the fetal presentation to vertex (crown of the head) presentation after 36 weeks of gestation. Use of epidural anesthesia is *controversial* in external cephalic version

because the degree of maternal discomfort guides the obstetrician during the manipulations. In some more recent reports, an increased number of successful versions have been accomplished without an increase in morbidity under epidural anesthesia.
- Delivery of the fetus in breech presentation under any circumstance is a strong relative indication for epidural anesthesia. This potentially difficult delivery may require obstetrical manipulation of the fetus, instrumental intervention, or cesarean delivery.
- There are many types of vertex malpresentations. The primary complicating factor associated with these presentations is that a larger cephalic diameter is presenting for delivery, resulting in increased maternal discomfort and prolonged labor.
- Cesarean delivery is necessary for a shoulder presentation or transverse lie.

17. When should maternal hemorrhage be anticipated?

Six diagnoses should signal potential maternal hemorrhage to the practitioner (see the following table):

Anesthesia Implications Associated with Maternal Hemorrhage

Obstetrical Problem	Anesthesia Implications
Placenta previa	Estimation of blood loss is difficult because it can be internal and external Monitor vital signs closely
Abruptio placentae	Thromboplastin release can activate the coagulation cascade; monitor for signs of coagulopathy Couvelaire uterus (myometrium infiltrated with blood) = uterine atony
Placenta accreta, increta, or percreta	Anticipate gravid hysterectomy Transfusion is usually necessary
Uterine rupture	Breakthrough abdominal pain occurs even with adequate labor epidural Aggressively treat maternal hypotension or shock Fetal distress General anesthesia required; rapid delivery Surgical intervention for hemorrhage control
Retained placenta	Uterine relaxation is necessary; volatile anesthetic agent or nitroglycerin, 50–100 mcg IV, may be used Maternal analgesia is required for manual exploration
Uterine atony	Correct hypovolemia quickly Uterine massage Uterotonics: oxytocin (Pitocin), 5 units, IV bolus, up to 40 units/L IV infusion; hypotension with rapid administration; methylergonovine (Methergine), 0.4 mg IM × 2, as needed (alpha adrenergic agonist); prostaglandin $F_{2\alpha}$ (Hemabate), 0.25 mg IM or intramyometrially, up to 1 mg; side effects: systemic and pulmonary vasoconstriction, bronchoconstriction

- Placenta previa—abnormal placental implantation at or over the cervical os
- Abruptio placentae—premature separation of a normally implanted placenta
- Placenta accreta, increta, or percreta—an abnormal placenta missing the basalis layer, which implants onto the myometrium (accreta), into the myometrium (increta), or into the abdominal structures (percreta)
- Uterine rupture
- Retained placenta
- Uterine atony

In all of these cases, primary attention must be directed toward rapid fluid and blood replacement and supplemental oxygen.

18. How should the practitioner proceed with resuscitation in a pregnant patient?

Cardiac arrest occurs in 1 in 30,000 pregnancies. Advanced life support should be instituted with careful attention given to left uterine displacement. A uterus greater than 20 weeks' gestation functionally impedes venous return. If there is a viable fetus (24 weeks), immediate cesarean delivery greatly improves maternal outcome. The best outcomes have been reported when delivery occurs within 5 minutes of cardiopulmonary resuscitation initiation.

 Key Points

- More than 25% of parturients are obese (>300 lb at delivery).
- Preeclampsia and eclampsia are differentiated by the degree of hypertension, proteinuria, and edema. Eclampsia is differentiated further as it is associated with possible impaired liver function, neurological problems, and hematological problems.
- HELLP syndrome is hemolysis, elevated liver enzymes, and low platelets.
- PIH complicates 6% to 10% of all pregnancies. The definitive treatment for PIH is delivery of the fetus.
- Anesthetic considerations in parturients with PIH include glottic edema, hypertension, hydration status, epigastric pain, and seizure activity.
- Diabetes mellitus is the most common complication affecting pregnant women.
- Epidural anesthesia decreases circulating catecholamines, improves placental blood flow, and facilitates instrumental or emergent delivery.
- A multiple-gestation pregnancy changes the physiology of pregnancy proportional to the number of gestations.
- Breech presentation is the most common abnormal presentation.
- Cesarean delivery is necessary for a shoulder presentation or transverse lie.
- Six diagnoses signal potential maternal hemorrhage—placenta previa; placental abruption; placenta accreta, increta, or percreta; uterine rupture; retained placenta; and uterine atony.

Internet Resources

Nurse Anesthesia.com:
http://www.nurse-anesthesia.com/

Update in Anesthesia: Practical Procedures Cumulative Index:
http://www.nda.ox.ac.uk/wfsa/html/pages/up_sect.htm

Med Matrix Web Portal:
www.medmatrix.com

GASNet Search: Obstetrical Anesthesia:
http://www.gasnet.org/about/search.php?p1=obstetrical+anesthesia

Hypertextbook of Regional Anaesthesia for Obstetrics:
http://www.manbit.com/oa/oaindex.htm

The University of Chicago Departement of Anesthesia and Critical Care: Anesthesia for the
Pregnant Patient:
http://daccx.bsd.uchicago.edu/manuals/obstetric/obanesthesia.html

Bibliography

American College of Obstetricians and Gynecologists: ACOG technical bulletin: hypertension in pregnancy,
Int J Gynecol Obstet 53:175-183, 1996.

Carlan SJ, Marshall JD, Huckaby T, et al: The effect of epidural anesthesia on safety and success of external
cephalic version at term, *Anesth Analg* 79:525-528, 1994.

Chestnut D: *Obstetric anesthesia, principles and practice,* ed 2, St. Louis, 1999, Mosby.

Dewan D, Hood D: *Practical obstetric anesthesia,* Philadelphia, 1997, WB Saunders.

Fawcett WJ, Haxby EJ, Male DA: Magnesium: physiology and pharmacology, *Br J Anaesth* 83:302-330, 1999.

Honor MW, Gross TL: Obesity in pregnancy, *Clin Obstet Gynecol* 37:596-604, 1994.

Hood D, Dewan D: Anesthetic and obstetrical outcome in morbidly obese parturients, *Anesthesiology*
79:1210-1218, 1993.

Norris M: *Obstetric anesthesia,* ed 2, Philadelphia, 1999, Lippincott Williams & Wilkins.

Palmer C, D'Angelo R, Paech M: *Handbook of obstetric anesthesia,* Oxford, UK, 2002, BIOS Scientific
Publishers Limited.

Neonatal Anesthesia

Susan Kathleen Tomso

1. Define preterm infant, term infant, postterm infant, and neonate.

- *Preterm infant:* an infant born before 37 weeks' gestation
- *Term infant:* an infant born between 37 and 42 weeks' gestation
- *Postterm infant:* an infant born after 42 weeks' gestation
- *Neonate:* an infant less than 30 days of age

2. What are two cardiac shunts present in fetal circulation? What causes functional closure of these shunts after birth, and when does anatomical closure occur?

The *foramen ovale* shunts blood from the right atrium to the left atrium. The *ductus arteriosus* shunts blood from the right ventricle into the descending aorta. Closure of the shunts is initiated by clamping of the umbilical cord and the first breath. After expansion of the lungs, pulmonary vascular resistance decreases, and pulmonary blood flow increases. The increase in blood flow to the left heart increases left atrial pressures, functionally closing the foramen ovale. The closure of the ductus arteriosus is stimulated by the increase in arterial oxygen tension, in addition to other chemical mediators, such as bradykinins and prostaglandins. The ductus arteriosus permanently closes 10 to 14 days after birth. The foramen ovale may take 18 months to close permanently. In approximately 20% to 30% of infants, the foramen ovale never anatomically closes.

If a neonate experiences hypoxia or acidosis during the first few days after birth, the transition from fetal to extrauterine circulation can be inhibited or reversed, leading to persistent pulmonary hypertension. If this occurs, pulmonary vascular resistance is increased, right-sided heart pressures remain high, and right-to-left shunting across the ductus arteriosus and foramen ovale continues. This situation can rapidly lead to poor outcomes for the neonate and must be treated expediently.

3. What is surfactant, why is it important, and at what gestational age does it develop?

Surfactant is a glycoprotein secretion of the alveoli that reduces alveolar surface tension, decreasing the pressure for alveolar collapse. Type II pneumocytes begin producing surfactant at 24 weeks of gestation. An adequate concentration of surfactant for extrauterine life is usually present by 34 to 38 weeks of gestation.

4. **Explain how the mechanics of breathing differs in the neonate.**

The neonate consumes three times as much oxygen (7 to 9 mL/kg/min) as the typical adult. The neonate also has higher closing volumes that are in the lower range of his or her normal tidal volume and a high minute ventilation-to-functional residual capacity ratio (5:1). Consequently the neonate has a low respiratory reserve and is prone to precipitous drops in arterial oxygen saturation.

At birth, the neonate has approximately half of the slow-twitch, high oxidative type I muscle fibers in the diaphragm that are necessary to sustain respiratory effort. Pliable ribs, low lung compliance (due to small alveoli), and an immature diaphragm all contribute to decreased functional residual capacity and decreased oxygen reserve. For these reasons, the neonate experiences respiratory fatigue easily during any alterations in pulmonary function. The diaphragm does not mature fully until 8 months of age, and the intercostal muscles do not reach maturity until 2 months of age. Alveoli mature in late childhood.

5. **Cardiac output of the neonate is dependent on which variable; why?**

Cardiac output depends on heart rate because stroke volume is fixed. An immature left ventricle limits the ability of the neonate to increase myocardial contractility. In an immature heart, cardiac output maximally increases only 30% to 40% above normal resting rate compared with an increase of 300% in the mature heart.

6. **What is the most common cause of bradycardia in the neonate?**

Hypoxia always should be suspected first during unexplained bradycardia in the newborn. The neonate's high rate of oxygen consumption, combined with high closing volumes, can precipitate rapid desaturation.

7. **What are the normal vital signs of the neonate?**

The neonate has faster respiratory and cardiac rates and lower blood pressure than the adult. Normal values fall near the following:

Respiratory rate	40 breaths/min
Heart rate	140 beats/min
Blood pressure	65/40 mm Hg

8. **Describe temperature regulation in the neonate.**

Because of their higher surface area-to-body weight ratio, neonates are much more susceptible to losing body heat to the environment. Many factors in the perioperative setting further compound this problem, including cold operating rooms, intravenous fluid administration, inhaled gas administration, and the direct effect of anesthetic agents on temperature regulation. The neonate's main method for heat production is metabolism of brown fat (located primarily in the back of the neck, the axilla, and between the scapulae) a process called *nonshivering thermogenesis*. This mechanism of temperature management is a sympathetic nervous system response initiated in the hypothalamus. Brown fat contains thermogenin, which combines with free fatty acids released by norepinephrine, resulting in combustion and heat production. Special attention to temperature control must be taken with infants who are sick or premature because their stores of brown fat may be significantly lower.

9. **Describe the anatomical differences of the neonatal airway compared with the adult airway and their effects on airway management.**

   Anatomical differences of the neonatal airway are summarized in the following table.

Neonatal Airway Differences

Anatomic Difference	Effect
Prominent occiput	Affects positioning during intubation; placing a shoulder roll is frequently helpful to establish proper positioning
Large tongue	Airway is easily obstructed; contributes to obligate nasal breathing
Long and narrow epiglottis	More difficult to lift epiglottis with laryngoscope blade
Prominent adenoids and tonsils	Can obstruct view during laryngoscopy
Cricoid cartilage is narrowest part of airway	An endotracheal tube that passes through the vocal cords may not pass through the subglottic region of the cricoid cartilage or may be tight-fitting, increasing the risk of airway edema
Larynx is at C3-4 and positioned high	Makes larynx appear more anterior
Narrow nasal passages	Must be taken into consideration if attempting nasal intubation; neonates are obligate nasal breathers, and obstruction can lead to respiratory distress

10. **Discuss two common postanesthetic complications in neonates.**

    Postintubation croup reportedly occurs in 0.1% to 1% of children. The anesthetist can minimize this complication through several important interventions. The endotracheal tube should be of small enough diameter to allow an air leak at less than 25 cm H_2O pressure. Other factors that contribute to postintubation croup include changes in patient position during intubation, any position other than supine, multiple attempts at intubation or a traumatic intubation, surgery lasting longer than 1 hour, coughing while intubated, and any previous history of croup. Management of this complication includes treatment with a racemic epinephrine nebulizer, humidified oxygen, and steroids administered intravenously or by nebulizer.

    Laryngospasm after extubation is another common complication and is caused by stimulation of the superior laryngeal nerve. This complication is best avoided by delaying extubation until the neonate is completely awake or by extubating "deep." Other preventive measures include thorough suctioning of the oropharynx before extubation and instituting a side-lying position during postoperative transport to prevent stimulation of the superior laryngeal nerve by secretions.

11. What postoperative complication is a premature infant (<50 to 60 weeks postconception) at high risk for?

This special population of neonates is at high risk for obstructive and central apnea for 24 hours after surgery. Some guidelines suggest that elective surgery should be postponed for premature infants until they are older than this age range. If surgery cannot be delayed, postoperative monitoring should be implemented for at least 12 hours. Other guidelines include avoidance of narcotics intraoperatively, intravenous caffeine (10 mg/kg), and judicious use of regional anesthesia when possible.

12. Describe the Hering-Breuer reflex and the role it plays in regulation of neonatal respiration.

Stimulation of stretch receptors in the lungs initiates the Hering-Breuer reflex. This reflex prevents overdistention of the alveoli by inhibiting excessive tidal volumes and decreasing the rate of breathing by causing transient apnea. Conversely, it increases respiratory effort when the lungs are deflated and may be responsible for periodic deep "sighs" to prevent atelectasis. This reflex may play a large role in regulation of respiration in neonates while other regulatory systems are still immature. The Hering-Breuer reflex declines in activity after the first month of life and does not seem to affect adult respiration.

13. Why do neonates respond differently to some medications?

Neonates respond differently to drugs for four main reasons:
- Neonates have less drug protein binding because they have lower total serum protein and albumin.
- A larger proportion of the neonate's body weight is water, and there is a greater volume of distribution for water-soluble medications.
- The neonate has a smaller proportion of body weight in the form of fat and muscle. This leaves less tissue for redistribution of drugs, leading to prolonged effects of some drugs that depend on redistribution.
- Immature liver and kidney function can prolong metabolism and excretion of drugs that depend on these systems.

14. Do neonates need more or less muscle relaxant per kilogram than adults?

Because succinylcholine is a water-soluble drug, a larger dose is needed for neonates because of their larger volume of distribution. In addition, neonates have an immature neuromuscular junction; either fewer nicotinic receptors are present, or the receptors may not be as sensitive to acetylcholine. Both cases require more succinylcholine to depolarize an adequate number of receptors to achieve muscle relaxation. Conversely, neonates are relatively sensitive to nondepolarizing muscle relaxants.

15. How does intraoperative fluid maintenance differ for the neonatal population?

A common fluid maintenance formula for neonates is: 4 mL/kg for the first 10 kg, 2 mL/kg for the second 10 kg, plus 1 mL/kg for the remaining weight. Because of the small amounts required, fluid administration must be monitored carefully to avoid overloading the infant. Using a burette set to control the volume of fluid administered is recommended. One method for replacing a fluid deficit is to replace half of the total deficit plus maintenance requirements in the first hour, one fourth of the deficit plus maintenance in the second hour, and the last fourth of the deficit plus maintenance in the third hour.

16. List the six most common surgical procedures that occur in the first month of life.

The six most common surgical procedures include:
- Exploratory laparotomy for necrotizing enterocolitis
- Inguinal hernia repair
- Correction of pyloric stenosis
- Patent ductus arteriosus ligation
- Shunt procedure for hydrocephalus
- Placement of a central venous catheter

17. Which vasopressor is frequently used during the treatment of necrotizing enterocolitis and why?

Dopamine infusions are frequently necessary for an infant with necrotizing enterocolitis. These infants are usually hypovolemic, are septic, and have metabolic acidosis and prerenal azotemia. Dopamine supports cardiac output, while improving renal and intestinal perfusion.

18. Describe the electrolyte and volume status of a patient with pyloric stenosis.

These patients may be hypovolemic, hypokalemic, and hypochloremic from protracted vomiting. The kidneys respond to the resulting metabolic alkalosis by excreting an alkaline urine, which compounds the hypokalemia. Because of these problems, intravascular volume repletion and electrolyte correction are primary concerns.

19. Identify two complications associated with patent ductus arteriosus ligation.

Injuries to the recurrent laryngeal nerve or a chylothorax resulting from injury to the thoracic duct are complications of this procedure. The anesthetist should be aware of nearby structures, such as the left pulmonary artery, the descending aorta, and the carotid artery, and the potential for accidental puncture or ligation of these vessels.

20. Describe anesthetic considerations for the patient undergoing shunt placement for hydrocephalus.

- Anesthetic goals include controlling intracranial pressure (ICP) and protecting the airway.
- Patients who are actively vomiting should be induced with a rapid-sequence technique with cricoid pressure applied.
- Anesthetic agents that increase ICP (e.g., ketamine) should be avoided in these patients; however, the risk of increasing ICP is small because of the compliance of the neonate's skull, which is still unfused.
- Hyperventilation and barbiturates help reduce ICP.
- Venous air embolism is possible during placement of the distal end of a ventriculoatrial shunt.
- If an external ventricular drainage system is present, the height of the drainage bag should remain stable in relation to the patient's head to avoid dramatic changes in ICP.
- Infants who exhibited periods of apnea or bradycardia before the operation should remain intubated with positive end-expiratory pressure postoperatively.

 Key Points

- An infant is considered preterm if it is born before 37 weeks of gestation. A term infant is one born between 37 and 42 weeks of gestation. A postterm infant is one born after 42 weeks of gestation. A neonate is any infant less than 30 days of age.
- The foramen ovale and the ductus arteriosus are two cardiac shunts present at birth. These shunts close immediately after clamping of the umbilical cord and the first breath.
- If a neonate experiences hypoxia or acidosis during the first few days after birth, the transition from fetal to extrauterine circulation can be inhibited or reversed, leading to persistent pulmonary hypertension.
- Surfactant is a glycoprotein secretion of the alveoli that reduces alveolar surface tension, decreasing the pressure for alveolar collapse. Type II pneumocytes begin producing surfactant at 24 weeks of gestation.
- Hypoxia always should be suspected first during unexplained bradycardia in a newborn.
- The neonatal airway differs from the adult airway in the following ways:
  - Relative macroglossia
  - Prominent occiput
  - Larynx location and orientation
- Premature infants are at higher risk for obstructive and central apnea for 24 hours after surgery.

Key Points *continued*

- Neonates respond differently to drugs for four main reasons:
  - Neonates have less drug protein binding because they have lower total serum protein and albumin.
  - A larger proportion of the neonate's body weight is water, and there is a greater volume of distribution for water-soluble medications.
  - The neonate has a smaller proportion of body weight in the form of fat and muscle. This leaves less tissue for redistribution of drugs, leading to prolonged effects of some drugs that depend on redistribution.
  - Immature liver and kidney function can prolong metabolism and excretion of drugs that depend on these systems.
- Fluid management in neonates follows the 4-2-1 rule: 4 mL/kg for the first 10 kg, 2 mL/kg for the second 10 kg, plus 1 mL/kg for the remaining weight.

Internet Resources

The Virtual Anaesthesiologist: Pediatric anesthesia:
http://www.anesthesiology.de/Links/Pediatric_anesthesia/pediatric_anesthesia.htm

Virtual Anaesthesia Textbook:
http://www.virtual-anaesthesia-textbook.com/

Nurse-Anesthesia.com:
http://www.nurse-anesthesia.com/

Update in Anaesthesia: Paediatric anaesthesia review:
http://www.nda.ox.ac.uk/wfsa/html/u08/u08_003.htm

GASNet Video Library:
http://www.gasnet.org/videos/index.php

Images.md: Pediatric anesthesia:
http://images.md/users/explore_chapter.asp?ID=ACA0701-05&colID=ACA0701&coltitle=Pediatric+Anesthesia

Cincinnati Children's Hospital Medical Center: Neonatal anesthesia:
http://www.cincinnatichildrens.org/health/info/anesthesia/anesthesia-neonatal.htm

Metrohealth Anesthesia: Pediatric anesthesia:
www.metrohealthanesthesia.com/presentations/pediatricAnesthesia.ppt.

GASNet: Neonatal anesthesia:
http://gasnet.med.yale.edu/gta/chapters/neonatal.php

Bibliography

Aker J: Pediatric anesthesia. In Nagelhout JJ, Zaglaniczny KL, editors: *Nurse anesthesia*, ed 2, Philadelphia, 2001, WB Saunders, pp 1132-1168.

Berry FA: Neonatal anesthesia. In Barash PG (ed): *Clinical anesthesia,* ed 3, Philadelphia, 1996, Lippincott-Raven, pp 1091-1113.

Blake WW, Murray JA: Heat balance. In Merenstein GB, Gardner SL, editors: *Handbook of neonatal intensive care,* ed 4, St. Louis, 1998, Mosby-Year Book, pp 100-115.

Cote CJ, Lugo RA, Ward RM: Pharmacokinetics and pharmacology of drugs in children. In Cote CJ, Todres ID, Goudsouzian NG, Ryan JF, editors: *A practice of anesthesia for infants and children,* ed 3, Philadelphia, 2001, WB Saunders, pp 121-171.

Eldridge EA, Sulpicio GS, Rockoff MA: Pediatric neurosurgical anesthesia. In Cote CJ, Todres ID, Goudsouzian NG, Ryan JF, editors: *A practice of anesthesia for infants and children,* ed 3, Philadelphia, 2001, WB Saunders, pp 493-521.

Goudsouzian NG: Muscle relaxants in children. In Cote CJ, Todres ID, Goudsouzian NG, Ryan JF, editors: *A practice of anesthesia for infants and children,* ed 3, Philadelphia, 2001, WB Saunders, pp 196-215.

Mallampati SR: Airway management. In Barash PG, Cullen BF, Stoelting RK, editors: *Clinical anesthesia,* ed 3, Philadelphia, 1997, Lippincott-Raven, pp 573-594.

Strafford MA: Management of the patient with repaired or palliated congenital heart disease. In Cote CJ, Todres ID, Goudsouzian NG, Ryan JF, editors: *A practice of anesthesia for infants and children,* ed 3, Philadelphia, 2001, WB Saunders, pp 415-460.

Todres ID, Cronin JH: Growth and development. In Cote CJ, Todres ID, Goudsouzian NG, Ryan JF, editors: *A practice of anesthesia for infants and children,* ed 3, Philadelphia, 2001, WB Saunders, pp 5-24.

Wheeler M, Cote C, Todres ID: Pediatric airway. In Cote CJ, Todres ID, Goudsouzian NG, Ryan JF, editors: *A practice of anesthesia for infants and children,* ed 3, Philadelphia, 2001, WB Saunders, pp 79-120.

Yaster M: Evaluation of the neonate. In Longnecker DE, Tinker JH, Morgan GE, editors: *Principles and practice of anesthesiology,* ed 2, St. Louis, 1998, Mosby, pp 426-437.

Pediatric Anesthesia

Sherry H. Owens

1. **Describe the fundamental characteristics of the pediatric cardiovascular system.**
   - The myocardium of the infant is noncompliant, and its ability to increase stroke volume and contractility is limited.
   - Cardiac output is heart rate dependent.
   - Infants possess increased parasympathetic tone. Profound bradycardia with resulting diminished cardiac output can be caused by activation of the parasympathetic nervous system, hypoxia, or anesthetic overdose.
   - Baroreceptor reflexes are immature.
   - Vasoconstriction in response to hypovolemia is poorly developed. The primary sign of volume depletion in infants is hypotension without tachycardia.

2. **What conditions precipitate reversion to fetal circulation?**

   Because anatomical closure of the foramen ovale and ductus arteriosus may take 4 months after birth, certain conditions can favor blood flow through these shunts, as follows:
   - Hypoxemia and acidosis: These two derangements lead to increased pulmonary vascular resistance, which can produce a right-to-left shunt, with blood flow through the foramen ovale and ductus arteriosus. A vicious cycle ensues as this results in hypoxemia.
   - Hypothermia: Norepinephrine production and nonshivering thermogenesis lead to pulmonary vasoconstriction. Vasoconstriction causes an increase in pulmonary vascular resistance, potentially leading to a right-to-left shunt.
   - Reductions in systemic vascular resistance.

3. **Summarize normal vital signs in children.**

   The table on page 394 summarizes vital signs in children.

4. **Discuss characteristics of the pediatric respiratory system that differentiate it from the adult respiratory system.**

   Immature musculature of the infant chest is susceptible to easy fatigability. Alveoli are small, immature, and few in number, resulting in reduced lung compliance. The horizontal orientation of the infant's cartilaginous rib cage makes

Age-Appropriate Vital Signs (Mean Values)

Age	Heart Rate (beats/min)	Systolic Blood Pressure (mm Hg)	Diastolic Blood Pressure (mm Hg)	Respiratory Rate
Neonate	140	65	50	40
1 yr	125	95	60	30
3 yr	100	100	70	25
9 yr	80	105	70	20
12 yr	75	115	75	20

the chest wall compliant. This quality makes a small contribution to chest expansion, promotes paradoxical chest movements during inspiration, and promotes low residual expiratory volumes. The result is decreased functional residual capacity and a predisposition to hypoxemia. This effect is exaggerated by the infant's high metabolic oxygen consumption, which is twice that of the adult.

5. List anatomical characteristics of the pediatric airway.

The pediatric airway is characterized by the following:
- Large head and tongue
- Anterior and cephalad larynx
- Larynx is adjacent to the C4 vertebra compared with C6 in the adult; it assumes an adult orientation by age 6
- Nasal passages are narrow; neonates and infants are obligate nose breathers
- Cricoid cartilage is narrowest part of the airway
- Right main stem bronchus branches from midline in a more acute fashion (55 degrees) than the adult bronchus (25 degrees)

6. What size guidelines should one follow in selecting an endotracheal tube (ETT)?

ETT size guidelines are presented in the table on page 395.

7. What is the appropriate ETT insertion depth?

The ETT can be inserted to a depth three times the internal diameter of the tube. An alternate method is to perform a right main stem bronchus intubation, then withdraw the tube until breath sounds are equal bilaterally.

8. What is an acceptable ETT leak?

An ETT acceptable leak, which allows adequate ventilation and prevents operating room pollution, is 15 to 20 cm H_2O pressure. An ETT that does not allow a leak

Age-Appropriate Endotracheal Tube Sizes

Age	Internal Diameter (mm) in Uncuffed Tube
Neonate	3.0–3.5
1 yr	4.0
2 yr	4.5
4 yr	5.0
6 yr	5.5

OR

[Age (yr) + 16] ÷ 4

A tube a $\frac{1}{2}$ size larger and a $\frac{1}{2}$ size smaller than predicted should be available.

until 30 cm H_2O pressure should be exchanged for a smaller tube to prevent postintubation airway edema.

9. **Pediatric patients are especially vulnerable to which two anesthetic complications?**

   Pediatric patients are especially vulnerable to *laryngospasm* and *postintubation croup*.

10. **List contributing factors to the development of postintubation croup.**

    The following factors contribute:
    • Early childhood (age 1 to 4 years)
    • Multiple intubation attempts
    • Prolonged surgery
    • Head and neck procedures
    • Large ETTs
    • Excessive movement of ETT

11. **How is postintubation croup treated?**

    Postintubation croup is treated with nebulized racemic epinephrine (0.25 to 0.5 mL of a 2.25% solution in 2.5 mL of normal saline).

12. **What anatomical characteristics of the pediatric patient make heat conservation problematic?**

    Pediatric patients are susceptible to intraoperative heat loss primarily because of their *large body surface area-to-weight ratio*. Other contributory factors include decreased insulating tissue mass and a narrow thermoregulatory range that is easily influenced by the environment.

13. Describe temperature regulating mechanisms in the infant.

An infant can increase heat production by three mechanisms:
- Physical activity
- Shivering
- Nonshivering thermogenesis

In infants younger than 3 months, the shivering response is virtually absent. Nonshivering thermogenesis increases heat production without muscular effort. Brown fat metabolism is the principal mechanism through which non-shivering thermogenesis occurs. Infants respond to cold stress through increased production of norepinephrine, which promotes brown fat metabolism.

14. Where is brown fat found?

Comprising 2% to 6% of an infant's total body weight, brown fat contains a rich blood supply and sympathetic nerve endings. It is found primarily between the scapulae, in the neck, in the mediastinum, and around the kidneys and adrenal glands.

15. How can normothermia be maintained intraoperatively in children?

The following aid in maintenance of normothermia:
- Increase operating room temperature: The major source of heat loss in the anesthetized patient is through radiation. An ambient temperature of 26° C has been shown to be necessary to maintain normothermia.
- Warming mattresses: Use of a warming mattress can minimize conductive heat loss effectively in newborns and infants. This method is less effective in older children because only a small fraction of their body surface area comes in contact with the mattress.
- Convective forced-air warmers.
- Plastic head covering: Because an infant's head contributes to a large portion of its body size, covering the head with plastic reduces evaporative heat losses.

16. Describe renal function in the infant.

Immature nephrons have an impaired ability to filter urine. Glomerular filtra-tion capability matures by 1 year of age. Infants have difficulty with fluid loads because of the decreased excretory power of the kidneys. This capability reaches adult levels by the end of the first year. Concentrating and diluting ability does not mature before 2 to 3 years of age.

17. Discuss key pharmacokinetic principles of intravenous agents in the pediatric patient.

- Infants possess reduced plasma albumin levels. Their albumin differs qualitatively from albumin in adults and has a decreased affinity for drugs.
- Reduced levels of alpha$_1$-acid glycoprotein contribute to a larger volume of distribution for numerous drugs, particularly opioids.

Doses for Commonly Used Induction Agents

Agent	Route	Dose
Ketamine	IV	1–2 mg/kg
	IM	6–10 mg/kg
	Rectal	10 mg/kg
Propofol	IV	2–3 mg/kg
	Maintenance infusion	60–300 mcg/kg/min
Thiopental	IV	5–6 mg/kg
Methohexital	IV	1–2 mg/kg
	IM	10 mg/kg
	Rectal	25–30 mg/kg

Commonly Used Nondepolarizing Muscle Relaxants

Agent	Dose (mg/kg)
Atracurium	0.5
Cisatracurium	0.1–0.2
Mivacurium	0.2–0.3
Pancuronium	0.1
Rocuronium	0.6–1.2
Vecuronium	0.1

- Infants and children possess increased total body water, extracellular fluid volume, and blood volume (per weight basis). These characteristics lead to a greater volume of distribution. Larger doses of some drugs are required (see the tables above).
- The distribution of cardiac output to vessel-rich groups is higher in the pediatric patient. Smaller muscle mass and fat stores limit the reservoir capacity of these sites. As a result, drug plasma concentrations are prone to be higher.
- The activity of biotransformation pathways is reduced in the neonate. At 3 months of age, enhanced metabolic activity in the form of increased phase I reactions is seen. This quality peaks at 2 to 3 years, then declines to adult values after puberty.

18. Children are more prone to which side effects associated with succinylcholine administration?

Children are more prone to *hyperkalemia* and *cardiac dysrhythmias*.

19. **Which two cardiac dysrhythmias are commonly seen after succinylcholine administration in the absence of atropine pretreatment in children?**

    Bradycardia and *sinus node* arrest are commonly seen.

20. **How is uptake and distribution of inhaled anesthetic agents affected in the pediatric patient?**

    Uptake and distribution of inhaled anesthetic agents is more rapid in infants and children than in adults. This effect may be due to several factors, including more rapid respiratory rate, increased cardiac index, and distribution of a larger proportion of the cardiac output to the vessel-rich group.

21. **Is the minimal alveolar concentration (MAC) higher or lower in the pediatric patient?**

    MAC of inhaled agents generally is inversely proportional to age. An increased MAC is particularly apparent in infants age 1 to 6 months.

22. **List emotional factors in children that contribute to psychological preparation for anesthesia and surgery.**

    Children exhibit anxiety associated with hospitalization in several areas:
    • Fear of separation from parents
    • Fear of physical harm or pain
    • Fear of the unknown
    • Uncertainty about the limits on behavior
    • Fear regarding loss of control

23. **Name drugs commonly used to premedicate the pediatric surgical patient.**

    Premedication should be tailored to suit the child's maturation and development and the medical condition; see the following table.

Commonly Used Pediatric Premedicants

Drug	Dose/Route
Midazolam	0.25–0.75 mg/kg (oral) 0.1–0.2 mg/kg (nasal) 0.75–1.0 mg/kg (rectal) 0.1–0.2 mg/kg (IM)
Ketamine	3–6 mg/kg (oral) 2–10 mg/kg (IM) 6 mg/kg (rectal) 3 mg/kg (nasal)

Commonly Used Pediatric Premedicants	*continued*
Drug	**Dose/Route**
Methohexital	10mg/kg (IM) 20–30 mg/kg (rectal)
Transmucosal fentanyl	10–15 mcg/kg (oral)
Sufentanil	2 mcg/kg (nasal)

24. What is the estimated blood volume (EBV) in pediatric patients?

The following table lists EBV values.

Estimated Blood Volume (EBV)	
Age	**EBV (mL/kg)**
Premature	100
Newborn	90
≤ 1 year	75
> 1 year	70

25. Discuss pediatric perioperative fluid management.

Maintenance fluid requirements can be determined by the 4-2-1 rule:
- 4 mL/kg/hr for the first 10 kg of weight
- 2 mL/kg/hr for the second 10 kg
- 1 mL/kg/hr for each remaining kg

Fluid deficit is ascertained by multiplying the hourly maintenance by the number of hours the patient was NPO (nothing by mouth) status. It is replaced by one half in the first hour and one quarter in the second and third hours.

Third space losses should be replaced as follows:

Surgical Trauma	mL/kg/hr
Minimal	3 to 4
Moderate	5 to 6
Severe	7 to 10

A balanced salt solution, such as lactated Ringer's solution, is recommended. Glucose-containing solutions should be used when indicated, such as circumstances involving a premature infant, an infant of a diabetic mother, a diabetic child who has received a portion of daily insulin, or a child who has received hyperalimentation.

26. How does the nurse anesthetist determine allowable blood loss (ABL)?

ABL should be based on the patient's medical condition, the surgical procedure, and the patient's overall cardiopulmonary function. Premature infants and neonates have a tendency toward postoperative apnea at a hematocrit (Hct) less than 30%. The following formula can be used to calculate ABL:

$$ABL = [EBV \times (starting\ Hct - lowest\ acceptable\ Hct)] \div average\ Hct$$

$$Average\ Hct = (starting\ Hct + lowest\ acceptable\ Hct) \div 2$$

Example: A 2-year-old child weighing 12 kg has an EBV of 840 mL; starting Hct is 40%; lowest acceptable Hct is 30%

$$840 \times (40 - 30) = 8400$$

$$8400 \div 35 = 240\ mL\ ABL$$

27. How is blood loss replaced?

Using balanced salt containing crystalloid solutions for blood replacement calls for infusing 3 mL for every 1 mL of blood lost. Colloid solutions are administered using a 1:1 ratio.

28. How does the anesthetist calculate the volume of packed red blood cells (PRBCs) to be infused?

$$PRBCs\ (mL) = [(blood\ loss - ABL) \times desired\ Hct] \div Hct\ of\ PRBCs$$

$$Hct\ of\ PRBCs = 75\%$$

Example: A 12-kg toddler with an allowable blood loss of 240 mL has an intraoperative blood loss of 350 mL; desired Hct is 30%.

$$[350 - 240] \times 30 = 3300$$

$$3300 \div 75 = 44\ mL\ to\ be\ infused$$

29. Identify anesthetic implications for premature infants.

Premature infants (<50 to 60 weeks' postconceptual age) are prone to episodes of postoperative obstructive and central apnea. This risk can last for 24 hours postoperatively. Risk factors for postoperative apnea include the following:
- Low gestational age at birth
- Hct <30%
- Hypothermia
- Sepsis
- Neurological abnormalities

Outpatient procedures should be delayed until 50 weeks' postconception.

There is an increased incidence of congenital anomalies.

30. When should children be made NPO in preparation for anesthesia?

Children should be made NPO based on the following:

Type of Food	Time Frame (before anesthesia)
Solids	6 or more hours
Formula	6 hours
Breast milk	4 hours
Clear liquids	2 hours

CONTROVERSY

31. Should surgery be canceled if a child presents with a cold?

Whether or not one should anesthetize a child who presents with a cold is a controversial topic. The following points should be considered when making the decision:
- A child with an active or resolving respiratory tract infection possesses a highly reactive airway and is prone to developing atelectasis, mucous plugging of the airways, postoperative hypoxemia, and laryngospasm.
- In the case of lower respiratory tract infection, airway reactivity can persist 6 to 8 weeks from the onset of symptoms.
- Elective surgery should be postponed if a child has a sore throat and cough accompanied by a fever.

32. List signs and symptoms of congenital diaphragmatic hernia (CDH).

Signs and symptoms of CDH include:
- Hypoxia
- Scaphoid abdomen
- Evidence of bowel in the thorax
- Malrotation of intestines

33. Name pulmonary derangements that are consistent with CDH.

Pulmonary derangements consistent with CDH are *pulmonary hypoplasia* and *pulmonary hypertension*.

34. Discuss anesthetic implications associated with CDH.

- Visceral distention caused by gas insufflation increases the mass effect in the thorax. For this reason, mask ventilation should be avoided. Awake intubation is recommended.
- Because infants with CDH have air in the gastrointestinal tract and are prone to hypoxia, nitrous oxide is contraindicated.

- Gastric distention should be alleviated by nasogastric suctioning.
- Adequate muscle relaxation is crucial to allow replacement of the gastrointestinal tract into the peritoneal cavity and to facilitate closure.
- When the abdominal contents have been returned, the anesthetist should avoid aggressive attempts to expand the hypoplastic lung. This action could result in pneumothorax on the contralateral side, which presents with a sudden decrease in compliance, blood pressure, or oxygenation.

35. What is the most common type of tracheoesophageal fistula (TEF)?

Occurring in 90% of cases, the most common type consists of the upper esophagus that ends in a dilated, blind pouch and the lower esophagus that connects to the trachea.

36. Are there any additional congenital defects associated with TEF?

Cardiac anomalies and the *VATER* association (vertebral abnormalities, imperforate anus, tracheosophageal fistula, esophageal atresia, and radial and renal dysplasia) are common.

37. Name two key concepts when managing the airway of a patient with TEF.

- Positive-pressure ventilation before intubation should be avoided because of the impairment of expansion from gastric distention and the risk of aspiration.
- The tip of the ETT ideally should be placed between the fistula and the carina.

38. Describe the similarities and differences between omphalocele and gastroschisis.

Both disorders involve a defect that allows herniation of abdominal viscera. Omphaloceles are enclosed by a membranous sac. Infants with omphalocele may have coexisting cardiac, urological, and metabolic abnormalities, whereas gastroschisis is often an isolated presentation. In both conditions, patients may present with impaired blood supply to the herniated organs, intestinal obstruction, and major intravascular fluid deficits.

39. Describe anesthetic considerations associated with omphalocele and gastroschisis.

- The stomach should be decompressed before induction.
- Nitrous oxide should be avoided.
- Muscle relaxation facilitates reduction of the eviscerated organs.
- Volume resuscitation should be aggressive. Balanced salt solution and 5% albumin are recommended.

40. List the pathophysiological problems associated with left-to-right intracardiac shunts.

Pathophysiological problems associated with left-to-right intracardiac shunts include:
- Volume overload of the pulmonary circuit
- Increased left ventricular workload
- Increased pulmonary vascular resistance

41. Describe the pathophysiology of right-to-left intracardiac shunts.

Right-to-left shunting occurs when pulmonary vascular resistance exceeds systemic vascular resistance. Cyanosis and hypoxemia are the result of the mixing of oxygenated and deoxygenated blood flowing through the shunt.

Key Points

- The fundamental characteristics of the pediatric cardiovascular system include:
  - Noncompliant myocardium
  - Cardiac output heart rate dependent
  - Increased parasympathetic tone
  - Immature baroreceptors
  - Poorly developed vasoconstrictive response to hypovolemia
- ETT insertion depth is three times the internal diameter of the ETT.
- Pediatric patients are susceptible to intraoperative heat loss primarily because of their large body surface area-to-weight ratio.
- An infant can increase heat production by three mechanisms:
  - Physical activity
  - Shivering
  - Nonshivering thermogenesis
- Brown fat metabolism is the principal mechanism through which nonshivering thermogenesis occurs.
- Key pharmacokinetic principles of intravenous agents in pediatric patients are:
  - Reduced plasma albumin levels
  - Larger volume of distribution
  - Larger portion of cardiac output to vessel-rich groups
  - Decreased enzymatic processes in the liver
- Children are more prone to hyperkalemia and cardiac dysrhythmias when succinylcholine is used.
- Uptake and distribution of inhaled anesthetic agents is more rapid in infants and children than in adults.

Continued

Key Points   *continued*

- The following formula can be used to calculate allowable blood loss:
  - ABL = [EBV × (starting Hct – lowest acceptable Hct)] ÷ average Hct
- To calculate the volume of PRBCs to be infused, the following formula can be used:
  - PRBCs (mL) = [(blood loss – ABL) × Desired Hct] ÷ Hct of PRBCs
- NPO requirements for children are 6 or more hours for solids, 6 hours for formula, 4 hours for breast milk, and 2 hours for clear liquids.
- The decision to anesthetize a child with an upper respiratory infection is based on the status of the infection, the reactivity of the airway, and the presence of a febrile state.

Internet Resources

Virtual Anaesthesia Textbook:
http://www.virtual-anaesthesia-textbook.com/

University of Wisconsin Department of Anesthesiology. Pediatric Anesthesiology: The Basics:
http://www.anesthesia.wisc.edu/med3/Peds/pedshandout.html

GASNet Search: Pediatric Anesthesia:
http://www.gasnet.org/about/search.php?p1=pediatric+anesthesia

Nurse-Anesthesia.com:
http://www.nurse-anesthesia.com/

Update in Anesthesia: Practical Procedures Cumulative Index:
http://www.nda.ox.ac.uk/wfsa/html/pages/up_sect.htm

Bibliography

Aker J: Pediatric anesthesia. In Nagelhout J, Zaglaniczny K, editors: *Nurse anesthesia*, Philadelphia, 2001, WB Saunders, pp 1132-1168.

American Society of Anesthesiologists: Practice guidelines for preoperative fasting and the use of pharmacological agents to reduce the risk of pulmonary aspiration: application to healthy patients undergoing elective procedures, *Anesthesiology* 90:896-905, 1999.

Cote CJ, Goudsouzian NG, Ryan JF, et al, editors: *A practice of anesthesia for infants and children*, Philadelphia, 2001, WB Saunders.

Davis JD, Motoyama EK, editors: *Smith's anesthesia for infants and children*, St. Louis, 1996, Mosby.

Morgan GE, Mikhail MS, Murray MJ: *Clinical anesthesiology*, New York, 2002, Lange Medical Books/McGraw-Hill.

Anesthesia for the Geriatric Patient

Dianna M. Heikkila

1. Describe the anesthetic implications of a prolonged circulation time in elderly patients.

A *reduced cardiac output* prolongs the circulation time in elderly patients and causes delayed perfusion to organs such as the brain, heart, and liver. A *prolonged circulation time* may delay the onset of drug effects. Consequently, there may be a delayed induction time and a delay in the onset of intravenous drug action.

2. What are the effects of reduced arterial compliance in the elderly?

- Increased afterload occurs.
- Left ventricular hypertrophy is present.
- Systolic blood pressure is elevated.
- General loss of elasticity is seen throughout the arterial vasculature, resulting in an increased peripheral vasculature resistance.

An increased afterload increases the amount of pressure needed in the left ventricle to pump effectively to the body, and the chronic increase in pressure eventually leads to left ventricular hypertrophy. The reduction in arterial compliance results in an elevated systolic blood pressure. Diastolic blood pressure remains unchanged or decreases, in the absence of coexisting disease.

3. Explain the effects of aging on the pulmonary system.

Aging is associated with reduced lung tissue elasticity. The loss of elasticity increases lung compliance and promotes alveolar overdistention. Age-induced parenchymal changes mimic emphysema, resulting in an increase in physiological shunt. The increased closing capacity associated with aging also contributes to the shunt. Consequently, the efficiency of oxygen exchange is reduced.

4. How is the resting arterial oxygen tension (Pao_2) affected by aging?

The Pao_2 normally decreases with age. The following equation can be useful when predicting a "normal" resting Pao_2 for an elderly patient:

$$Pao_2 \text{ (mm Hg)} = 100 - (0.4 \times \text{age in years})$$

As a general rule, the Pao_2 decreases from 0.35 to 0.5 mm Hg per year.

5. Why are elderly patients more prone to develop acute postoperative respiratory failure?

The elderly are more likely to develop apnea and respiratory depression after administration of opioids and benzodiazepines, suggesting the need for higher inspired oxygen concentrations and supplemental oxygen in the postoperative period.

6. Is the minimal alveolar concentration (MAC) of inhalational anesthetic agents increased or decreased in the elderly?

The MAC is significantly lower for the elderly. In addition, the median effective dose is reduced for many other anesthetic agents, including local anesthetics, opioids, barbiturates, and benzodiazepines.

7. Describe the effects of aging on the renal system.

The elderly have decreased renal blood flow and a decreased glomerular filtration rate (GFR). The reduction in renal blood flow is caused by decreases in cardiac output that accompany aging. There also is an associated decreased ability to conserve water and concentrate urine. The GFR declines about 6% to 8% every decade. Creatinine clearance reflects GFR and is a sensitive indicator of renal function in the elderly.

8. Discuss the anesthetic implications associated with reduced renal function in the elderly.

Decreased renal function, in combination with decreased cardiac reserve, makes a geriatric patient more prone to fluid overload. The anesthetist should keep urine output greater than 0.5 mL/kg/hr. In addition, anesthetic agents that depend on renal clearance should be monitored closely because their elimination may be prolonged in the elderly.

9. What are the consequences of loss of protective airway reflexes in the elderly?

The elderly have diminished protective laryngeal reflexes, placing them at increased risk for aspiration pneumonia. Insertion of a cuffed endotracheal tube and the use of cricoid pressure during induction is recommended.

10. Why are the elderly susceptible to decreases in temperature?

The elderly have a decreased ability to retain and generate body heat. When exposed to the cool environment of the operating room, they experience a significant decrease in temperature. Some of the reasons for this decline include:
- Slowed blood circulation
- A blunted vasoconstrictor response
- Less lean muscle mass and less effective shivering
- Decreased basal metabolic rate
- Thinner skin

11. How does the body composition change in the elderly?

As people age, there is a loss of lean body mass or skeletal muscle and an increase in body fat. The blood volume decreases by 20% to 30%, producing a higher than anticipated initial plasma concentration after intravenous drug administration. Increased lipid storage sites account for enhanced deposition of lipid-soluble anesthetic agents. As a result, lipid-soluble agents may have prolonged effects in an elderly patient.

12. Is regional anesthesia duration different in the elderly?

There is a prolongation of spinal and epidural anesthesia in elderly patients secondary to a decreased vascular absorption of local anesthetics.

13. Is isoflurane a good anesthetic choice for the geriatric patient?

There is no evidence that one volatile agent is better than the other; however, isoflurane might be a prudent choice for the geriatric patient for the following reasons:
- Isoflurane decreases systemic vascular resistance, which decreases the work of the heart.
- It undergoes little metabolism.
- The tachycardia produced by isoflurane is attenuated in the elderly.
- It has low solubility in the blood, producing rapid onset and offset.
- It produces minimal depression of cardiac output and left ventricular ejection fraction.

14. Why do elderly patients have a reduced response to beta-adrenergic agonists?

Elderly patients have changes in autonomic function referred to as *physiological beta blockade*. Possible explanations for the decreased response to beta adrenergic agonists include the following:
- A reduced number of beta receptors
- Abnormal receptor affinity for beta-adrenergic agonists
- Reduced cyclic adenosine monophosphate production after activation of the beta receptor

 Key Points

- A reduced cardiac output prolongs the circulation time in the elderly and causes delayed perfusion to organs such as the brain, heart, and liver. The result may be a delayed onset of drug effects.
- PaO_2 normally decreases with age:
  - PaO_2 (mm Hg) = $100 - (0.4 \times age\ in\ years)$

Continued

Key Points   *continued*

- The MAC of inhalational agents is significantly lower for the elderly. In addition, the median effective dose is reduced for many other anesthetic agents, including local anesthetics, opioids, barbiturates, and benzodiazepines.

- The elderly have decreased renal blood flow and a decreased GFR. There is also an associated decreased ability to conserve water and concentrate urine.

- Decreased renal function, in combination with decreased cardiac reserve, makes a geriatric patient more prone to fluid overload, and anesthetic agents that depend on renal clearance should be monitored closely because their elimination may be prolonged in the elderly.

- The elderly have diminished protective laryngeal reflexes, placing them at increased risk for aspiration pneumonia.

- Elderly patients are susceptible to decreases in body temperature due to slowed blood circulation, a blunted vasoconstrictor response, less lean muscle mass, decreased basal metabolic rate, and thinner skin.

- There is a prolongation of spinal and epidural anesthesia in elderly patients secondary to a decreased vascular absorption of local anesthetics.

Internet Resources

Virtual Anaesthesia Textbook:
http://www.virtual-anaesthesia-textbook.com/

GASNet: Survey of Anesthesiology:
http://www.gasnet.org/sa/2001/06/

Aging and Anesthetic Pharmacology:
http://www.cucrash.com/Handouts/aging_shafer.pdf

American Society of Anesthesiologists: Syllabus on geriatric anesthesiology, palliative care in geriatric anesthesia:
http://www.asahq.org/clinical/geriatrics/palliative.htm

Society for the Advancement of Geriatric Anesthesia:
http://societywebsite.com/saga/

The Deep Blue Book: History of anesthesia:
http://www.arss.org/book/deepblue.htm

Nurse-Anesthesia.com:
http://www.nurse-anesthesia.com/

Bibliography

Martin-Sheridan D: Geriatrics and anesthesia practice. In Nagelhout JJ, Zaglaniczny KL, editors: *Nurse anesthesia*, ed 2, Philadelphia, 2001, WB Saunders, pp 1169-1176.

Morgan GE, Mikhail MS: *Clinical anesthesiology*, ed 2, Stamford, CT, 1996, Appleton & Lange, pp 743-748.

Muravchick S: Anesthesia for the geriatric patient. In Barash PG, Cullen BF, Stoelting RK, editors: *Clinical anesthesia*, ed 3, Philadelphia, 1997, Lippincott-Raven, pp 1125-1136.

Muravchick S: Anesthesia for the elderly. In Miller RD, editor: *Anesthesia*, ed 5, New York, 2000, Churchill Livingstone, pp 2140-2156.

Stoelting RK, Dierdorf SF: *Anesthesia and co-existing disease*, ed 4, New York, 2002, Churchill Livingstone, pp 739-756.

Outpatient Anesthesia

Jennifer Burd

1. Where does ambulatory surgery take place?

Most often, ambulatory (or "outpatient") surgery is performed in the hospital. Specific areas often are designated for the screening, admission, preoperative holding, operative care, and postoperative care of primarily ambulatory surgical patients. Satellite surgery centers may perform solely outpatient surgeries. Increasingly, more surgical procedures take place in physician offices, dentistry clinics, and plastic surgery offices.

2. Describe the types of surgical procedures performed in the ambulatory surgery setting.

Acceptable procedures include cases that are relatively brief and minimally invasive. Criteria for acceptable procedures should focus on the type of surgical case, the proposed length of the case, the anticipated blood loss and physiological fluid shifts, and the need for aggressive postoperative pain control measures. Few intraoperative or postoperative complications should be anticipated, and the ability for postoperative care to take place at home should be considered. Commonly performed procedures include:
- Laparoscopic cholecystectomy
- Laparoscopic tubal ligation
- Arthroscopy
- Hernia repair
- Breast biopsy
- Vaginal hysterectomy
- Select ear, nose, and throat procedures

3. Discuss the advantages of ambulatory surgery.

Economics is a driving force in ambulatory surgery. Outpatient surgical procedures provide cost savings for the patient and third-party payers. Hospitals also benefit, seeing more beds available for patients who require inpatient care. Patients not only reduce their medical costs, but also decrease the risk of nosocomial infection associated with hospital stay. Social concerns, such as child care or postoperative home care, are minimized. Psychological confusion created by child separation from parents or unfamiliarity among geriatric patients is reduced.

411

4. Are patients satisfied with ambulatory surgery and anesthesia?

A study by Tong et al showed that 98% of patients would return to the ambulatory surgical setting in the future. Convenience, faster physiological recovery, fewer complications, and an earlier return to daily activities compared with inpatient procedures make ambulatory surgery attractive.

5. Describe the disadvantages of ambulatory anesthesia.

Because patients are not admitted into the hospital setting preoperatively, they may be asked to visit the ambulatory surgical center a few days before surgery to be evaluated by the anesthesia team. This may require more than one trip for the patient and subsequent arrangements for child care or time off work. In the center, children and the elderly have limited time to adapt to their surroundings. At times, arrangements must be made for postoperative care, which may be difficult for individuals living alone.

6. Are only certain American Society of Anesthesiologists (ASA) classifications considered candidates for ambulatory surgery?

In the early days of ambulatory anesthesia, preference was given to ASA I and ASA II patients almost exclusively. Now, with major advances in safety through monitoring and pharmaceutical agents, outpatient surgery and anesthesia can be offered to medically stable ASA III and ASA IV patients. Patients with complex medical conditions require careful history and physical assessment, including medication review and appropriate laboratory and physical testing, to determine their suitability for outpatient surgery. If required, outside consultations may be requested before surgery. In general, minor surgical procedures are performed for ASA III and ASA IV patients, especially when hospitalization may increase the risk of postoperative complications (e.g., Hickman catheter insertion for immunocompromised patients).

7. What is the age limit for ambulatory anesthesia in the elderly?

Chronological age alone does not determine whether an elderly patient is suitable for outpatient anesthesia. Most medical problems in the elderly are related to organ dysfunction rather than age. Consideration should be given to the physiological, rather than the chronological, age of the patient. Careful examination, including a complete history and physical assessment of the patient, determines the patient's suitability for ambulatory anesthesia. Assessment should be conducted in person, paying special attention to cardiopulmonary reserve and disease.

8. Can premature infants be considered for ambulatory anesthesia?

Infants born at 37 or less weeks of gestational age or who are younger than 50 weeks' postconceptual age are at greater risk for postoperative complications and generally are not appropriate candidates for outpatient anesthesia. Specifically the immature development of the respiratory system and brainstem in premature infants places them at an increased risk for postoperative apnea and hypoxia. Anemia (hematocrit $<$ 30%), common among premature infants, increases this risk. Underdeveloped gag reflexes and brainstem temperature control mechanism enhance the risk for aspiration and hypothermia.

9. Who should *not* have outpatient anesthesia?

Every patient should be assessed by the anesthesia provider to determine his or her specific eligibility for outpatient anesthesia. Certain patient populations are not candidates for surgery at outpatient facilities, however, because their physiological or psychological state mandates the prolonged attention of an inpatient facility. These groups include:
- Infants less than 37 weeks' gestational age at birth or less than 50 weeks' postconceptual age
- Infants with respiratory or cardiac disease
- Infants with a positive family history of sudden infant death syndrome
- Patients with active substance abuse
- Patients with psychosocial difficulties
- Patients with poorly controlled convulsive disorders
- Patients with poorly controlled diabetes mellitus
- Patients with symptomatic sleep apnea
- Patients under sepsis/infectious disease/isolation precautions in centers that lack isolation facilities.

10. How is a preoperative assessment performed for patients undergoing outpatient anesthesia?

Preoperative assessments in ambulatory surgical centers are usually done in one of two ways. For healthy, uncomplicated patients, *telephone interviews,* performed before the day of surgery, can adequately obtain the history required for anesthesia evaluation. If laboratory tests or further screening are necessary, visiting the surgical center for this purpose would be necessary. Telephone screening increases patient convenience, but carries the risk that not all necessary patient data are obtained.

Elderly patients and patients with preexisting complex disease may require an *in-house patient assessment* at least 1 week before surgery. Early assessment provides time for preoperative testing, laboratory work, necessary consultations, and changes to medication regimens.

11. What laboratory tests should be performed for ambulatory surgery patients?

Physical testing and laboratory studies should be performed as necessary, providing the same level of assessment as for inpatients.

12. Are the same NPO (nothing by mouth) status and aspiration prophylaxis measures used in the ambulatory surgery setting as in the inpatient setting?

Patients should be instructed to follow NPO guidelines outlined by the practice guidelines for preoperative fasting, set forth by the American Society of

Anesthesiologists. NPO guidelines for a healthy patient undergoing elective surgery are summarized in the following table. To simplify this regimen, adult patients are often instructed to remain NPO after midnight. Patients with risk factors for pulmonary aspiration (e.g., obesity, diabetes, hiatal hernia, postpartum status, gastroesophageal reflux) should receive appropriate pharmaceutical agents to reduce the risk of pulmonary aspiration.

Fasting Guidelines to Reduce the Risk of Pulmonary Aspiration

Ingested Material	Minimum Fasting Period (hr)
Clear liquids (e.g., water, fruit juices without pulp, clear tea, black coffee, carbonated beverages)	2
Breast milk	4
Infant formula	6
Nonhuman milk*	6
Light meal (e.g., toast and clear liquids)†	6

*Nonhuman milk is similar to solids in gastric emptying time. The amount ingested must be considered when determining an appropriate fasting period.
†The amount and type of foods ingested must be considered when determining an appropriate fasting period. Fried or fatty foods or meat may prolong gastric emptying time.

13. Should an ambulatory surgical patient receive less anxiolytic premedication to avoid prolonged postoperative sedation?

If administered judiciously, short-acting agents should not prolong the post-operative stay and recovery. Premedication should be administered, as necessary, in the appropriate dosages. Midazolam (Versed) (0.07 to 0.1 mg/kg intravenously [IV]) and fentanyl (0.5 to 1.5 mcg/kg IV) are commonly administered pre-medicants in the outpatient setting.

14. Is general anesthesia performed the same way in the ambulatory setting as in the inpatient setting?

General anesthesia is induced and maintained with the same standards of care as in the inpatient setting. Special consideration may be given, however, to the time limitation of the surgical procedure and the associated use of appropriate shorter acting anesthetic agents.

Propofol (1 to 3 mg/kg IV) may be an appropriate agent for the induction of general anesthesia. Its short half-life and antiemetic qualities make it a suitable agent for procedures of any length. Sevoflurane and desflurane, volatile agents with low blood gas coefficients and rapid onset and recovery profiles, are ideal agents in the outpatient setting. For muscle relaxation, succinylcholine is often used when rapid-sequence induction is indicated and may be used for procedures of short duration. Short-acting nondepolarizng muscle relaxants, such as rocuronium and mivacurium, are ideal for standard inductions and during maintenance of anesthesia, and do not have the adverse effects profile associated with succinylcholine. The use of nitrous oxide is controversial, owing to the increased incidence of postoperative emesis with its use. Nitrous oxide is useful, however, as an accompaniment to inhalational induction in children. Remifentanil and alfentanil infusions are used successfully in the outpatient setting, capitalizing on their rapid recovery profiles.

15. Is regional anesthesia acceptable for outpatient surgical procedures; what are the advantages and disadvantages?

Regional anesthesia, using short-acting agents with rapid onset and offset (e.g., procaine, lidocaine, ropivacaine), is ideal for outpatient procedures. Regional anesthesia provides postoperative pain relief, while decreasing the sedation and nausea associated with general anesthesia. Spinal and epidural anesthesia, peripheral nerve blocks, and intravenous regional anesthesia all may be used.

A potential disadvantage to regional anesthesia in the outpatient setting is the time required to perform the block. Delayed discharge can result from urinary retention, hypotension, and prolonged motor and sensory blockade associated with spinal or epidural anesthesia. Care must be taken postoperatively to protect extremities with residual blockade.

16. List criteria for discharge from the outpatient surgical facility.

Discharge criteria are as follows:
- No abnormal swelling or bleeding from the operative site
- Vital signs stable
- Able to take oral fluids without nausea or vomiting; able to swallow
- Able to ambulate unassisted
- Controlled pain
- Able to urinate after urological procedure or neuraxial blockade
- No respiratory distress
- Discharge instructions explained, and written guidelines provided to a responsible caregiver. The caregiver should be instructed to stay with the patient overnight.

17. How is nausea and vomiting managed in the ambulatory surgical setting?

Nausea, with or without vomiting, delays discharge more often than any other postoperative symptom and may contribute to unanticipated admission into an inpatient facility. The prevention and treatment of nausea are imperative in the outpatient setting. Postoperative nausea and vomiting can be preemptively treated by administering antiemetics before surgery. Metoclopramide (10 mg

IV), droperidol (0.0625 to 0.125 mg IV), dexamethasone (170 mcg/kg IV), and scopolamine (patch) have been used successfully. Aggressive fluid therapy should be instituted perioperatively. Before skin closure, ondansetron (4 to 8 mg IV) may be given. Rescue postoperative nausea relief may be provided by one or more of the above-mentioned agents.

18. What are the ideal agents for pain control in this setting?

Surgical pain should be treated quickly and effectively in the ambulatory setting to maintain patient satisfaction and to prevent delayed discharge. Local nerve block, opioids, and nonsteroidal antiinflammaotry drugs (NSAIDs) are used successfully in preventing postoperative pain. Carefully titrated intravenous doses of short-acting opioids, such as fentanyl 0.5 to 1.5 mcg/kg, are often effective in controlling postoperative pain. NSAIDs, such as ketorolac (30–60 mg, IV or IM), provide pain relief and reduce the dosage requirements for opioids. NSAIDs are devoid of the respiratory depression, nausea, or vomiting associated with opioids. Children may receive an elixir of acetaminophen with codeine (120 mg acetaminophen and 12 mg codeine per 5 mL) or an ibuprofen elixir for pain relief. As an alternative, an acetaminophen suppository (10–15 mg/kg, PR) may be inserted before emergence.

19. Can malignant hyperthermia (MH)–susceptible patients be cared for in the ambulatory surgical setting?

Patients susceptible to MH can receive care in the appropriate outpatient setting when necessary preparatory measures are taken. Patients at risk for MH include:
- A patient with a previous MH episode
- A patient with a first-degree relative with a history of an MH episode or a positive muscle biopsy test
- A patient with a positive muscle biopsy test

Measures to prepare for a possible event involve early scheduling of the procedure; standard monitoring; and immediate availability of all treatment drugs, monitors, and equipment needed for an MH episode. Dantrolene sodium must be on hand. If an event does not occur, the patient may be discharged home with standard follow-up procedures.

20. Are tonsillectomies appropriate procedures for the outpatient setting; which patients should not have tonsillectomies performed as outpatients?

Tonsillectomies are successfully performed in the ambulatory surgical setting. Hesitancy in the past has centered on the high risk for postoperative bleeding after this procedure. Tonsillectomies should be scheduled early in the day to allow for adequate postoperative monitoring. Some centers require a minimum 23-hour stay.

Adequate preoperative and intraoperative hydration must account for pre-operative, intraoperative, and anticipated postoperative volume deficits. Close postoperative monitoring is imperative to assess for bleeding.

The American Association of Otolaryngology-Head and Neck Surgery suggests that tonsillectomies should be performed as inpatients for patients younger than 3 years old or if geographical or social factors inhibit the patient's prompt return to an emergency department. Patients scheduled for tonsillectomy who have associated obstructive sleep apnea, craniofacial or airway disorders, or peritonsillar abscess should have the procedure performed as inpatients.

Key Points

- ASA I and ASA II patients are acceptable candidates for ambulatory surgery as are medically stable ASA III and ASA IV patients.
- Physiological age, not chronological age, should determine suitability for the ambulatory setting in the elderly patient.
- Infants born at 37 or less weeks of gestational age, or who are younger than 50 weeks' postconceptual age, are at greater risk for postoperative complications and are generally not appropriate candidates for outpatient anesthesia.
- NPO and aspiration prophylaxis measures are the same as the inpatient setting.
- Regional anesthesia, using short-acting agents with rapid onset and offset (e.g., procaine, lidocaine, ropivacaine) are ideal for outpatient procedures.
- Nausea, with or without vomiting, delays discharge more often than any other postoperative symptom and may contribute to unanticipated admission into an inpatient facility.

Internet Resources

GASNet Search: Amublatory Surgery:
http://www.gasnet.org/about/search.php?p1=ambulatory+surgery

Update in Anesthesia: Cumulative Index:
http://www.nda.ox.ac.uk/wfsa/html/pages/up_issu.htm#1

Virtual Anaesthesia Textook:
http://www.virtual-anaesthesia-textbook.com/

Nurse-Anesthesia.com:
http://www.nurse-anesthesia.com/

Bibliography

Barash PG, Cullen BF, Stoelting RK: *Clinical anesthesia,* ed 3, Philadelphia, 1997, Lippincott Williams & Wilkins.

Hurford WE, Bailin MT, Davison JK, et al: *Clinical anesthesia procedures of the Massachusetts General Hospital,* ed 6, Philadelphia, 2002, Lippincott Williams & Wilkins.

Morgan GE, Mikhail MS, Murray MJ: *Clinical anesthesiology,* ed 3, New York, 2002, McGraw-Hill.

Nagelhout JJ, Zaglaniczny KL: *Nurse anesthesia,* ed 2, Philadelphia, 2001, WB Saunders.

Sa Rego M, Watcha MF, White PF: The changing role of monitored anesthesia care in the ambulatory setting, *Anesth Analg* 85:1020-1036, 1997.

Song D, Joshi GP, White PF: Fast-track eligibility after ambulatory anesthesia: a comparison of desflurane, sevoflurane, and propofol, *Anesth Analg* 86:267-273, 1998.

Steward DL, Lerman J: *Manual of pediatric anesthesia,* ed 5, New York, 2001, Churchill Livingstone.

Tong D, Chung F, Wong D: Predictive factors in global and anesthesia satisfaction in ambulatory surgical patients, *Anesthesiology* 87:856-864, 1997.

Warner MA, Caplan RA, Epstein BS, et al: Practice guidelines for preoperative fasting and the use of pharmacologic agents to reduce the risk of pulmonary aspiration: application to healthy patients undergoing elective procedures. Report by the American Society of Anesthesiologists, (1999); available online: http://www.asahq.org/publicationsandservices/NPO.pdf.

Chapter 46

Trauma

Anne B. Harrington

1. Summarize the statistics regarding trauma in the United States.

In the United States, trauma is the leading cause of death in individuals younger than age 40, and it is the third leading cause of death regardless of age. Prehospital care continues to improve, and the number of trauma victims reaching the hospital alive is increasing.

Currently, one third of all hospital admissions can be attributed to trauma. In patients who survive the critical "golden hour," aggressive resuscitation, stabilization, and perioperative care can minimize later morbidity and mortality. Because emergency surgery is required for many trauma victims, anesthetists play a pivotal role in the initial resuscitation and management of these patients.

2. List items to include in a trauma operating room setup.

In addition to the standard operating room setup, it is important to have the following items readily available:
- A difficult airway cart that includes a fiberoptic bronchoscope
- Standard emergency drugs, including vasopressors, inotropes, atropine, calcium chloride, and sodium bicarbonate
- Readily available crystalloid solutions, colloid solutions, and blood products
- Multiple large-bore intravenous catheters and equipment for central venous access
- Rapid infusion devices
- Several intravenous tubings, infusion pumps, blood filters, and pressure bags
- Arterial line kits, transducers, and pressure cables
- Forced air warming blanket and fluid warmers

3. Discuss unique considerations regarding anesthesia induction in a trauma patient.

FULL STOMACH
Because trauma delays gastric emptying, all patients require full-stomach precautions, regardless of the last oral intake. If a nasogastric tube is present, it should be placed to suction; however, this does not ensure an empty stomach. The airway should be secured with a rapid-sequence induction while maintaining cricoid pressure.

CERVICAL INSTABILITY

Neck immobilization in the neutral position is advised during intubation if the patient is unconscious or complains of neck pain or if pain is present that could mask cervical tenderness. Before attempting intubation, manual in-line axial stabilization, with the anterior portion of the cervical collar removed, should be applied. Use of a Bullard laryngoscope may facilitate intubation with decreased head and neck extension compared with intubation with a Miller or Macintosh blade. Awake fiberoptic intubation with topical anesthesia and carefully titrated sedation before anesthesia induction may be used for a cooperative trauma patient with known cervical injury.

DRUG OR ALCOHOL USE

Intoxication with alcohol or street drugs occurs in 30% to 50% of all trauma patients. Patients with illicit drug ingestion before surgery may show increased or decreased anesthetic requirements, labile blood pressure, delayed recovery, and postoperative hallucinations.

HYPOVOLEMIA

A contracted intravascular blood volume reduces the volume of distribution, causing a higher plasma concentration of intravenous drugs. Decreased hepatic and renal blood flow slows metabolism of many drugs so that their effects are prolonged. Small incremental dosing is suggested.

4. Which induction drugs are appropriate for a hypotensive trauma patient?

Hypotension in the trauma patient suggests uncompensated hypovolemia. Induction presents a challenge because administration of anesthetics invariably worsens the degree of circulatory compromise. Aggressive restoration of intravascular volume should be attempted before induction. If severe hemorrhage prevents establishment of euvolemia, small doses of hypnotic agents should be used.

The myocardial depressive and vasodilatory effects of thiopental sodium and propofol can cause severe hemodynamic compromise in patients who are not adequately fluid resuscitated even when given in reduced dosages. Because of its sympathomimetic effects, *ketamine* can be a useful agent in hypovolemic trauma patients; however, its direct cardiac depressant properties can be unmasked in patients who already have maximal sympathetic stimulation. Ketamine increases intracranial pressure and should be avoided in patients with suspected head injury. Etomidate causes minimal circulatory deterioration and is often an appropriate choice for a hypotensive trauma patient. Opioids such as fentanyl and sufentanil have minimal cardiovascular or baroreflex activity but can aggravate hypotension by attenuating sympathetic tone.

5. In which patients should nasal intubation be avoided?

Maxillofacial injury and head trauma, particularly basilar and midface skull fractures, can compromise the integrity of the cribriform plate of the ethmoid bone. Cerebrospinal fluid otorrhea and rhinorrhea and the presence of blood behind the eardrum indicate a basilar fracture. With these types of injuries, nasal intubation is contraindicated because the nasal endotracheal tube can aberrantly enter the orbital fossa or cranium. Nasal endotracheal tube placement also can contaminate cerebrospinal fluid with nasal flora, leading to bacteremia or meningitis. Similarly, insertion of a nasogastric tube or nasal airway should be avoided in these patients.

6. Why are trauma patients at high risk for recall, and what can be done to minimize awareness?

Severe hemodynamic instability may preclude the maintenance of anesthesia at levels appropriate to prevent patient recall. Scopolamine, 5 to 10 mcg/kg, is a useful amnestic agent with minimal cardiac effects. Redosing should be considered in young patients having surgery lasting more than 4 hours. Alternatively, intermittent doses of midazolam can be given and may be especially appropriate when there is a concern regarding anticholinergic hypersensitivity.

7. In what situations would using nitrous oxide be deleterious to a trauma patient?

The high diffusibility of nitrous oxide allows expansion of air-filled cavities or an increase in pressure in airspaces surrounded by a rigid wall. It is contraindicated in patients with the following:
- Pneumothorax
- Closed head injury
- Pneumocephalus
- Bowel injury
- Presence of air emboli.

In addition, use of nitrous oxide has limited value in a patient requiring high inspired oxygen concentrations (e.g., patient with lung contusion). When used in conjunction with opioids, nitrous oxide may reduce cardiac output and exaggerate hypotension. For these reasons, many practitioners routinely avoid nitrous oxide during acute trauma management.

8. What is Beck's triad, and what does it indicate?

The components of Beck's triad are jugular venous distention, hypotension, and muffled heart tones. Cardiac tamponade, the result of accumulation of blood in the pericardial sac, causes these characteristic symptoms. Tachycardia, a narrow pulse pressure, pulsus paradoxus (a decrease in systolic blood pressure by >10 mm Hg with spontaneous inspiration), and electrical alternans are additional manifestations of cardiac tamponade. Because these findings are difficult to appreciate in a hypovolemic trauma patient, definitive diagnosis is made by echocardiography. Cardiac tamponade is life-threatening. Pericardiocentesis and surgical decompression offer immediate treatment.

9. **A patient with a known pericardial tamponade presents for a thoracotomy. What mnemonic describes your anesthetic goals?**

Fast, full, and tight. Blood in the pericardial sac restricts diastolic filling, decreases stroke volume, and leads to an overall reduction in cardiac output. These effects are magnified with general anesthesia and positive-pressure ventilation. It is often preferable to have the tamponade evacuated under local anesthesia before definitive surgical repair, if possible. Anesthetic management is aimed at maintaining chronotropism, contractility, and preload by preventing vasodilation and myocardial depression. Ketamine is the induction agent of choice for these reasons.

10. **How does a tension pneumothorax present under general anesthesia?**

The initiation of positive-pressure ventilation can transform a simple pneumothorax to a tension pneumothorax. Under these circumstances, air forced into the pleural space with inspiration is unable to escape with expiration, causing collapse of the ipsilateral lung. As air accumulates in the pleural space, it displaces the mediastinum to the opposite side, impairing venous return and expansion of the unaffected lung. Tachycardia, hypotension, tracheal deviation, neck vein distention, and loss of unilateral breath sounds result. Positive-pressure ventilation shows an increase in peak inspiratory pressures. Hypoxemia, cyanosis, and cardiovascular collapse can occur if left untreated. Placement of a large-bore (14-gauge) needle into the second intercostal space at the midclavicular line on the affected side allows for immediate decompression until a chest tube can be placed.

11. **Differentiate between a pericardial tamponade and a tension pneumothorax.**

The following table presents signs of pericardial tamponade and tension pneumothorax.

Pericardial Tamponade and Tension Pneumothorax		
Sign	**Pericardial Tamponade**	**Tension Pneumothorax**
Tachycardia	+	+
Hypotension	+	+
Neck vein distention	+	+
Loss of unilateral breath sounds	−	+
Muffled heart tones	+	−

12. **A trauma patient presents to the operating room with a pelvic fracture. What is noteworthy about this injury?**

Pelvic fractures are associated with a high mortality rate. Laceration of arteries and veins that exit the pelvis can cause several liters of blood to escape and accumulate in the retroperitoneal space before tamponade occurs. Anesthetic management includes ongoing fluid resuscitation. Fat emboli syndrome and an associated hypoxic respiratory failure may occur in these patients as a result of seeding of marrow fat into the venous circulation. Additionally, patients with pelvic injury are at high risk for deep vein thrombosis.

13. **A patient was involved in an industrial crush accident and is undergoing a revascularization procedure of his arm; his urine is dark amber. Why should you be concerned?**

Myoglobin is released from damaged muscle cells after a crush injury. It produces a characteristic tea-colored urine and can lead to acute renal failure unless treated. Vigorous fluid administration is advised to maintain renal perfusion and a high urine output. Mannitol also may be used to promote tubular flow and induce diuresis. Hyperkalemia, hypotension, and metabolic acidosis also are seen in patients with crush injuries.

14. **Define shock and describe the treatment goals for a trauma patient in shock.**

Shock is an abnormal circulatory state characterized by inadequate tissue perfusion and oxygenation. The leading cause of shock in trauma patients is hemorrhagic hypovolemia. The reduction in effective circulating blood volume leads to organ hypoperfusion and ultimately cellular death. The initial management is directed at restoration of cellular and organ perfusion with adequately oxygenated blood. Fluid resuscitation must be rapid and aggressive.

15. **A trauma patient loses 30% of his blood volume. Describe the associated signs and symptoms.**

An adult accident victim who has lost 30% of his blood volume is anxious, restless, and possibly confused. The patient may complain of thirst, and his skin is cool and pale. When 30% of the blood volume is lost, compensatory hemodynamic mechanisms are taxed, and blood pressure decreases. Vital signs show tachycardia, tachypnea, and a narrowed pulse pressure. The elderly have limited ability to increase their heart rate in response to hypovolemia and a normal heart rate gives little indication of the severity of volume depletion in these patients. Children have strong cardiac reserve and typically do not show deterioration until a 30% to 40% acute volume loss.

16. **Outline the physiological changes seen with progressive blood loss in a 70-kg patient; how does this guide fluid resuscitation?**

Physiological changes and fluid replacement guidelines are outlined in the table on page 424.

Physiological Changes Observed with Progressive Blood Loss in 70-kg Patient				
Factors	*Blood Loss*			
	<15%	**15–30%**	**30–40%**	**>40%**
Blood loss (mL)	Up to 750	750–1500	1500–2000	>2000
Heart rate (beats/min)	<100	>100	>120	>140
Blood pressure	Normal	Normal	Decreased	Decreased
Respiratory rate	Normal	Slight tachypnea	Moderate tachypnea	Rapid
Urine output (mL/hr)	>30	20–30	5–15	Negligible
Mental status	Slightly anxious	Mildly anxious	Anxious/confused	Confused/ lethargic
Fluid replacement	Crystalloid (3:1 rule*)	Crystalloid (3:1 rule*)	Crystalloid + blood	Crystalloid + blood

*3:1 rule = 3 mL of crystalloid administration for 1 mL of blood lost.
Adapted from the American College of Surgeons.

17. What is the most common cause of coagulopathy in a trauma patient?

Dilutional thrombocytopenia occurs most frequently as a result of massive fluid and blood administration. With massive blood transfusion (generally defined as one to two times the patient's blood volume), the patient's blood increasingly resembles bank blood, which contains few functional platelets and low levels of factors V and VIII. It is recommended to consider platelet replacement when 1.5 to 2 times the patient's blood volume has been transfused, when the platelet count is less than 50,000/mm³, or when the platelet count is less than 70,000/mm³ with ongoing bleeding. Coagulation studies should guide fresh frozen plasma and specific coagulation factor replacement.

CONTROVERSY

18. Should crystalloids or colloid infusions constitute the mainstay of fluid resuscitation in trauma?

The debate over which solution should be used for resuscitation is ongoing and controversial, owing to conflicting data whether one has improved outcomes versus the other. Colloid (e.g., albumin, dextran, starch) solutions contain large molecules that remain in the intravascular compartment longer. This osmotic effect results in less volume shift into the interstitial fluid. Because of this, fluid resuscitation with colloids is purportedly more rapid and effective. Colloid solutions are expensive, however, and some solutions can contribute to coagulopathy.

Larger volumes of crystalloid solutions are needed for intravascular volume resuscitation in trauma patients because the fluid is rapidly redistributed to the interstitial space. This may contribute to the development of tissue and pulmonary edema. Advantages of crystalloids are that they are inexpensive and cause few adverse reactions. The use of both solutions is often advocated to restore intravascular volume, but until definitive data exist to support a specific fluid therapy regimen, the debate will continue.

Key Points

- Trauma is the leading cause of death in individuals younger than age 40, and it is the third leading cause of death regardless of age.
- Unique considerations regarding anesthesia induction in the trauma patient include:
  - Full stomach
  - Cervical instability
  - Drug or alcohol use
  - Hypovolemia
- Ketamine is a good induction drug in a trauma patient due to its sympathomimetic effects.
- Etomidate causes minimal circulatory deterioration and is often an appropriate choice for a hypotensive trauma patient.
- Maxillofacial injury and head trauma, particularly basilar and midface skull fractures, are contraindications to nasal intubation.
- Nitrous oxide is contraindicated in a trauma patient with pneumothorax, closed head injury, pneumocephalus, bowel injury, or the presence of air emboli. When used in conjunction with opioids, nitrous oxide may reduce cardiac output and exaggerate hypotension.
- Jugular venous distention, hypotension, and muffled heart tones are the components of Beck's triad, caused by cardiac tamponade, which is life-threatening. Pericardiocentesis and surgical decompression offer immediate treatement.
- *Fast, full, and tight* describe the anesthetic goals in a patient with cardiac tamponade.
- A tension pneumothorax presents under general anesthesia as tachycardia, hypotension, tracheal deviation, neck vein distention, and loss of unilateral breath sounds. Hypoxemia, cyanosis, and cardiovascular collapse can occur if a pneumothorax is left untreated.
- Dilutional thrombocytopenia is the most common cause of coagulopathy in a trauma patient.

Internet Resources

GASNet Search: Trauma and Anesthesia:
http://gasnet.med.yale.edu/about/search.php?p1=trauma+anesthesia

Virtual Anesthesia Textbook.com:
http://www.virtual-anaesthesia-textbook.com/

Update in Anesthesia: Cumulative Update:
http://www.nda.ox.ac.uk/wfsa/html/pages/up_issu.htm#1

Nurse-Anesthesia.com:
http://www.nurse-anesthesia.com/

The WorldWide Anaesthetist: Anaesthetic Techniques:
http://www.anaesthetist.com/anaes/tech/index.htm

Bibliography

Barton CR: Trauma anesthesia. In Nagelhout JJ, Zaglaniczny KL, editors: *Nurse anesthesia*, ed 2, Philadelphia, 2001, WB Saunders, pp 824-844.

Capan LM, Miller SM: Trauma and burns. In Barash PG, Cullen BF, Stoelting RK, editors: *Clinical anesthesia*, ed 3, Philadelphia, 1997, Lippincott-Raven, pp 1173-1200.

Chapman NN, Cullen BF: Anesthesia induction and maintenance, *Anesthesiol Clin North Am* 14:173-190, 1996.

Domino KB: Pulmonary function and dysfunction in the traumatized patient, *Anesthesiol Clin North Am* 14:59-80, 1996.

Grande CM, Smith CE, Stene JK: Trauma anesthesia. In Longnecker DE, Tinker JH, Morgan GE, editors: *Principles and practice of anesthesiology,* vol II, ed 2, St. Louis, 1998, Mosby, pp 2138-2161.

International Trauma Anesthesia and Critical Care Society: *More about trauma,* accessed June 2, 2002; available online: http://www.trauma.itaccs.com/more/more.htm.

Morgan GE Jr, Mikhail MS, Murray MJ: Anesthesia for the trauma patient. In: *Clinical anesthesiology,* ed 3, New York, 2002, Lange Medical Books/McGraw-Hill, pp 793-800.

Stene JK, Grande CM: Anesthesia for trauma. In Miller R, editor: *Anesthesia,* New York, 1994, Churchill Livingstone, pp 2157-2172.

Stoelting RK, Miller RD: *Basics of anesthesia,* ed 4, Philadelphia, 2000, Churchill Livingstone, pp 239, 437-438.

Burn Patients

Joseph Anthony Joyce

1. What are common causes of burn injury?

Boiling water, high-voltage wires, sulfuric acid, motor vehicle accidents, fire, hot grease, sodium hydroxide, electrical outlets, and "dry ice" all produce significant burn injuries.

2. Define commonly used terms related to the care and treatment of burn injuries.

- *Allograft*—skin graft obtained from a human source other than the patient; usually obtained from cadavers.
- *Autograft*—skin graft obtained from uninjured areas of the patient's skin.
- *Carboxyhemoglobin*—biological compound formed by carbon monoxide and hemoglobin.
- *Circumferential*—involving the entire circumference of a body part (e.g., hands, feet, arms, legs, torso, head, and neck).
- *Dermis*—second layer of skin within which are contained sweat glands, nerve endings, and hair follicles.
- *Débridement*—removal of devitalized tissue from a burn injury to the point of exposure of healthy, viable tissue.
- *Donor site*—area from which healthy skin is harvested (obtained) for use in grafting (autografting).
- *Epidermis*—outermost layer of skin.
- *Eschar*—tough, sometimes leathery, nonviable tissue that is produced in full-thickness burn injuries.
- *Heterograft*—grafting material obtained from another animal species, usually porcine; also called *xenograft*.

3. Burns used to be called first, second, or third degree; what is the current method for classifying burn injuries?

Burns were formally classified by a "degree system." That classification system poorly described the extent of damage to the skin that occurred and has been replaced with a more accurately descriptive system.

- *Superficial partial-thickness* injuries involve predominantly the epidermis, sometimes extensively. Occasionally the injury can extend down to the level of the dermis. Numerous Americans experience this type of burn when sun bathing too long. Although it can be painful, the discomfort experienced is neither agonizing nor constant.

- *Deep partial-thickness* burns consume the epidermal layer entirely and extend well into, but not through, the dermal layer. Burned areas become edematous with bodily fluids being lost via "weeping" of the denuded areas. *Dermal inclusions* (i.e., sweat glands, nerve endings, and hair follicles) are not destroyed at this depth of injury. As a result of this injury, the nerve endings are exposed and constantly stimulated/hyperactive, which produces the characteristic hyperesthesia associated with this depth of injury. Skin grafting usually is not required for wound closure, although it is an option for this depth burn injury.
- *Full-thickness* burns are more serious. The entire thickness of the skin, the epidermis and the dermis, is consumed or destroyed. By definition, with the entire skin being destroyed, the dermal inclusions also are destroyed or obliterated. The wound is relatively dry and pain-free. The area of injury is edematous and pale or ashen or black in color; there is no blanching or capillary refill. The injured area has the look and feel of leather or the sole of a shoe. There is no elasticity in full-thickness burns. As a result, circumferential burns require escharotomy to release the pressure built up by edema formation to maintain circulation to tissues deep to the burn injury. In cases in which full-thickness burns occur circumferentially to the chest/torso, escharotomy is required to allow expansion of the chest wall during respiration. Extensive surgical débridement and skin grafting are required to achieve wound closure; that is, this depth of injury leaves no remnant of skin tissue whereby "spontaneous" regeneration of skin tissues can occur.
- *Fourth degree* is the last remaining vestige of the former classification system. This depth burn injury destroys the entire epidermis, dermis, and subcutaneous layers and extends well into, often through, the muscle layer and may damage the bone. The devitalized tissue must be excised completely. Often this complete excision occurs in the form of amputation of the extremity involved. If the extremity eventually survives, its function is severely limited.

4. Explain what constitutes a minor versus a major burn.

Classification of the seriousness of a burn injury incorporates many factors along with the depth of the burn injury itself. Other contributing factors include, but are not limited to:

- Age
- Overall percentage of the total body surface area (%TBSA) involved
- Portion of the %TBSA that is deep partial thickness
- Portion of the %TBSA that is full thickness
- Presence of associated traumatic injury
- Coexisting disease processes
- Presence of burns to special care areas (i.e., eyes, ears, face, hands, feet, genitalia/perineum, and joints)

See the table on page 429 for the American Burn Association classification of major versus minor burn injury.

Minor, Moderate, and Major Burns

Minor Burn	Superficial partial thickness <15% TBSA (adult) or <10% TBSA (pediatric) Full thickness burn <2% TBSA without special care area involvement Absence of electrical injury, inhalational injury, associated trauma, or poor risk classification (extremes of age, concurrent disease process)
Moderate Burn	Superficial partial thickness to 15–25% TBSA (adult) or 10–20% TBSA (pediatric) Full thickness <10% TBSA without special care area involvement Absence of electrical injury, inhalational injury, associated trauma, or poor-risk classification
Major Burn	Superficial partial thickness to >25% TBSA (adult) or >20% TBSA (pediatric) Full-thickness >10% TBSA All burns to special care areas All electrical injuries, inhalational injuries, presence of associated trauma, and all poor-risk patients

TBSA, total body surface area.

5. What are the consequences of the disruption of the skin?

The skin is the largest organ of the body. Some of its primary functions are to exclude infectious organisms and help regulate the balances of bodily fluids and temperature. Intact skin is the first barrier to infectious organisms. Whenever this barrier is broken, wound and systemic infections are major concerns throughout the course of recovery.

Intact skin also functions to help preserve the balances of the body's fluid compartments. Superficial partial-thickness burns do not result in the loss of interstitial fluids. Deep partial-thickness burns are characterized by blisters and "weeping" wounds; this is the loss of interstitial fluids and proteins. As a result, plasma fluids and proteins shift into the interstitium, where they are subsequently lost. The fluid and protein shifts reduce the circulatory volume resulting in hypovolemia and can spiral downward to burn shock and potentially fatal circulatory collapse. The fluid shifts and losses contribute to electrolyte shifts and imbalances. Finally, the fluids lost through the weeping wounds evaporate to a considerable extent. Because of the evaporative cooling that occurs, hypothermia is an ongoing concern with burn patients.

6. Define burn shock.

Burn shock is a form of hypovolemic shock relatively peculiar to burn-injured patients, which can culminate in cardiovascular collapse and death. Within minutes of a burn injury, edema begins to form in affected and unaffected tissues. Intravascular volume is depleted by seepage of fluids and plasma

proteins into the interstitium, where they are lost by weeping from the denuded body surfaces. The shift of fluids and proteins into the interstitium occurs as the result of at least four factors:
- Increased intravascular hydrostatic pressure
- Decreased interstitial fluid hydrostatic pressure
- Increased interstitial osmotic pressure
- Loss of endothelial cell barrier function

7. What constitutes fluid resuscitation in a burn patient?

To maintain intravascular volume, aggressive fluid replacement must be initiated on arrival to the emergency department, if not at the site of the injury. Several formulas have been developed and employed over many years for fluid resuscitation of burn-injured patients. The following table lists some formulas that are used for the adult burn patient. No matter which resuscitation formula is used, it is crucial that calculations for the infusions be predicated on the time of the actual injury, *not* on the time of arrival to the emergency department.

Adult Burn Resuscitation Formulas

Initial 24 Hours

Formula	Crystalloid	Colloid	Glucose in water
Evans	Normal saline 1 mL/kg/%TBSA	1 mL/kg/%TBSA	2000 mL
Brooke	Lactated Ringer's 1.5 mL/kg/%TBSA	0.5 mL/kg/%TBSA	2000 mL
Parkland	Lactated Ringer's 4 mL/kg/%TBSA		
Modified Brooke	Lactated Ringer's 2 mL/kg/%TBSA		
Second 24 Hours			
Evans	50% of first 24-hr requirement	50% of first 24-hr requirement	2000 mL
Brooke	50–75% of first 24-hr requirement	50–75% of first 24-hr requirement	2000 mL
Parkland		20–60% of calculated plasma volume	Titrate to maintain urine output
Modified Brooke		0.3–0.5 mL/kg/%TBSA	Titrate to maintain urine output

Adapted from Yowler CJ, Fratianne RB: Current status of burn resuscitation, Clin Plast Surg 27: 1-10, 2000.

8. How is the percentage of the TBSA calculated?

Body surface area is measured in square meters. The amount of the TBSA involved in a burn injury can be estimated quickly by using the *rule of nines*. The rule of nines divides the body into areas consisting of 9%, or multiples of nine, of the TBSA. For example, each arm, from shoulder to finger tips, represents 9% TBSA (see the following figure). This method of calculating the %TBSA is typically used in the field to communicate to emergency departments the estimate of the extent of the burn injury.

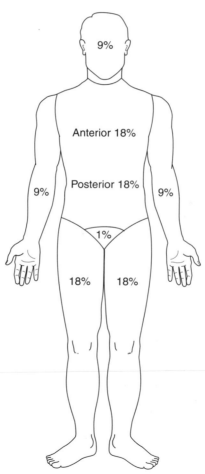

The rule of nines. Estimated percentage of body surface area (BSA) in an adult is arrived at by sectioning the body surface into areas with a numerical value related to nine. In burn victims, the total estimated percentage of BSA injured is used to calculate the patient's fluid replacement needs.

Another estimate often used in the field, particularly for burns that are not contiguous, is the *number of palms*. The palm of the hand is considered to represent approximately 1% TBSA. The number of palms used to "cover" the areas of burn injury approximates the overall %TBSA that has been injured.

On arrival to the emergency department or specialized burn care unit, more precise determination of the extent of the %TBSA involved is undertaken using the Lund and Browder chart (see the following figure). Precise calculation/estimation of the %TBSA is an integral piece of information for the calculation of fluid resuscitation requirements.

Area	Birth–1 yr	1–4 yr	5–9 yr	10–14 yr	15 yr	Adult
Head	19	17	13	11	9	7
Neck	2	2	2	2	2	2
Ant. Trunk	13	13	13	13	13	13
Post. Trunk	13	13	13	13	13	13
R. Buttock	$2^1/_2$	$2^1/_2$	$2^1/_2$	$2^1/_2$	$2^1/_2$	$2^1/_2$
L. Buttock	$2^1/_2$	$2^1/_2$	$2^1/_2$	$2^1/_2$	$2^1/_2$	$2^1/_2$
Genitalia	1	1	1	1	1	1
R. U. Arm	4	4	4	4	4	4
L. U. Arm	4	4	4	4	4	4
R. L. Arm	3	3	3	3	3	3
L. L. Arm	3	3	3	3	3	3
R. Hand	$2^1/_2$	$2^1/_2$	$2^1/_2$	$2^1/_2$	$2^1/_2$	$2^1/_2$
L. Hand	$2^1/_2$	$2^1/_2$	$2^1/_2$	$2^1/_2$	$2^1/_2$	$2^1/_2$
R. Thigh	$5^1/_2$	$6^1/_2$	8	$8^1/_2$	9	$9^1/_2$
L. Thigh	$5^1/_2$	$6^1/_2$	8	$8^1/_2$	9	$9^1/_2$
R. Leg	5	5	$5^1/_2$	6	$6^1/_2$	7
L. Leg	5	5	$5^1/_2$	6	$6^1/_2$	7
R. Foot	$3^1/_2$	$3^1/_2$	$3^1/_2$	$3^1/_2$	$3^1/_2$	$3^1/_2$
L. Foot	$3^1/_2$	$3^1/_2$	$3^1/_2$	$3^1/_2$	$3^1/_2$	$3^1/_2$

Lund and Browder burn estimate diagram as modified by the U.S. Army Institute of Surgical Research. Area of head and lower extremities is proportional to age. Numbers represent the percentage of BSA as the individual grows. *(Data from U.S. Army Institute of Surgical Research.)*

9. Discuss features specific to electrical burns.

Electrical burns are extraordinarily deceptive. The outward appearance of the injury may seem to involve considerably less than 1% TBSA of the victim. Electrical energy flows from one pole to the other via the path of least resistance, however. When the conduit for the flow of electrical energy is the human body, this path follows the water and electrolyte content of the body. The bones contain the least percentage of water, whereas, the viscera, muscles, and other tissues have high water and electrolyte content. Within the various fluid compartments, the dissolved electrolytes—ions—transmit the electrical energy that is received. As a result, the true nature or extent of an electrical injury may not be appreciated on initial examination; it may take 12 to 24 hours to manifest itself fully. Depending on the path taken by the electrical current, the heart may be damaged, producing ischemia, infarction, or ventricular fibrillation. The muscles may be extensively damaged and result in compartment syndrome, which must be treated with a fasciotomy to relieve the pressure and prevent further ischemic damage to the underlying tissues and possibly loss of limb.

Occasionally, contact with sources of electricity produces arcing, which can ignite the victim's clothing resulting in extensive cutaneous burns. The contact with electricity may produce intense spasmodic muscular contraction or unconsciousness and result in other traumatic injuries. The entry and exit wounds may be obscured on initial examination.

Because of the deceptive nature of electrical burns, often fluid resuscitation may be inadequate, being initially based on the small observable tissue damage. For fluid resuscitation of electrical burns, more so than other types of burns, urine output is more the end point of the treatment regimen. Common output goals are 0.5 to 1.5 mL/kg/hr. The urine output must be screened for the presence of myoglobin, which can precipitate out in the renal tubules and result in acute renal failure. For positive myoglobinuria, the fluid resuscitation is aimed at achieving the higher output goal of 1.5 mL/kg/hr.

10. What are the cardiovascular effects associated with burn injuries?

The cardiovascular response to burn injuries is described as an *ebb and flow* pattern. The "ebb" end of the spectrum is characterized by dramatic decreases in cardiac output that are accompanied by significant increases in systemic and pulmonary vascular resistances. Intravascular volume can decrease 20% to 50% over the course of the first few hours postinjury. Fluid shifts and subsequent losses reduce ventricular filling pressures, and the heart is faced with falling preload and increased afterload, culminating in dramatically reduced cardiac output. Afterload changes occur in part as a result of the continuous overproduction of catecholamines. The ebb phase can last 24 to 72 hours.

When fluid resuscitation is adequate and the degree of hypovolemia is maintained to a minimum, the cardiovascular response begins to convert or shift to the "flow" end of the spectrum. The flow phase is characterized by increases in cardiac output and peripheral blood flow. This phase also is characterized by hyperdynamic circulatory conditions, during which volume of oxygen use may increase by 200%. The cardiac index dramatically increases and systemic vascular resistance is reduced. The flow phase, similar to the ebb phase, is mediated in part by the continuous overproduction of endogenous catecholamines.

11. In what way is the respiratory system affected by burn injuries?

The lungs are susceptible to edema formation even without direct/inhalational injury. As discussed earlier, edema formation occurs in the injured tissues and in uninjured tissues owing to microvascular changes. The susceptibility to pulmonary edema formation is enhanced further by increases in pulmonary and systemic vascular resistances combined with the dramatic reduction in cardiac output. Any edema that does form within the lungs is an excellent growth medium for pathogens; pulmonary infection and adult respiratory distress syndrome are continuous concerns.

12. How are inhalational injuries diagnosed?

The physical appearance of the patient and knowledge of the circumstances of the burn injury are initial indicators of the presence of an inhalational injury. The presence of carbonaceous deposits (sootlike material) in or around the nostrils or mouth or both; extensive deep partial-thickness or full-thickness burns, especially to the face; and singed facial or nasal hair all are highly suspicious of inhalational injury and warrant further, more invasive investigation measures. Burns that occur within enclosed spaces, whether thermal or chemical, also suggest the presence of inhalational injury. Inhalational injury occurs when there is exposure to superheated air, steam, or the end products of combustion, which can include sulfur dioxide, ammonia, and nitrogen dioxide. These vectors produce physical damage to the tissues of the airway. Along with the direct injury comes tissue edema formation in the same manner as cutaneous burns. Edema formation in the upper airways can deteriorate rapidly to a mechanical obstruction of the airway and prompt emergency interventions (i.e., endotracheal intubation or tracheostomy).

Lower airway injury is characterized by wheezing, rales, rhonchi, or bronchospasm and warrants further investigation. Direct visualization for pulmonary carbon deposits can be accomplished via bronchoscopy. Xenon-enhanced computed tomography also detects the presence of pulmonary injury.

13. Describe the signs and symptoms of carbon monoxide (CO) poisoning.

Carbon monoxide is a clear, odorless gas produced by incomplete combustion of carbon-containing fuels. It binds to oxygen-binding sites on the hemoglobin molecule with a tenacity 200 to 250 times greater than oxygen itself. The signs and symptoms of carbon monoxide poisoning vary with the amount of carbon monoxide inhaled. The table on page 435 lists commonly occurring physical signs and symptoms of different levels of carbon monoxide poisoning.

Manifestations of Carbon Monoxide Poisoning

Percentage of COHb in blood	Signs and Symptoms
0–10	Minimal symptoms
10–20	Nausea, headache
20–30	Drowsiness, weakness
30–40	Confusion, agitation
40–50	Coma, respiratory depression
>50	Death

Adapted from Yowler CJ, Fratianne RB: Current status of burn resuscitation, Clin Plast Surg 27: 1-10, 2000.

One parameter that is of no help in determining the adequacy of oxygenation when carbon monoxide poisoning is present is pulse oximetry. The molecule formed by carbon monoxide and hemoglobin is indistinguishable from that formed by oxygen and hemoglobin. Carboxyhemoglobin (COHb) produces a left shift of the oxygen hemoglobin dissociation curve. Supplemental oxygen should be administered via facemask at the highest possible percentage with a nonrebreathing system. The additional oxygen increases the rate at which COHb dissociates and produces a relative right shift of the oxygen hemoglobin dissociation curve.

14. What are the effects incurred by the renal system as a result of burn injury?

The initial period of lower cardiac output due to the burn injury delivers less blood flow to the kidneys. The massive fluid shifts during the initial hours to days postinjury contribute to the decreased renal blood flow. One of the goals of fluid resuscitation is to help preserve renal function, as determined by the hourly urine output goals of the resuscitation assessment.

Acute renal failure has been reported to be 1% to 30% in burn patients with an associated mortality range of 73% to 100%. Prolonged acute hypovolemia can produce renal failure, as can the so-called high-output phase. The key to avoiding renal failure is adequate perfusion, which is directly reflective of the adequacy of fluid resuscitation.

15. Describe the effects of burn injuries on the gastrointestinal system.

Similar to other traumatic events/injuries, initially the gastrointestinal system becomes paralyzed (i.e., paralytic ileus), which leads to gastric distention, nausea, and vomiting and increases the potential for aspiration. Gastric distention can be alleviated by placement of a nasogastric tube connected to intermittent low suction. The nasogastric tube may produce an erosional ulceration of the stomach or duodenum—a Curling ulcer. The nasogastric tube is indicated until there is spontaneous return of bowel sounds. The stomach may be the last portion of the gastrointestinal system to experience the return of peristaltic function. As a result of the dramatically high caloric requirements of burn patients and the potentially rapid decline into a caloric deficit that can occur, enteral feedings or supplementation or both are needed to maintain the healing process.

16. What hematological effects occur as the result of burn injuries?

The initial observed effects on the hematological system are increases in hematocrit and blood viscosity secondary to the loss of fluids and proteins to the interstitial compartment. During recovery, anemia is a persistent concern, in part due to blood loss during surgical procedures, but also because the half-life of red blood cells is reduced as the result of burn injuries. Platelet concentrations typically decline partially as a dilutional phenomenon during the resuscitation phase, but also secondary to the formation of microaggregates within the damaged areas.

The burn injury and the ensuing resuscitation cause clotting factors to be activated and consumed at a more rapid pace. The large volumes of fluid that must be infused also dilute the concentration of the clotting factors. Disseminated intravascular coagulation is a devastating complication that can occur.

17. Discuss important considerations during the preoperative assessment.

The *extent and depth of the burn injury* are important to the planning of an anesthetic, as is the elapsed time since the injury. The extent and depth of the injury contribute significantly to the fluid requirements for each patient. A patient with larger burns requires higher ambient temperatures and warming of infusions to maintain relative normothermia. Additionally, the anesthetist must be aware of any coagulation or electrolyte imbalances that may be present.

The remaining parameters of preoperative assessment differ slightly compared with healthy patients. The *assessment of the patient's airway* may be more tedious. True Mallampati classification may be obscured by facial burns and dressings, edema, scars, or contractures. An otherwise normal patient airway, Mallampati class I, may be transformed into a class III or IV by the nature or extent of the burn injury.

NPO (nothing by mouth) status is a dynamic consideration. The anesthetist must consider the risks of aspiration with induction of general anesthesia; however, these concerns must be tempered by the knowledge of the extremely high nutritional/caloric requirements of the patient to heal the wounds. At least one study suggested no increased risk of aspiration when supplemental enteral feedings via duodenal feeding tubes are continued even during the surgical procedure/anesthesia.

Familiarity with the proposed *area for harvesting skin for grafting* is important. Some potential donor sites necessarily require special positioning during the procedure or creativity in the placement of monitoring devices.

18. What preoperative laboratory tests are indicated for burn-injured patients?

Based on all the previously described considerations, basal metabolic panels, coagulation parameters, complete blood counts, and arterial blood gas analysis all are important, with consideration of the stage of the patient's recovery and underlying state of health. Any acid-base or electrolyte imbalances should be corrected as nearly as possible before the initiation of anesthesia. Patients burned in enclosed spaces especially should be screened for carbon monoxide poisoning by testing for carboxyhemoglobin. The concentration of carboxy-hemoglobin present has a significant impact on the planning and implementation of an anesthetic plan.

19. Discuss appropriate monitoring for burn patients during anesthesia.

Core temperature monitoring is important. Temperature regulation is one of the skin's several important functions. The denuded flesh weeps fluids, which evaporate, producing temperature loss; hypothermia is a great concern for the anesthetist.

Patients with large %TBSA injury scheduled for extensive excision or grafting or both may benefit from direct arterial blood pressure monitoring and placement of a pulmonary artery catheter to obtain more accurate beat-to-beat pressures and monitoring of the adequacy of fluid balances over the course of the surgical procedure. Large excisions with multiple donor sites produce large amounts of blood loss, which may be greater if coagulopathies are present.

20. Discuss two alterations in drug response that can be anticipated with burn patients.

The first drug response alteration concerns *opioid analgesics*. Patients with deep partial-thickness burns are in constant pain, even when not engaged in any activity. The nerve endings are exposed and constantly stimulated. These patients require relatively large amounts of opiates to approach some level of comfort, and they may develop a tolerance to the actions of opioid analgesics, requiring increased doses to produce the desired effect.

The second alteration concerns *drugs with a high degree of protein binding*. Plasma proteins are lost extensively over the course of the first few days post-injury. The fraction of unbound drug plays a significant role in the efficacy of many drugs used in anesthesia. Decreased protein binding may enhance drug effects.

21. How does the response to muscle relaxants change in burn patients?

The response to depolarizing muscle relaxants and nondepolarizing muscle relaxants (NDMRs) changes in burn patients. The theoretical cause of these alterations is the proliferation of acetylcholine receptors. These receptors seem to develop not only just deep to the actual injury, but also at uninvolved sites removed from the actual injury. As a result, burn patients are sensitive to depolarizing muscle relaxants and have a high potential for hyperkalemia if depolarizing muscle relaxants are administered.

Patients with large %TBSA (>30% TBSA) exhibit a marked resistance to NDMRs. The resistance to NDMRs generally appears within 1 week of injury and has been documented to persist for 18 months postinjury. The anesthetist can assume that larger doses will be required to produce the desired results and that these doses will have a shorter than expected duration of action than would be observed in healthy patients.

22. Identify appropriate medications for induction of general anesthesia in burn patients.

Traditionally, *ketamine* has been used with adult and pediatric burn patients with unqualified success. The analgesic and dissociative properties produced by ketamine and the preservation of adequate blood pressure are highly desirable qualities for burn patients. *Etomidate* also is efficacious for burn patients because it has minimal effects on the patient's blood pressure.

 Key Points

- Burns are classified as superficial partial thickness (predominantly the epidermis), deep partial thickness (consumes the epidermal layer entirely and extends well into, but not through, the dermal layer), full thickness (the entire thickness of the skin, the epidermis and the dermis, is consumed or destroyed), and fourth degree (this depth burn injury destroys the entire epidermis, dermis, subcutaneous layers, and extends well into, often through, the muscle layer and may damage the bone).

- When the skin integrity is disrupted, wound and systemic infections are major concerns, along with the balances of the body's fluid compartment, and hypothermia.

- Burn shock is a form of hypovolemic shock relatively peculiar to burn-injured patients.

- Intravascular volume is depleted by seepage of fluids and plasma proteins into the interstitium, where they are lost by "weeping" from the denuded body surfaces.

- Calculations for fluid resuscitation in the burn patient should be predicated on the time of the actual injury *not* on the time of arrival to the emergency department.

- The amount of the TBSA involved in a burn injury can be estimated quickly by using the rule of nines. The rule of nines divides the body into areas consisting of 9%, or multiples of 9, of the total body surface area.

- The outward appearance of an electrical burn injury may seem to involve considerably less than 1%TBSA of the victim. Electrical energy flows from one pole to the other via the path of least resistance, however. When the conduit for the flow of electrical energy is the human body, this path follows the water and electrolyte content of the body.

- With fluid resuscitation of electrical burns, more so than other types of burns, urine output is more the end point of the treatment regimen.

Key Points   *continued*

- Cardiovascular changes in the "flow" phase are increases in cardiac output and peripheral blood flow and hyperdynamic circulatory conditions.
- Edema formation in the upper airways can deteriorate rapidly to a mechanical obstruction of the airway and prompt emergency interventions (i.e., endotracheal intubation or tracheostomy).
- Acute renal failure has been reported at 1% to 30% in burn patients with an associated mortality range of 73% to 100%. Prolonged acute hypovolemia can produce renal failure, as can the so-called high-output phase.
- Initially after the injury, the gastrointestinal system becomes paralyzed (i.e., paralytic ileus), which leads to gastric distention, nausea, and vomiting and increases the potential for aspiration.
- Important preoperative considerations are fluid requirements, maintenance of body temperature, electrolyte and coagulation profiles, airway evaluation, NPO status, and monitoring sites.
- Burn patients are sensitive to depolarizing muscle relaxants and have a high potential for hyperkalemia if depolarizing muscle relaxants are administered.
- Patients with large %TBSA (>30% TBSA) burns exhibit a marked resistance to NDMRs.

Internet Resources

Virtual Anaesthesia Textbook:
http://www.virtual-anaesthesia-textbook.com/

GASNet: Survey of anesthesiology:
http://www.gasnet.org/sa/2001/06/

Nurse-Anesthesia.com:
http://www.nurse-anesthesia.com/

Bibliography

Carleton SC, Tomassoni AJ, Alexander JK: The cardiovascular effects of environmental traumas: cardiac problems associated with burns, *Cardiol Clin* 13:257-262, 1995.

Chrysopoulo MT, Jeschke MG, Dziewulski P, et al: Acute renal dysfunction in severely burned adults, *J Trauma* 46:141-144, 1999.

Flowers-Byers J, LaBorde PJ: Management of patients with burn injury. In Smeltzer SC, Bare BG, editors: *Brunner and Suddarth's textbook of medical-surgical nursing,* ed 9, Philadelphia, Lippincott Williams & Wilkins, 2000, pp 1501-1535.

Jaehde U, Sorgel F: Clinical pharmacokinetics in patients with burns, *Clin Pharmacokinet* 29:15-28, 1995.

Jenkins ME, Gottschlich MM, Warden GD: Enteral feedings during operative procedures in thermal injuries, *J Burn Care Rehabil* 15:199-205, 1994.

MacLennan N, Heimbach D, Cullen BF: Anesthesia for major thermal injury, *Anesthesiology* 89:749-770, 1998.

Shirani KZ, Vaughan GM, Mason AD Jr, et al: Update on current therapeutic approaches in burns, *Shock* 5:4-16, 1996.

Yowler CJ, Fratianne RB: Current status of burn resuscitation, *Clin Plast Surg* 27:1-10, 2000.

Obesity

Grace A. Simpson

1. Define ideal body weight (IBW).

IBW is a measurement of height and body mass with the statistically highest life expectancy. It is often used to calculate drug dosages in obese patients.

2. Calculate IBW using the Broca index.

Males: weight (kg) = height (cm) − 100
Females: weight (kg) = height (cm) − 105

Example: IBW calculated for a woman, 5 feet, 8 inches:

Convert inches to centimeters: 68 inches × 2.54 cm = 172.72 cm
172.72 cm − 105 = 67.72 kg IBW

3. Classify obesity in terms of IBW.

- Body weight that is 20% greater than IBW is classified as *obese*.
- Body weight that is greater than 100 pounds (45.3 kg) over IBW in an adult or greater than two times IBW is classified as *morbidly obese*.

4. Define body mass index (BMI).

BMI is a ratio of weight to height. BMI is the internationally recognized system for classifying obesity in adults.

5. Calculate BMI using the Quetelet index.

Metric conversion formula:

$$\text{BMI} = \frac{\text{weight (kg)}}{\text{height (m)}^2}$$

Example: BMI calculated for a person weighing 79 kg and 177 cm (1.77 m) tall:

$$\frac{79}{(1.77)^2} = 25$$

Nonmetric conversion formula:

$$BMI = \frac{\text{weight (lb)}}{\text{height (inches)}^2} \times 703$$

Example: BMI calculated for a person weighing 164 lb and 5 feet, 8 inches tall:

$$\left[\frac{164}{(68)^2} \right] \times 703 = 25$$

6. Classify obesity in terms of BMI.

See the following table for classification of obesity based on BMI.

Body Mass Index (BMI) Classification for Adults

BMI	Classification
18.5–24.9	Ideal weight
25–29.9	Overweight
>30	Obese
35–40	Morbidly obese

7. List cardiovascular system changes associated with obesity.

The following changes occur:
- Expansion of vasculature and increased absolute blood volume
- Decreased proportion of blood volume to body weight
- Increased basal metabolic demand
- Increased oxygen consumption
- Increased cardiac output
- Increased stroke volume in proportion to body weight; leads to left ventricular dilation and hypertrophy
- Increased carbon dioxide production; causes pulmonary vasoconstriction and pulmonary hypertension; leads to right ventricular dilation and hypertrophy
- Increased risk of systemic hypertension with increased cardiac output and normal systemic vascular resistance

8. List the respiratory system changes associated with obesity.

The following changes occur:
- Increased work of breathing due to increased oxygen consumption and increased carbon dioxide production
- Decreased chest wall compliance
- Restrictive pulmonary disease pattern on pulmonary function tests

- Decreased vital capacity, total lung capacity, expiratory reserve volume, and functional residual capacity
- Functional residual capacity becomes less than closing capacity causing premature airway closure, increased carbon dioxide retention, and ventilation-perfusion mismatch

9. Identify two respiratory syndromes experienced by some obese patients.

Obstructive sleep apnea syndrome has periods of airflow cessation lasting 10 seconds or more. There is abnormal relaxation of the genioglossus muscle, normally pulling the tongue forward, and relaxation of the pharyngeal muscles causing upper airway obstruction. Breathing effort is present, but airway movement is absent.

Obesity hypoventilation syndrome occurs in morbidly obese patients and is synonymous with *Pickwickian syndrome*. The cardinal manifestation of obesity hypoventilation syndrome is hypercapnia. The etiology is unclear; however, respiratory drive is consistently blunted. Associated characteristics include sudden somnolence, sleep apnea, hypoxia, polycythemia, and right-sided heart failure.

10. List gastrointestinal system changes associated with obesity.

The following changes occur:
- Increased intragastric pressure in proportion to weight
- Increased acidity of gastric fluid
- Increased incidence of gastroesophageal reflux and hiatal hernia
- Decreased gastric emptying

11. List hepatobiliary system changes associated with obesity.

The following changes occur:
- Liver function tests are usually elevated in obese patients, but they do not always reflect the degree of liver dysfunction.
- Fatty infiltrates may disrupt hepatocytes, obstruct bile canaliculi, and cause inflammation and necrosis of hepatic lobules resulting in fibrosis.
- Decreased serum albumin, increased partial thromboplastin time, and increased serum transaminase may indicate liver dysfunction.
- Increased prevalence of gallstones due to increased cholesterol in bile and increased ratio of bile salts to lecithin

12. What endocrine system changes are associated with obesity?

There is a high incidence of type 2 diabetes mellitus as a result of impaired insulin receptor sensitivity and hyperinsulinemia.

13. What is the inhaled anesthetic of choice for obese patients and why?

Desflurane is preferred. Among the halogenated anesthetics, it is the most resistant to hepatic metabolism.

14. How are pharmacokinetics of intravenous anesthetics altered in obese patients?

Lipophilic drugs (e.g., opioids, benzodiazepines, barbiturates) have increased volumes of distribution and prolonged elimination half-lives. Fentanyl and remifentanil are exceptions because they exhibit similar pharmacokinetics in obese and nonobese patients. *Hydrophilic drugs* have similar volumes of distribution, elimination half-lives, and clearance rates in obese and nonobese patients. Enhanced pseudocholinesterase activity may require increased *succinylcholine* doses (1.2 to 1.5 mg/kg). *Nondepolarizing muscle relaxants* exhibit pharmacokinetic variability. Initial doses should be calculated using IBW. Neuromuscular function should be monitored with a peripheral nerve stimulator.

15. Describe preoperative anesthesia considerations for obese patients.

- Premedicate with H_2-receptor antagonist and metoclopramide due to the increased risk of aspiration pneumonia.
- Avoid premedication with respiratory depressant drugs.
- Avoid intramuscular premedication due to unpredictable absorption.
- Have phenylephrine hydrochloride available to reverse intraoperative hypotension if patient reports use of weight-reducing drugs, which deplete catecholamines.
- Explain anticipated technical difficulties to the patient as appropriate to allay anxiety (e.g., awake fiberoptic intubation, central and peripheral venous access, arterial access, regional techniques).
- Review test results and laboratory data anticipating pathophysiological changes of an obese patient.
- Complete the physical examination with particular attention to the patient's airway. There is no direct correlation between BMI and laryngoscopic view of the patient's larynx, but more complex airway management should be anticipated in an obese patient.

16. Describe intraoperative anesthesia considerations for obese patients.

- Decrease local anesthetic dose by 20% to 25% for spinal and epidural techniques due to epidural fat and distended epidural veins producing a smaller epidural and subarachnoid space.
- For general anesthesia, the airway should be secured with an endotracheal tube. Mechanical ventilation should incorporate larger tidal volumes (15 to 20 mL/kg IBW) based on IBW.
- Anticipate difficulty in obtaining and maintaining a mask airway.
- Avoid allowing the patient to breathe spontaneously during general anesthesia because hypoxia and hypercarbia result from inadequate respirations.
- Allow time for adequate preoxygenation because functional residual capacity decreases further with induction of general anesthesia.
- Use an appropriate-size noninvasive blood pressure cuff (see the table on page 445).
- Determine that the operating room table can accommodate the patient's weight and size. It may be necessary to position the patient on two tables. Have additional padding materials available for pressure point padding.

Blood Pressure Cuff Sizing

Bladder Cuff	Circumference of Extremity
Width	40%
Length	80%

17. What position maximizes respiratory function in an obese patient?

The lateral decubitus position maximizes respiratory function. Abdominal weight and pressure is kept off the chest.

18. Describe postoperative anesthesia considerations for obese patients.

- Respiratory failure is the major postoperative problem for obese patients.
- Delay extubation until the patient is fully awake.
- Avoid postoperative hypoxemia by administering supplemental oxygen and monitoring oxygen saturation.
- Use continuous positive airway pressure at 10 to 15 cm H_2O if the patient has a history of sleep apnea syndrome.
- Keep the head of the bed elevated 30 to 45 degrees to maximize respiratory function.
- Avoid intramuscular analgesics because of unpredictable absorption.
- IBW should be used to calculate intravenous patient-controlled analgesia and epidural local anesthetics or opioids.
- There is an increased incidence of deep vein thrombosis due to polycythemia, immobility, and increased abdominal pressure. To decrease the incidence of deep vein thrombosis, consider use of antiembolic stockings, pneumatic compression boots, subcutaneous heparin injections (5000 units twice daily), and early ambulation. Maintain adequate hydration.

 Key Points

- IBW is a measurement of height and body mass with the statistically highest life expectancy.
- IBW can be calculated using the Broca index:
  - Males: weight (kg) = height (cm) − 100
  - Females: weight (kg) = height (cm) − 105
- Body weight that is 20% greater than IBW is classified as obese.
- Body weight that is greater than 100 lb over IBW or greater than two times IBW is classified as morbidly obese.

Continued

Key Points   *continued*

- The Quetelet index can calculate BMI:

  - Metric: $BMI = \dfrac{weight(kg)}{height\ (m)^2}$

  - Nonmetric: $BMI = \dfrac{weight\ (lb)}{height\ (inches)^2} \times 703$

- An endocrine system change associated with obesity is the high incidence of type 2 diabetes mellitus due to impaired insulin receptor sensitivity and hyperinsulinemia.
- Pharmacokinetic factors of intravenous anesthetics are altered in the obese patient.
  - Lipophilic drugs have increased volumes of distribution
  - Hydrophilic drugs have similar volumes of distribution
- Preoperative considerations in obese patients include:
  - Premedicate with an H_2-receptor antagonist and metoclopramide; avoid respiratory depressant drugs
  - Explain anticipated technical difficulties to patient, specifically airway problems
- Intraoperative considerations in obese patients include:
  - Difficulty obtaining and maintaining a mask airway
  - Avoid spontaneous ventilation
  - Preoxygenate
  - Size-appropriate equipment

Internet Resources

Virtual Anaesthesia Textbook:
http://www.virtual-anaesthesia-textbook.com/

GASNet: The Global Textbook of Anesthesiology, Table of contents:
http://gasnet.med.yale.edu/gta/

Nurse-Anesthesia.com:
http://www.nurse-anesthesia.com/

Update in Anaesthesia Cumulative Index:
http://www.nda.ox.ac.uk/wfsa/html/pages/up_issu.htm

Bibliography

Base-Smith V: Obesity and anesthesia practice. In Nagelhout JJ, Zaglaniczny KL, editors: *Nurse anesthesia*, ed 2, Philadelphia, 2001, WB Saunders, pp 971-986.

Buckley P, Martay K: Obesity and gastrointestinal disorders. In Barash PG, Cullen BF, Stoelting RK, editors: *Clinical anesthesia*, ed 4, Philadelphia, 2001, Lippincott Williams & Wilkins, pp 1035-1041.

Ogunnaike BO, et al: Anesthetic considerations for bariatric surgery, *Anesth Analg* 95:1793-1805, 2002.

Perloff D, et al: Human blood pressure determination by sphygmomanometry: scientific statement from the American Heart Association, *Circulation*, 88:2460-2467, 1993.

Pi-Sunyer FX, et al: *Clinical guidelines on the identification, evaluation, and treatment of overweight and obesity in adults: the evidence report*, NIH publication no. 98-4083, 1998.

Pories WJ: The surgical treatment of obesity. In Besser M, et al, editors: *Endotext.com*, 2002; available online: www.endotext.org, 2002.

Stoelting RK, Dierdorf SF, editors: Nutritional diseases and inborn errors of metabolism. In: *Anesthesia and co-existing disease*, ed 4, Philadelphia, 2002, Churchill Livingstone, pp 441-451.

Section VI

Regional Anesthesia and Pain Management

Subarachnoid Block

Donna Landriscina Johnson

1. Describe the anatomy of the vertebral column and spinal cord.

The *vertebral column* provides structural support and protection to the spinal cord and its nerve roots. The vertebral column consists of cervical (7), thoracic (12), lumbar (5), sacral (5 fused), and coccygeal (4 fused) vertebrae. Each vertebra normally has one vertebral body, two pedicles, and two laminae. Also, each vertebra has a midline spinous process and two transverse processes. Four articular processes serve as synovial joints between vertebrae. Notches from adjacent vertebrae form intervertebral foramina. Nerve roots exit the spinal column via the intervertebral foramina. The vertebral segments L2-S2 have spinous processes that are shorter and less angled, allowing for the most direct access to the subarachnoid space.

The *spinal column* is shaped with the cervical and lumbar regions convex anteriorly and the thoracic and sacral regions concave anteriorly. Ligaments and muscle provide structural support to the spinal column.

The *spinal canal* consists of the spinal cord, fatty tissue, and a venous plexus. Dorsal and ventral nerve roots emerge from segmental spinal cord levels and combine to form 31 pairs of spinal nerves. A dural sheath covers most nerve roots for a small distance after they exit the spinal canal. The spinal cord is cylindrical in shape with the thickest portion in the cervical and lumbar regions.

2. What anatomical differences exist between the spinal canal of an infant compared with an adult?

In recent years, subarachnoid block (SAB) has been recommended for high-risk infants to prevent postoperative apnea associated with general anesthesia. At birth, the neonatal spinal cord extends from the foramen magnum to T12 to L3 (see the figure on page 452). In an adult, the spinal cord typically ends at L1. Performing a lumbar SAB below L1 in an adult or L3 in a child should avoid needle trauma to the spinal cord. The approximate depth of the subarachnoid space in infants is 1 to 1.5 cm from the skin. A 1.5-inch needle is recommended for infants and children weighing 15 kg or less. The volume of the cerebrospinal fluid (CSF) in a full-term newborn is approximately 50 mL compared with 140 mL in adults. The dural sac and the subarachnoid space usually extend to S3 or S4 in children compared with S2 in adults.

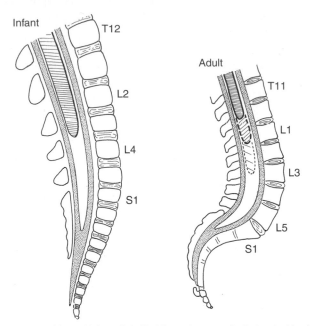

Anatomical differences between adults and infants that affect the performance of spinal and epidural anesthesia; an infant's sacrum (*left*) is flatter and narrower than an adult's (*right*). The tip of the spinal cord in a neonate ends at L3 and does not achieve the normal adult position (L1-2) until approximately 1 year of age. *(From Polaner DM, Suresh S, Coté C: Pediatric regional anesthesia. In Coté C, Todres ID, Goudsouzian NG, et al, editors: A practice of anesthesia for infants and children, ed 3, Philadelphia, 2001, WB Saunders, p 642.)*

3. **The spinal cord is covered with three membranes, called the meninges; name the three meninges, and provide a brief explanation of the structural and functional role of each.**

- *Pia mater:* The pia mater is a thin, delicate, and highly vascular membrane. It surrounds the spinal cord and terminates at the filum terminale. The filum terminale functions to secure the cord to the upper portion of the coccyx.
- *Arachnoid mater:* The arachnoid mater is a thin, avascular, cobweb-like membrane covering the brain and spinal cord. The subarachnoid space and CSF lie immediately beneath the arachnoid mater. The CSF functions to insulate and protect the spinal cord. The arachnoid mater and dura mater continue beyond the level of the cord and form a cylindrical-shaped column, the dural sac, ending at the level of S2.
- *Dura mater:* The dura mater is a tough outer membrane that extends from the foramen magnum to S2, then tightly adheres to the filum terminale as it runs to the coccyx. The fibers of the dura mater run longitudinally along the spine. When placing a needle for a spinal anesthetic, the needle pierces the dura mater and arachnoid mater before accessing CSF.

4. List and describe the most important ligaments encountered when performing a subarachnoid block.

The vertebrae are structurally supported and held in position by several important ligaments. The supraspinous ligament, interspinous ligament, and ligamentum flavum are of particular importance for identification during spinal and epidural anesthesia techniques (see the figure below). The supraspinous and interspinous ligaments may become calcified with age, in which case a paramedian approach to SAB may be indicated.

- *Supraspinous ligament:* The supraspinous ligament is a tough ligament that connects the apices of spinous processes from C7 to the sacrum.
- *Interspinous ligament:* The interspinous ligament is a thin ligament that is attached to the spinous processes. The interspinous ligament is fused zposteriorly with the supraspinous ligament and anteriorly with the ligamentum flavum. Movement through the interspinous ligament is difficult to discern with needle advancement to the subarachnoid space.
- *Ligamentum flavum:* The ligamentum flavum is a tough, elastic ligament that connects the anterior and inferior aspects of one lamina to the posterior and superior aspects of the lamina below. Small blood vessels penetrate the ligamentum flavum and may be a source of blood return during spinal needle aspiration.

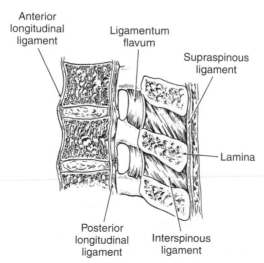

Sagittal section of vertebral column, showing ligaments. *(From Bridenbaugh PO, Greene NM, Brull SJ: Spinal (subarachnoid) neural blockade. In Cousins MJ, Bridenbaugh PO, editors: Neural blockade in clinical anesthesia and management of pain, ed 3, Philadelphia, 1998, Lippincott-Raven, p 205.)*

5. Discuss the mechanism of action for local anesthetics in the subarachnoid space.

Spinal anesthesia is initiated by the injection of local anesthetic into the CSF. Anesthesia results from temporarily interrupting the transmission of impulses along sensory, autonomic, and motor nerve fibers in the anterior and posterior nerve roots. The goal is to bathe the nerve fibers with local anesthetic within the subarachnoid space.

Typically the initial response observed with onset of an SAB is a sympathetic blockade, followed by a sensory blockade, and finally motor blockade. Generally the sympathetic blockade is two dermatome segments higher than the sensory block, and the sensory block is two segments higher than the motor blockade. Preganglionic sympathetic blockade results in vasodilation, especially of venous capacitance vessels, producing decreased venous return to the heart and decreased cardiac output.

6. List contraindications to SAB.

ABSOLUTE CONTRAINDICATIONS
- Patient refusal
- Septicemia or bacteremia
- Unstable central nervous system disease
- Infection at the site of needle insertion
- Increased intracranial pressure
- Severe hypovolemia
- Preexisting severe stenotic valvular heart disease or asymmetrical septal hypertrophy
- Bleeding diathesis
- Patients on full anticoagulation therapy
- Allergy to local anesthetics

RELATIVE CONTRAINDICATIONS
- Untreated, chronic hypertension
- Severe deformities of the spinal column
- Minor abnormalities of blood clotting, secondary to long-term aspirin therapy or mini-dose heparin administration
- Chronic headache or backache

7. Summarize the technique for lumbar puncture for a SAB.

Placement of a SAB is carried out in three principal positions: (1) lateral decubitus (see the figure on page 455), (2) sitting, and (3) prone. A key factor in positioning the patient for lumbar puncture is the ability to identify easily the midline for needle placement and to correct for existing lumbar lordosis. In some instances, such as with obese patients or patients with scoliosis, the sitting position can facilitate identification of the midline. The sitting position allows maximal anterior flexion of the spinal column (see the figure on page 456). The prone jackknife position is primarily used when a hypobaric technique is desired

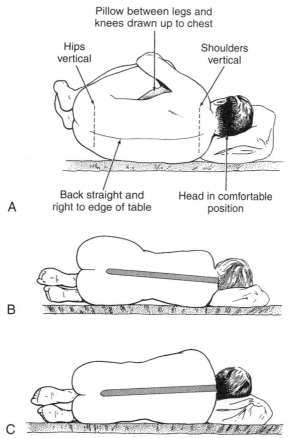

Pillow between legs and
knees drawn up to chest

Hips
vertical

Shoulders
vertical

Back straight and
right to edge of table

Head in comfortable
position

A

B

C

A, Lateral decubitus position for spinal anesthesia. **B** and **C**, Note skeletal differences of female (**B**) and male (**C**) on the level of the subarachnoid space. *(From Bridenbaugh PO, Greene NM, Brull SJ: Spinal (subarachnoid) neural blockade. In Cousins MJ, Bridenbaugh PO, editors: Neural blockade in clinical anesthesia and management of pain, ed 3, Philadelphia, 1998, Lippincott-Raven, p 230.)*

for surgical procedures involving the rectum or sacrum and is advantageous because it allows the patient to be positioned before placement of the SAB.

Identifying the correct site for lumbar puncture begins by mentally drawing a line between the top of both iliac crests to the associated vertebral body. This generally corresponds with the L4 or the L4-5 interspace. Identification of the most approachable interspace, most often L2-3 or L3-4, is followed with a skin wheal injection of local anesthetic and introduction of the selected spinal needle. An introducer placed into the supraspinous ligament may be used to facilitate advancement of a small-gauge spinal needle. As the needle passes through the supraspinous and interspinous ligaments and enters the tough ligamentum flavum, a change in resistance usually is noted, followed by a sudden loss of resistance as the epidural space is entered. After loss of resistance, the

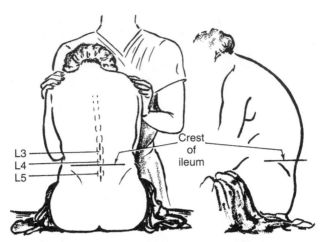

Correct sitting position for spinal anesthesia. *(From Bridenbaugh PO, Greene NM, Brull SJ: Spinal (subarachnoid) neural blockade. In Cousins MJ, Bridenbaugh PO, editors: Neural blockade in clinical anesthesia and management of pain, ed 3, Philadelphia, 1998, Lippincott-Raven, p 230.)*

needle is advanced further, and an increase in resistance is felt as the needle penetrates the dura mater. A second loss of resistance or "pop" is often noted when entering the subarachnoid space. Correct needle placement is confirmed by the free flow of CSF when the stylet is removed. Strict maintenance of aseptic conditions is mandatory during all steps of the technique.

8. Identify factors that affect local anesthetic spread in the subarachnoid space.

The spread of the local anesthetic solution is determined by four primary factors:
• Volume of local anesthetic solution injected
• Rate of injection
• Effects of gravity
• Volume of the spinal subarachnoid space.

9. What is the significance of local anesthetic baricity?

Baricity defines the ratio between the density of the local anesthetic solution and the density of the CSF (1.004 to 1.008). The relationship between local anesthetic baricity and patient position is as follows:
• A hypobaric solution produces the greatest anesthetic effect on the nondependent side.
• An isobaric solution tends to remain at the level of injection.
• A hyperbaric solution moves with gravity and produces the greatest effect on the dependent side.

- A hyperbaric solution is the most frequently selected local anesthetic for SAB and has a density greater than that of the CSF (density > 1.008). A hypobaric solution has a density less than that of the CSF (<1.008). A hypobaric solution may be desirable for surgical procedures in the prone jackknife position (hemorrhoidectomy) or lateral position (femur fractures). The density of isobaric solutions closely approximates the CSF. Isobaric spinal anesthetics are particularly useful for procedures requiring an anesthetic level at or lower than T10.

10. Anatomical landmarks or dermatomes are used to identify the level of neuraxial blockade; name the most common anatomical references, and briefly summarize each.

- *S2-5, saddle block:* This block anesthetizes structures that normally would be in contact with a "saddle," including the perineum, perianal area, and external genitalia. Minimal effect is noted on the autonomic nervous system. Motor blockade includes muscles of the sacral plexus.
- *T10, umbilicus:* Anesthesia to this dermatomal level involves the sacral nerves and the lower lumbar roots. Surgical areas covered include the perineum, perianal area, external genitalia, urethra, vagina, and cervix. This level also is desirable for vaginal delivery, including forceps or suction-assisted delivery; cystoscopy; transurethral resection of the bladder or prostate; and lower extremity vascular and orthopedic procedures. A T10 level of blockade affects some preganglionic sympathetic fibers. Vasodilation of the lower extremities and decreased venous blood return create the potential for hypotension.
- *T4, nipples:* In addition to the above-mentioned surgical procedures, this level provides sufficient anesthesia for orthopedic procedures of the lower extremity requiring a pneumatic tourniquet, upper abdominal procedures, testicular surgery, inguinal herniorrhaphy, appendectomy, ovarian cystectomy, cesarean delivery, and vaginal or abdominal hysterectomy. Afferent innervation of most intraabdominal tissues originates from a spinal level several segments higher than the anatomical location of the surgical site. A higher level of anesthetic blockade is needed for the patient to remain comfortable.
- *C8, little finger:* Dermatomal level of blockade above T2 is undesirable for SAB. If the level of the block rises above C8, the patient often perceives difficulty in breathing and may need reassurance or ventilatory support. Cardiac accelerator fibers, which arise from spinal cord levels T1-4, are affected. When this occurs, the patient is at risk for bradycardia and hypotension. Anticipation and immediate intervention with elevation of the lower extremities or placement in a slightly head-down position, intravenous fluids, vasopressors, and atropine help to minimize a potentially catastrophic event. A slight head-down position does not cause extracephalad spread in most patients. The phrenic nerve arises from spinal cord level C3-5. If the local anesthetic block is high enough to block the phrenic nerve, respirations are compromised. Immediate respiratory and circulatory support is required.

11. Identify factors that influence the duration of SAB.

Local anesthetics are not metabolized at the site of injection, but rather in the liver (amides) or by plasma cholinesterase (esters). Three factors contribute to the decline in local anesthetic concentration in spinal fluid:
• Spread of local anesthetic in the CSF
• Tissue uptake
• Vascular absorption of the local anesthetic from the subarachnoid space
Local anesthetic duration varies and depends primarily on the following:
• Local anesthetic dose
• Type of local anesthetic used (i.e., lipid solubility)
• Spread of the solution
• Baricity
• Perfusion at the site of action

If a vasoconstrictor is added to the solution, the local anesthetic effect may be prolonged, depending on the local anesthetic agent selected.

12. Discuss the physiology, diagnosis, and treatment of post-dural puncture headache (PDPH).

PDPH occurs when transdural leakage of CSF through a dural puncture hole allows the brain to lie lower within the cranium, resulting in traction on pain-sensitive intracranial vessels. Diagnosis of PDPH is a process of exclusion. A hallmark clinical feature is the relationship of headache to change in posture. A PDPH occurs when assuming an erect or semierect position and resolves quickly on resumption of the supine position.

The most important factor determining the likelihood of a PDPH is the choice of spinal needle. A small-diameter, noncutting (blunt or rounded point) spinal needle reduces the incidence of PDPH. The incidence is increased in younger age groups and is more common in women than men, especially during pregnancy. In addition, a higher incidence of PDPH is associated with early ambulation, particularly in ambulatory surgery patients sent home the same day of the procedure.

Conservative treatment modalities include bed rest, analgesics, and hydration. For more recalcitrant headaches, an autologous epidural blood patch, epidural saline, or intravenous or oral caffeine may be employed.

Autologous epidural blood patch remains the most definitive treatment for PDPH. When performing an autologous epidural blood patch, it is advisable to select a spinal interspace lower than the original puncture site and inject approximately 12 to 15 mL of aseptically acquired autologous blood. A high relapse rate limits the usefulness of epidural saline.

13. List possible complications associated with SAB.

The table on page 459 lists complications associated with SAB.

Complications Assoiciated with Subarachnoid Block

Cardiovascular	Respiratory	Neurological	Gastrointestinal
Hypotension	Respiratory depression	Backache	Nausea
Bradycardia	Atelectasis	Paresthesia/	Vomiting
Venous and arterial dilation	Pneumothorax (thoracic	transient paresis	Decreased gastric
Myocardial ischemia	subarachnoid block)	Paraplegia	motility
Ventricular arrhythmias	Intercostal muscle	Anterior spinal	Hiccough
Congestive heart failure	paralysis (inability	artery syndrome	
Cardiac arrest	to cough or clear	Subarachnoid or	**Other**
	secretions)	epidural hematoma	Decreased uterine,
	Phrenic nerve paralysis	Septic meningitis	renal, hepatic
	Delayed respiratory	Chemical meningitis	blood flow
	arrest (neuraxial	Epidural abscess	Urinary retention
	narcotics)	Cauda equina	
		syndrome	
		Neuropathy/brain	
		damage	
		Exacerbation of	
		herpes simplex	

14. **An elective cesarean section is scheduled in a parturient known to be HIV positive. The patient has been following the protocol for prevention of maternal-to-fetal transfer of HIV. Is SAB an option for anesthetic management of this patient?**

Studies indicate that treatment with zidovudine and nevirapine and delivery by elective cesarean section are effective in decreasing the risk of mother-to-infant transmission of HIV infection. Regional anesthesia has been administered safely to parturients infected with HIV. Several studies in this subpopulation indicated that there were no changes in the immunological parameters studied and that HIV-1 disease remained stable in the peripartum period. Elective cesarean section under SAB for women infected with HIV-1 was not associated with intraoperative or postoperative complications.

Key Points

• The vertebral column provides structural support and protection to the spinal cord and its nerve roots. The vertebral column consist of cervical (7), thoracic (12), lumbar (5), sacral (5 fused), and coccygeal vertebrae (4 fused).

Continued

Key Points *continued*

- The differences in the infant and adult spinal canal are in:
  - Length, L3 in the infant and L1 in the adult
  - Depth, 1 to 1.5 cm from skin in the infant and 3 to 4 cm in the adult
  - Volume of CSF, 50 mL in the newborn and 140 mL in the adult
  - End of dural sac, S3-4 in the child and S2 in the adult.
- The spinal cord is covered with three layers of meninges: pia mater, arachnoid mater, and dura mater.
- Onset of a SAB shows an initial sympathetic blockade, followed by a sensory blockade, and finally motor blockade.
- The spread of the local anesthetic solution is determined by four primary factors:
  - Volume of local anesthetic solution injected
  - Rate of injection
  - Effects of gravity
  - Volume of the spinal subarachnoid space
- Anatomical landmarks or dermatomes are used to identify the level of neuraxial blockade:
  - S2-5, saddle block
  - T10, umbilicus
  - T4, nipples
  - C8, little finger
- If a vasoconstrictor is added to the solution, the local anesthetic effect may be prolonged, depending on the local anesthetic agent selected.
- PDPH occurs when transdural leakage of CSF through a dural puncture hole allows the brain to lie lower within the cranium, resulting in traction on pain-sensitive intracranial vessels.
- The most important factor determining the likelihood of a PDPH is the choice of spinal needle.

Internet Resources

New York School of Regional Anesthesia:
http://www.nysora.com/

Virtual Anaesthesia Textbook:
http://www.virtual-anaesthesia-textbook.com/

The University of Chicago, Anesthesia and Critical Care: Anesthesia manuals: common and not so common complications of epidural anesthesia:
http://daccx.bsd.uchicago.edu/manuals/epidural.html

Hypertextbook of regional anaesthesia for obstetrics:
http://www.manbit.com/oa/oaindex.htm

Internet Resources *continued*

Anesthesiology Info: Regional anesthesia:
http://anesthesiologyinfo.com/artregional.php

Update in anaesthesia:
http://www.nda.ox.ac.uk/wfsa/html/pages/up_issu.htm#1

Nurse-Anesthesia.com:
http://www.nurse-anesthesia.com/

Bibliography

Avidan MS, et al: Low complication rate associated with cesarean section under spinal anesthesia for HIV-1 infected women on antiretroviral therapy, *Anesthesiology* 97:320-324, 2002.

Bridenbaugh PO, Greene NM, Brull SJ: Spinal (subarachnoid) neural blockade. In Cousins MJ, Bridenbaugh PO, editors: *Neural blockade in clinical anesthesia and management of pain,* ed 3, Philadelphia, 1998, Lippincott-Raven, pp 203-241.

Caplan RA, et al: Unexpected cardiac arrest during spinal anesthesia: a closed claims analysis of predisposing factors, *Anesthesiology* 68:5-11, 1988.

Greene NM, Brull SJ: *Physiology of spinal anesthesia,* ed 4, Baltimore, 1993, Lippincott Williams & Wilkins.

Hughes SC, et al: Parturients infected with human immunodeficiency virus and regional anesthesia: clinical and immunologic response, *Anesthesiology* 82:32-37, 1995.

Kleinman W: Spinal, epidural, and caudal blocks. In Morgan GE, Mikhail MS, Murray M, editors: *Clinical anesthesiology,* ed 3, New York, 2002, Lange Medical Books/McGraw-Hill, pp 253-282.

Neal JM: Management of postdural puncture headache, *Anesthesiol Clin North Am* 10:163-178, 1992.

Polaner DM, Suresh S, Coté C: Pediatric regional anesthesia. In Coté C, Todres ID, Goudsouzian NG, et al, editors: *A practice of anesthesia for infants and children,* ed 3, Philadelphia, 2001, WB Saunders, pp 636-674.

Reese CA, Nicholson C, Wicks TC, editors: *Clinical techniques of regional anesthesia: spinal and epidural blocks,* ed 2, Chicago, 1996, AANA, pp 13-81.

Sinclair CJ, Scott DB, Edstrom HH: Effect of the Trendelenburg position on spinal anaesthesia with hyperbaric bupivacaine, *Br J Anaesth* 54:497, 1982.

Epidural Anesthesia and Analgesia

Joseph E. Pellegrini

1. What is the epidural space?

The epidural space is a potential space that lies just outside the subarachnoid space and extends from the base of the skull to the sacral hiatus. The epidural space contains nerve roots, lymphatic tissue, blood vessels, and fat. It can be entered using any spinal interspace, but is most commonly entered below the L2 vertebrae. Interspaces L2-3, L3-4, or L4-5 are often used for access to the epidural space because they are the easiest to identify and enter.

2. Describe landmarks used to identify the epidural space and the layers that the epidural needle must pass through to enter the epidural space.

The crests of the ileum correspond with the L4-5 vertebral level in most patients. Adding or subtracting from this intervertebral space allows the anesthetist to identify other interspaces. When using a midline approach to enter the epidural space, the epidural needle must pass through the skin, subcutaneous tissue, supraspinous ligament, interspinous ligament, and ligamentum flavum.

3. Explain the difference between epidural anesthesia and epidural analgesia.

Anesthesia is the elimination of all sensation (as required for surgical blockade). It can be achieved by the epidural administration of large-volume, high-concentration local anesthetic solutions (e.g., 2% lidocaine, 0.5% to 0.75% bupivacaine, 0.5% levobupivacaine, 0.75% to 1% ropivacaine). *Analgesia* is the elimination of pain perception but not the elimination of all sensation. It can be achieved by the epidural administration of a dilute concentration of local anesthetic (e.g., 0.0625% to 0.25% bupivacaine, 0.125% to 0.2 % ropivacainc), administered as a single bolus dose or continuous infusion. Epidural opioids can be used in conjunction with local anesthetic solutions to augment anesthesia or alone to provide analgesia.

4. What does the term segmental level of anesthesia mean, and how does the anesthetist determine the sensory level of anesthesia using cutaneous landmarks?

Segmental anesthesia is the level or height of sensory blockade as measured by dermatomal levels (see the table on page 464). Determining the height of

Key Levels of Dermatome Blockade

Cutaneous Landmark	Height of Sensory Blockade	Significance
Little finger	C8	Cardioaccelerator fibers (T1-4) blocked May manifest as profound hypotension and bradycardia
Inner portion of arm and forearm	T1 and T2	Some cardioaccelerator fibers blocked May manifest as hypotension and bradycardia
Nipple line	T4–5	Some cardioaccelerator fibers blocked; level needed for upper abdominal surgery and cesarean section Some hypotension
Tip of xyphoid	T6–7	Splanchnic nerve fibers blocked; level needed for lower abdominal surgery Some hypotension
Umbilicus	T10	Sympathetic block limited to lower extremities; level needed for hip surgery Usually well tolerated hemodynamically
Inguinal ligament	T12	Level needed for lower extremity surgery
Lower knee	L2–3	Level needed for foot surgery
Perineal	S2–5	Level required for rectal surgery

sensory blockade is important to ensure that the patient has an adequate level of anesthesia to facilitate surgery. Often the practitioner can predict physiological hemodynamic responses based on the height of the sensory blockade.

5. What determines the type of local anesthetic needed for epidural blockade?

The choice of local anesthetic is dictated primarily by the duration of anesthesia desired: 0.5% bupivacaine produces approximately three times the duration of anesthesia as 2% chloroprocaine.

6. How does the anesthetist determine how much local anesthetic solution to administer to achieve a desired sensory level?

To determine the appropriate volume for epidural anesthesia, the anesthetist can use the "5 foot rule." For an individual 5 feet in height, 1 mL of local anesthetic is administered for each segment requiring blockade. For every 2 inches above 5 feet, the volume per segment is increased by 0.1 mL.

7. **When should the anesthetist reinforce an epidural blockade to ensure that an adequate surgical level of anesthesia is maintained?**

The dose used to reinforce a block usually requires approximately one fourth the initial dose. The following table outlines common epidural anesthesia agents and reinforcement block guidelines commonly used in clinical practice.

Reinforcement Block Guidelines

Agent	mL/Segment	Reinforcement Time (min)	Maximal safe bolus dose (mg/kg)	
			Plain	With Epinephrine
Lidocaine 2%	1–1.6	45–60	4	NA
Lidocaine 2% with epinephrine		90	NA	7
Mepivacaine 2%	1–1.6	45–60	4	7
Bupivacaine 0.5%	1.1–1.5	90	2.5*	3.2*
Chloroprocaine 3%	1.0–1.4	25–35	11	14
Ropivacaine 0.5%†	1.0–1.7	60–90	4*	5.5*

*Epinephrine decreases systemic absorption and may not increase analgesic duration/efficacy.
†Ropivacaine can be used in concentrations of 0.75%, but limit single bolus dose to 200 mg
NA, not applicable.

8. **List factors that affect the height of epidural blockade and duration of anesthesia.**

- *Dosage:* The dose of the local anesthetic is a function of the volume injected and the concentration of the solution.
- *Interspace in which epidural needle is placed:* Epidural anesthesia can be achieved over a small area. To achieve thoracic anesthesia at the T4 level when the needle is placed at the T6 level, a volume of only 6 to 12 mL of local anesthetic may be required.
- *Age of the patient:* The dose decreases with age because of changes in the size and compliance of the epidural space. Geriatric patients achieve a higher cephalad spread of anesthesia from a given volume of local anesthetic than that observed in young adults.
- *Weight:* A correlation exists between a patient's weight and the cephalad spread of anesthetic. Morbidly obese and pregnant patients have a smaller epidural space. Doses may need to be decreased in these patients.
- *Vasoconstrictors:* Epinephrine augments anesthesia by decreasing the vascular uptake of local anesthetic from the epidural space. Secondarily, epinephrine may augment anesthesia due to its own local anesthetic properties.

9. **Summarize key differences between epidural anesthesia and spinal anesthesia.**

The following table summarizes the differences between epidural anesthesia and spinal anesthesia.

Spinal Anesthesia and Epidural Anesthesia	
Spinal Anesthesia	**Epidural Anesthesia**
Local anesthetic requirements: small volume/higher concentration (e.g., 2 mL of 0.75% bupivacaine)	Local anesthetic requirements: large volume/less concentration (e.g., 15–20 mL of 0.5% bupivacaine)
Onset of sympathetic blockade: fast (pronounced impact on hemodynamics)	Onset of sympathetic blockade: slow (less impact on hemodynamics)
Zone of differential sympathetic blockade: 2 dermatome levels above sensory level	Zone of differential sympathetic blockade: no differential zone (level of sympathectomy the same as level of sensory blockade)
Height of block: depends on local anesthetic volume and baricity, individual patient characteristics (age, height, weight), and patient position	Height of block: depends on local anesthetic volume
Needle size: small, 25- to 27-gauge	Needle size: large, 16- to 18-gauge
Length of anesthesia/analgesia: limited to amount of local anesthetic and/or opioid injected (single injection)	Length of anesthesia/analgesia: unlimited — with catheter placement, can supplement anesthesia and analgesia

10. **What are the advantages and disadvantages of using epidural anesthesia over a subarachnoid block (SAB)?**

EPIDURAL ADVANTAGES
- Segmental block can be focused on the area of surgery or pain or both
- Less hypotension
- Offers more flexibility regarding the density and duration of block
- Extended postoperative analgesia can be accomplished via an epidural catheter

EPIDURAL DISADVANTAGES
- Requires larger doses of local anesthetics, which can result in higher plasma levels of local anesthetics
- More predictable levels of anesthesia can be achieved with a single-injection SAB than with single-injection epidural injection
- Slower onset of anesthesia

- Less definable end point indicating proper placement within the epidural space (i.e., cerebrospinal fluid [SAB] versus loss of resistance [epidural])
- Requires larger needle for placement with higher incidence of post–dural puncture headache if accidental dural puncture is made

11. List contraindications for epidural anesthesia.

ABSOLUTE
- Patient refusal
- Sepsis—risk of epidural abscess formation in the epidural space
- Bacteremia
- Skin infection at injection site
- Coagulopathy—bleeding into the epidural space can result in catastrophic nerve damage
- Severe hypovolemia
- Increased intracranial pressure
- Therapeutic anticoagulation

RELATIVE
- Peripheral neuropathy
- Patient currently on or scheduled to receive mini-dose heparin, low-molecular-weight heparin, or heparinoids in the postoperative period
- Prior history of spinal surgery
- History of back pain or injury
- Aspirin use preoperatively
- Uncooperative or emotionally unstable patient
- Resistant surgeon

12. What preparatory actions must be taken before insertion of an epidural catheter?

- Have emergency resuscitative equipment available (Ambu-bag, laryngoscope, oxygen, suction, drugs to treat hypotension and bradycardia).
- Ensure proper monitoring equipment is available (electrocardiogram, pulse oximeter, blood pressure monitoring device).
- Ensure that a well-functioning intravenous line is in place, and initiate a bolus of crystalloid solution (usually 5 to 15 mL/kg).
- Position the patient in a sitting or lateral decubitus position.
- Provide sedation as necessary.
- Identify landmarks (iliac crests), and draw an imaginary line across the corresponding vertebral level to identify the L4 spinous process. Palpate and mark the L2-3, L3-4, and L4-5 interspaces, and select the widest interspace available.
- Don mask, hat, and sterile gloves. Prepare the skin from T10 to S1 with a povidone-iodine (Betadine) solution using aseptic technique. Place a sterile drape. Make a subcutaneous skin wheal over the desired interspace with 1% lidocaine solution.

13. How is the loss of resistance technique used to identify the epidural space?

- Insert the epidural needle midline through the skin wheal. Resistance is felt when the needle enters the intraspinous ligament (usually about 3 cm). When firmly within the intraspinous ligament, remove the needle stylet and attach a syringe containing 3 mL of either air or normal saline solution. If the needle is in the proper position, the practitioner should note that it is difficult to inject air or normal saline, and the syringe plunger should "spring back" to its original position when the plunger is tapped.
- Using a *loss of resistance* technique, tap the barrel of the syringe while advancing the needle. An increased resistance and a gritty or leathery "feel" is noted when the needle enters the ligamentum flavum. At this point, the needle should be advanced slowly (2 to 3 mm at a time), while maintaining continuous pressure on the plunger of the syringe.
- When the needle passes through the ligamentum flavum and enters the epidural space, the nurse anesthetist feels a "give" or a sudden loss of resistance to the pressure exerted on the plunger of the needle.
- Remove the syringe and inject a *test dose* of local anesthetic solution (see Question 15). After a negative test dose, the local anesthetic required for surgical blockade is administered in 5-ml increments at 5-minute intervals.

14. Describe the technique for placing an epidural catheter.

- An epidural catheter may be placed to facilitate repeated injections of local anesthetic into the epidural space.
- After determining loss of resistance in the epidural space, an epidural catheter is threaded 3 to 5 cm through the needle into the epidural space.
- After noting the centimeter mark at the hub of the needle, the needle is removed over the catheter. The catheter should be aspirated for the presence of cerebrospinal fluid and blood. If no cerebrospinal fluid or blood is noted, the test dose and dosing regimen are administered, and the catheter is taped in place.

15. What is a test dose?

The test dose is a trial injection of local anesthetic solution into the epidural space followed by a waiting period of 3 to 5 minutes to ensure that the injection is neither intravascular nor intrathecal. The two most popular local anesthetic solutions used as a test dose are 3 mL of lidocaine 1.5% with 1:200,000 epinephrine (5 mcg/mL) or 3 mL of 2% lidocaine solution. With intravascular injection of a test dose, the anesthetist may note the following:

- Increased heart rate (>20 beats/min)
- Increased blood pressure
- Circumoral pallor
- Palpitations
- Tremulousness

The increases in heart rate and blood pressure are more prevalent when epinephrine is used in the test dose. Some practitioners advocate not using epinephrine as part of the test dose with obstetrical patients. A "positive" intravascular test dose response typically occurs within 2 minutes after injection and may last only 15 to 30 seconds. Use of continuous electrocardiogram monitoring is mandatory. An intrathecal test dose may take 3 to 5 minutes before spinal anesthesia effects are seen. An epidural test dose is more reliable in young adults versus elderly adults, owing to a reduction in beta adrenergic responsiveness with aging.

16. List potential complications associated with epidural anesthesia.

Complications include the following:
- Hypotension may occur secondary to sympathetic blockade.
- Systemic toxicity may occur with accidental intravascular injection of local anesthetic. The central nervous system is particularly sensitive to the effects of local anesthetic toxicity. Symptoms include circumoral numbness, lightheadedness, dizziness, tinnitus, blurred vision, tremors, and disorientation.
- Accidental subdural or subarachnoid injection of local anesthetic should be suspected when profound hypotension or respiratory depression occurs after administration of a small amount of local anesthetic.
- Dural puncture and post–dural puncture headache may occur.
- Nerve damage may occur. Neurological deficits are usually due to trauma. The incidence after epidural blockade is approximately 0.04%.
- Epidural hematoma is a rare complication, but occurs at a higher frequency in patients with a coagulopathy or on anticoagulation therapy.

17. Discuss the advantages to coadministering an opioid with the local anesthetic solution in epidural anesthesia; what are some of the most commonly used opioids?

Opioids may be administered with a local anesthetic solution to augment and intensify the block and to facilitate analgesia, based on the knowledge that opioid receptors are present in the substantia gelatinosa of the spinal cord. Common epidural opioids include fentanyl, 50 to 100 mcg; morphine, 1 to 3 mg; and sufentanil, 15 to 30 mcg. The more lipophilic opioids (fentanyl, sufentanil) have a faster onset (about 5 minutes) but a shorter duration of action (about 2 to 4 hours). A more hydrophilic agent, such as morphine, has a slower onset (1 hour) and a longer duration of action (18 to 24 hours). There is a greater risk of rostral spread and respiratory depression after epidural administration of hydrophilic agents, such as morphine sulfate.

Opioids are often given in combination with local anesthetics as continuous infusions to facilitate analgesia. The two most commonly used agents for continuous epidural infusions are bupivacaine and ropivacaine. The table on page 470 outlines continuous infusions used in labor and delivery or for postoperative analgesia.

Continuous Infusions Used in Labor and Delivery or for Postoperative Analgesia

Infusion	Comments
0.0625% bupivacaine + 2 mcg/mL fentanyl at 5–15 mL/hr	Best suited for early-stage labor pain
0.0625% bupivacaine + 0.3–0.5 mcg/mL sufentanil at 5–12 mL/hr	Good for laboring analgesia and postoperative analgesia
0.125% bupivacaine + 1-2 mcg/mL fentanyl at 5–10 mL/hr	Ideal for labor analgesia and postoperative analgesia
0.125% bupivacaine + 0.2 mcg/mL sufentanil at 5–10 mL/hr	Good for labor analgesia and postoperative analgesia
0.1% ropivacaine + 1 mcg/mL fentanyl at 5–15 mL/hr	Better suited for early-stage labor pain
0.2% ropivacaine + 2 mcg/mL fentanyl at 5–15 mL/hr	Good for labor analgesia and postoperative analgesia
0.1% ropivacaine + 0.3-0.5 mcg/mL sufentanil at 5–10 mL/hr	Good for labor analgesia and postoperative analgesia
0.2% ropivacaine + 0.2 mcg/mL sufentanil at 5–10 mL/hr	Good for labor analgesia and postoperative analgesia

Key Points

- The epidural space is a potential space that lies just outside the subarachnoid space and extends from the base of the skull to the sacral hiatus.
- The crests of the ileum correspond with the L4-5 vertebral level in most patients.
- An epidural needle must pass through the skin, subcutaneous tissue, supraspinous ligament, interspinous ligament, and ligamentum flavum.
- Epidural anesthesia can be achieved by the epidural administration of large-volume, high-concentration local anesthetic solutions (e.g., 2% lidocaine, 0.5% to 0.75% bupivacaine, 0.5% levobupivacaine, 0.75% to 1% ropivacaine).
- Epidural analgesia can be achieved by the epidural administration of a dilute concentration of local anesthetic (e.g., 0.0625% to 0.25% bupivacaine, 0.125% to 0.2 % ropivacaine), administered as a single bolus dose or continuous infusion.
- To determine the appropriate volume for epidural anesthesia, in an individual 5 feet in height, 1 mL of local anesthetic is administered for each segment requiring blockade. For every 2 inches above 5 feet, the volume per segment is increased by 0.1 mL.

Key Points   *continued*

- The dose used to reinforce a block usually requires approximately one fourth the initial dose.
- The factors that affect the height of epidural blockade and duration of blockade are dosage, chosen interspace, age of patient, weight, and addition of vasoconstrictors.
- To identify the epidural space, a loss of resistance technique can be used. After insertion of the epidural needle, if in the epidural space, a sudden loss of resistance is felt on the plunger of the syringe attached to the needle.
- To place an epidural catheter, when loss of resistance is felt, an epidural catheter is threaded 3 to 5 cm through the needle, into the epidural space.
- A test dose is a trial injection of local anesthetic solution into the epidural space followed by a waiting period of 3 to 5 minutes to ensure that the injection is neither intravascular nor intrathecal.
- Potential complications with epidural anesthesia are hypotension, systemic toxicity from intravascular injection, accidental subdural or subarachnoid injection of local anesthetic, dural puncture and post–dural puncture headache, nerve damage, and epidural hematoma.

Internet Resources

GASNet Search: Epidural anesthesia:
http://www.gasnet.org/about/search.php?p1=epidural+anesthesia

Virtual Anaesthesia Textbook:
http://www.virtual-anaesthesia-textbook.com/

Nurse-Anesthesia.com:
http://www.nurse-anesthesia.com/

Update in Anaesthesia:
http://www.nda.ox.ac.uk/wfsa/html/pages/up_issu.htm

Medmatrix.org: Anesthesiology:
http://www.medana.unibas.ch/MMana.HTM

Anesthesiology Info: Regional Anesthesia:
http://anesthesiologyinfo.com/artregional.php

Online Regional Anesthesia Techniques: Do It Yourself!:
http://www.csen.com/blocks.htm

New York School of Regional Anesthesia:
http://www.nysora.com/

Bibliography

Beilin Y, et al: Quality of analgesia when air versus normal saline is used for identification of the epidural space in the parturient, *Reg Anesth* 25:596-599, 2000.

Cousins MJ, Veering BT: Epidural neural blockade. In Cousins MJ, Bridenbaugh PO, editors: *Neural blockade,* ed 3, Philadelphia, 1998, Lippincott Williams & Wilkins, pp 243-321.

Koff HD: Placenta praevia. In Yao FF, Artusio JF, editors: *Anesthesiology problem-oriented patient management,* ed 4, Philadelphia, 1998, Lippincott Williams & Wilkins, pp 654-681.

Stoelting RK: *Pharmacology and physiology in anesthetic practice,* ed 3, Philadelphia, 1999, Lippincott Williams & Wilkins, pp 158-181.

Tanaka M, Nishikawa T: Aging reduces the efficacy of the simulated epidural test dose in anesthetized adults, *Anesth Analg* 91:657-661, 2000.

Valentine SJ, Jarvis AP, Shutt LE: Comparative study of the effects of air or saline to identify the extradural space, *Br J Anaesth* 66:224-227, 1991.

Chapter 51

Intravenous Regional Anesthesia

J. Frank Titch

1. What is intravenous regional anesthesia (IVRA)?

IVRA was introduced by Bier in 1908 and, in his honor, is also called the *Bier block*. The technique involves injecting local anesthetic into the venous system of an extremity after it has been exsanguinated by compression and its circulation occluded with a pneumatic tourniquet. The technique is deceptively simple, easily learned, yet the least forgiving if not precisely administered. IVRA provides profound anesthesia and muscle relaxation.

2. Discuss the indications for IVRA.

This technique is well suited for a variety of extremity operations, including soft tissue and orthopedic procedures. IVRA may be used for surgery of the foot and lower leg but is used most often for operations on the hand and forearm. Onset of anesthesia usually ensues within 5 minutes and is effective for procedures lasting 90 to 120 minutes when a double tourniquet is used. Anesthetic duration is minimal beyond tourniquet release. If the surgeon wishes to achieve hemostasis with the tourniquet deflated, another technique should be selected.

3. Describe the technique for IVRA of the upper extremity.

The patient is prepared as for any anesthetic and should be resting supine with an intravenous line already established in the nonsurgical arm. Intravenous sedatives and narcotics are important for patient comfort. The location of the tourniquet on the surgical extremity is protected with linen stockinette (preferred) or cotton Webril (may wrinkle and cause areas of uneven pressure) before application of the double tourniquet. An appropriately sized double tourniquet is placed over the stockinette. An intravenous catheter is inserted in the operative extremity as distal as possible. This catheter acts as the injection port for the anesthetic solution in the operative extremity and should be 22-gauge or smaller to minimize leakage of the anesthetic solution when the catheter is removed.

The surgical extremity is elevated to enhance venous drainage. An Esmarch elastic bandage is wrapped tightly around the extremity, beginning distally, partially overlapping each wrap, with care being taken not to dislodge the intravenous catheter or cause too much pain. Asking the patient to grip a roll of cotton Webril facilitates wrapping the hand while the Esmarch bandage is applied. If the surgical procedure involves removal of a ganglion cyst, one must take care not to rupture the cyst. Adequate exsanguination facilitates local anesthetic filling the venous system.

After limb exsanguination, the distal tourniquet cuff is inflated, then the proximal cuff is inflated, and lastly the distal cuff is deflated. This action completes exsanguination of the extremity and allows for distribution of the local anesthetic solution under the distal cuff. If the patient begins to experience tourniquet pain later in the procedure, the anesthetist can inflate the distal cuff over the anesthetized area and deflate the proximal cuff.

Recommendations for tourniquet inflation range from 50 to 100 mm Hg above the patient's systolic blood pressure or 300 mm Hg for the adult arm and 400 mm Hg for the adult leg. When the cuff is inflated, its inflation should be checked by gently squeezing the cuff and monitoring the pressure gauge for fluctuations or "bounce." When proper inflation is verified, the Esmarch bandage is removed. Other methods of exsanguination for painful extremities include elevating the extremity for 4 to 5 minutes or using a zippered pneumatic splint.

After removal of the Esmarch bandage, and confirmation of adequate tourniquet inflation, 40 to 50 mL of lidocaine, 0.5% without vasoconstrictor, is injected into the venous catheter. The author prefers to occlude the extremity circumferentially just above the surgical site with one hand while injecting with the other. The patient should be monitored continually for signs of local anesthetic toxicity. The patient may complain of transient "hot," "burning," or "pins-and-needles" feelings in the extremity. The patient should be reassured that this sensation will pass as the arm becomes anesthetized. Onset of the block is usually within 5 minutes. If the extremity is elevated as the block progresses, the patient loses spatial orientation of the extremity regardless of its position and may complain of its perceived position.

After injection of the local anesthetic, the intravenous catheter in the operative extremity is removed. The individual preparing the surgical site is asked to hold pressure over the intravenous site.

4. List the manifestations of local anesthetic toxicity.

Manifestations of local anesthetic toxicity include the following:
- Tinnitus
- Circumoral numbness
- Tongue paresthesias
- Metallic taste
- Dizziness
- Dysrhythmias
- Apprehension
- Restlessness

- Nausea
- Blurred vision
- Seizures
- Apnea
- Cardiac arrest

5. A patient's surgery involves one or more fingers. How can the nurse anesthetist further promote digital exsanguination?

Before the Esmarch bandage is applied, digital exsanguination may be accomplished by wrapping the appropriate digits with a 5/8-inch Penrose drain. The goal of IVRA is to drain the venous system adequately, then fill it with local anesthetic solution.

6. Which local anesthetic should be used for IVRA?

Lidocaine 0.5% is the only solution for IVRA approved by the Food and Drug Administration in the United States. Vasoconstrictors should not be added to the local anesthetic solution.

7. What should the nurse anesthetist do if the patient begins to complain of tourniquet pain during IVRA?

Patients normally begin to complain of tourniquet pain after the tourniquet has been inflated 30 to 45 minutes. The double tourniquet is ideally suited for IVRA. When the patient begins to complain of tourniquet pain, the distal cuff is inflated over the anesthetized skin, and the proximal cuff is released. The distal cuff must be inflated (confirm by squeezing and monitoring the pressure gauge for fluctuations) before the proximal cuff is released. Proper sequencing is crucial to avoid premature release of local anesthetic solution into the circulation.

8. When surgery is complete, how should tourniquet deflation proceed?

When the tourniquet is released, local anesthetic solution floods into the systemic circulation. The tourniquet should not be released if the inflation time has been less than 20 minutes because excessive local anesthetic would be released into the circulation. At the end of the procedure, the patient should be informed that the tourniquet will be deflated. If 20 to 40 minutes have elapsed since local anesthetic injection, the tourniquet can be deflated briefly, then immediately reinflated. The patient should be observed for 1 minute and questioned regarding any symptoms of local anesthesia toxicity. If manifestations of systemic toxicity do not appear, the tourniquet again is deflated and immediately reinflated, and the patient again is assessed for signs of systemic toxicity. If none occur, the cuff can be deflated and the tourniquet removed. If 40 minutes or more have elapsed since local anesthetic injection, the tourniquet may be deflated slowly and the patient observed for any symptoms of systemic local anesthetic toxicity.

9. Discuss the complications associated with IVRA.

Premature release of the local anesthetic solution into the systemic circulation is the greatest complication; often this is associated with tourniquet failure. Systemic local anesthetic toxicity can progress to convulsions and apnea. If systemic toxicity occurs, the extremity should be quickly isolated, and patient ventilation and circulation should be supported. Careful monitoring of the patient is mandatory, especially after release of the tourniquet.

10. Can IVRA be used on the lower extremity?

Although IVRA is used most frequently on the upper extremity, it has been used for operations on the lower extremity. Technically the procedure is the same as that used for the upper extremity. Tourniquet placement can be either midthigh or on the calf. The midthigh technique requires larger volumes (60 to 80 mL) of local anesthetic solution. Placing the tourniquet at the calf reduces the required volume of local anesthetic to 40 to 50 mL.

 Key Points

- IVRA involves injecting local anesthetic into the venous system of an extremity after it has been exsanguinated by compression and its circulation occluded with a pneumatic tourniquet.
- Onset of IVRA anesthesia usually ensues within 5 minutes, and anesthesia is effective for procedures lasting 90 to 120 minutes when a double tourniquet is used.
- The manifestations of local anesthetic toxicity include tinnitus, circumoral numbness, tongue paresthesias, metallic taste, dizziness, dysrhythmias, apprehension, restlessness, nausea, blurred vision, seizures, apnea, and cardiac arrest.
- Lidocaine 0.5% is the only solution for IVRA approved by the Food and Drug Administration in the United States.
- After IVRA, the tourniquet should not be released if the inflation time is less than 20 minutes because excessive local anesthetic would be released into the circulation.
- Premature release of the local anesthetic solution into the systemic circulation is the greatest complication of IVRA; often this is associated with tourniquet failure.

Internet Resources

Virtual Anaesthesia Textbook:
http://www.virtual-anaesthesia-textbook.com/

Nurse-Anesthesia.com:
http://www.nurse-anesthesia.com/

Tourniquets.org: A North American Survey of Intravenous Regional Anesthesia:
http://www.interchange.ubc.ca/jamc/pdf/ivra.pdf

New York School of Regional Anesthesia: Intravenous Regional Block (Bier Block):
http://www.nysora.com/techniques/basic/bierblock/bierblock.html

Bibliography

Brown DL: *Atlas of regional anesthesia*, ed 2, Philadelphia, 1999, WB Saunders.

Ellis WE: Regional anesthesia. In Nagelhout JJ, Zaglaniczny K, editors: *Nurse anesthesia*, ed 2, Philadelphia, 2001, WB Saunders.

Eriksson E, editor: *Illustrated handbook in local anaesthesia*, ed 2, Philadelphia, 1989, WB Saunders.

Morgan GE, Mikhail MS, Murray MJ: *Clinical anesthesiology*, ed 3, New York, 2002, Lange Medical Books/McGraw-Hill.

Scott DB: *Techniques of regional anaesthesia*, Norwalk, CT, 1989, Appleton & Lange.

Winnie AP: *Plexus anesthesia: perivascular techniques of brachial plexus block*, Philadelphia, 1983, WB Saunders.

Zenz M, et al, editors: *Regional anesthesia*, ed 2, St. Louis, 1990, Mosby-Year Book.

Chapter 52

Peripheral Nerve Blocks

J. Frank Titch

1. Discuss potential complications associated with peripheral nerve block (PNB).

Systemic local anesthetic toxicity can occur from either inadvertent intravascular injection (immediate) or absorption of excessive amounts of local anesthetic (delayed). Local anesthetic toxicity produces varying effects on the central nervous system (numbness of tongue, convulsions, unconsciousness) and cardiovascular system (hypotension, refractory dysrhythmias, cardiovascular collapse). PNB success often depends on the volume of local anesthetic used, and the large volumes required frequently push the maximal acceptable limits for systemic local anesthetic toxicity. Epinephrine may be added in an attempt to slow systemic uptake. Rates of systemic uptake and peak plasma levels vary with the site of injection: tracheal > intercostal > caudal > epidural (lumbar) > brachial plexus > sciatic/femoral > subcutaneous.

Another potential complication of peripheral nerve block is *intraneural injection*. Intraneural injection occurs when the needle tip is located in the nerve itself, and it is characterized by sharp, shooting pain. If the patient complains of lancinating pain on injection, the needle must be repositioned before continuing local anesthetic injection. Continued intraneural injection risks inducing permanent nerve injury. Using short-bevel needles, not seeking paresthesias, and not injecting at stimulator settings less than 0.2 mA may reduce the risk of intraneural injection. Patients also may complain of dull, aching pain ("pressure paresthesia") when large volumes of local anesthetic are injected into the confined perivascular space. If this pain occurs, the anesthetist should slow the rate of injection, and the discomfort should pass.

2. Should a patient be medicated before placing a PNB?

Only a rare individual enjoys being fully lucid when punctured with a needle, especially when repeated attempts may be necessary. Nerve isolation with the nerve stimulator also may be uncomfortable. Preemptive pain control and sedation results in a cooperative and comfortable patient. Many practitioners heavily sedate patients, only to end up with an uncooperative patient, thrashing about during needle placement. Judicious administration of intravenous analgesics allows the patient to tolerate needle insertion and nerve isolation while remaining cooperative and conversant. The author prefers careful titration of 50 to 150 mcg of fentanyl combined with small amounts of midazolam before needle insertion.

3. Are patient monitoring devices necessary during PNB placement?

The patient's electrocardiogram, blood pressure, and oxygen saturation should be closely monitored before, during, and after PNB placement. Delayed systemic local anesthetic toxicity can occur 30 minutes after injection. Supplemental oxygen also is highly recommended. Resuscitation drugs and equipment should be readily available.

4. How is a nerve stimulator used to isolate the desired nerve/nerve plexus?

Low-output nerve stimulators capable of delivering 0.2 to 5 mA via the negative lead are available commercially. When combined with specially insulated needles, which permit current flow only at the tip, precise isolation of nerves is possible. When the needle has penetrated the skin, the current is increased to 1.5 to 2 mA, which allows approximation of the nerve to within 2 cm. When twitching of the desired nerve distribution is observed, the current is reduced while the needle's position simultaneously is adjusted until the current is reduced to 0.2 to 0.5 mA. Small, deliberate, delicate movements of the needle are used during this adjustment period. After confirming negative aspiration, injection of 1 to 2 mL of local anesthetic should cause the twitch to disappear rapidly, confirming the close proximity of the nerve to the needle tip. Increasing the volume of local anesthetic solution injected may compensate for deficiencies in accuracy.

5. Should the practitioner use commercially prepared local anesthetic solutions that contain epinephrine or prepare his or her own?

Local anesthetics commercially prepared with epinephrine contain stabilizing agents that lower the pH of the local anesthetic solution. Because local anesthetics possess a high pK_a, onset of anesthesia is slowed due to the low pH. It is preferable if epinephrine is added to the local anesthetic solution when the block is performed.

6. The technique calls for 40 mL of local anesthetic containing 1:400,000 epinephrine; how is this solution prepared?

Epinephrine is readily available in 1-mL ampules containing a 1:1000 solution. The ratio of 1:1000 indicates a solution containing 1 g of epinephrine dissolved in 1000 mL of diluent.

$$\frac{1 \text{ gram}}{1000 \text{ mL}} = \frac{1000 \text{ mg}}{1000 \text{ mL}} = \frac{1 \text{ mg}}{1 \text{ mL}}$$

The ampule of 1:1000 epinephrine contains 1 mg/mL.

The desired solution is 1:400,000 or:

$$\frac{1\ g}{400,000\ mL} = \frac{1000\ mg}{400,000\ mL} = \frac{1\ mg}{400\ mL} = \frac{0.0025\ mg}{1\ mL} = \frac{2.5\ mcg}{1\ mL}$$

Therefore,

$$40\ mL \times \frac{2.5\ mcg}{1\ mL} = 100\ mcg$$

or 0.1 mL of the 1:1000 epinephrine must be added to the 40 mL of local anesthetic to yield a 1:400,000 solution.

Concentration	Epinephrine
1:100,000	10 mcg/1 mL
1:200,000	5 mcg/1 mL
1:400,000	2.5 mcg/1 mL

7. The anesthetist wishes to use 40 mL of ropivacaine 0.5%; how many milligrams of ropivacaine are in the solution?

Local anesthetics are collectively expressed as a percent concentration or weight of solute per 100 mL of solution (grams per 100 mL solution). The percent concentration designates grams of active drug in 100 mL of the total preparation and is also known as *grams percent*.

Ropivacaine 0.5%:

$$\frac{0.5\ g}{100\ mL} = \frac{500\ mg}{100\ mL} = \frac{5\ mg}{1\ mL}$$

0.5% = 5 mg/1 mL.

Therefore,

$$40\ mL \times \frac{5\ mg}{1\ mL} = 200\ mg$$

of ropivacaine.

AXILLARY BRACHIAL PLEXUS BLOCK

8. Which surgical procedures are appropriate for the axillary approach to the brachial plexus block?

The axillary approach for block of the brachial plexus, *axillary block,* is well suited for operations distal to the elbow, especially those on the forearm and hand. This approach has limited application for procedures above the elbow.

9. Discuss the anatomical considerations for performing the axillary block.

The brachial plexus (principally C5, C6, C7, C8, and T1) extends from the neck to the axilla, passing between the clavicle and first rib. The nerves and primary blood vessels of the brachial plexus are surrounded by connective tissue, which forms a tube, the *perivascular sheath*. Local anesthetics injected into the perivascular sheath (tube) spread up and down the sheath, anesthetizing the nerves that lie within it. As the brachial plexus approaches the axilla, it divides into its terminal branches consisting of the musculocutaneous, median, radial, and ulnar nerves. The musculocutaneous nerve exits the perivascular sheath above the axilla and enters the coracobrachialis muscle just lateral to the pectoralis minor muscle. At the level of the axilla, the median, radial, and ulnar nerves lie in close proximity to the axillary artery within the fascial tube of the perivascular sheath. The axillary block involves injecting local anesthetic within the perivascular sheath to anesthetize musculocutaneous, median, radial, and ulnar nerves.

10. Identify contraindications for the axillary block.

Absolute contraindications include patient refusal, local infection at the injection site, coagulopathy, and lymphangitis (presumed infected axillary nodes). Coagulopathy is considered a contraindication due to the close proximity of the nerves to the axillary artery and possible incidental arterial puncture. Preoperative nerve injury to the extremity is a *relative contraindication*.

11. How is the patient positioned for an axillary block?

The patient is positioned supine with the arm abducted 45 degrees and the forearm flexed so that it is parallel to the patient's body. Hyperabduction should be avoided because it may obliterate the arterial pulse and impede local anesthetic spread up the sheath toward the musculocutaneous nerve.

12. Which local anesthetics should be used for an axillary block, and what is the appropriate volume?

The choice of local anesthetic depends on the length of anesthesia required (see the table on page 483). Also, success of the axillary technique is volume dependent and requires significant amounts of local anesthetic (sufficient to reach the musculocutaneous nerve). The musculocutaneous nerve is often spared if a volume less than 30 mL is used. Dividing the patient's height in inches by 2 provides a simple estimate for determining the appropriate volume (e.g., height 70 inches ÷ 2 = 35 mL). Large volumes often require adjusting the local anesthetic concentration to avoid local anesthetic overdosage.

13. What equipment does the anesthetist need to perform an axillary block?

An axillary block usually is carried out using the "immobile needle" system and requires two people (one to place the needle and one to aspirate/inject the syringes). The immobile needle, as described by Winnie, simply places intra-

Local Anesthetic and Length of Anesthesia

Local Anesthetic	Duration
Procaine 2%	20–30 min
Procaine 2% + epinephire 1:200,000	30–60 min
Chloroprocaine 2%	30–60 min
Chloroprocaine 2% + epinephire 1:200,000	60–90 min
Lidocaine 1%	60–90 min
Lidocaine 1% + epinephire 1:200,000	150–180 min
Mepivacaine 1%	150–180 min
Prilocaine 1%	3–4 hr
Tetracaine 0.15-0.2% + epinephire 1:200,000	5–6 hr
Bupivacaine 0.5%	≥10–12 hr
Ropivacaine 0.5%	5–8 hr
Mepivacaine 1% + epinephire 1:200,000 + tetracaine 0.2%	4–6 hr

venous extension tubing (18 to 20 inches) between the needle and the syringes (two 20-mL syringes) containing the local anesthetic. This system ensures stability of the needle while injecting the local anesthetic. The needle should be approximately 1.5 inches, 22-gauge or smaller, with a translucent hub, and preferably have a short bevel (B-bevel).

14. How is the axillary brachial plexus block performed?

Many different techniques are used to perform an axillary brachial plexus block. Common approaches include the transarterial technique, elicitation of paresthesias, four-quadrant approach, or use of a peripheral nerve stimulator and insulated needle. All of the techniques have some common elements:
- The axillary arterial pulse is palpated and followed as far proximally as possible.
- After skin preparation with an antiseptic solution, a skin wheal is raised over the pulse, and the needle is introduced slowly.
- The needle is advanced until, depending on the technique selected:
  - A paresthesia is elicited from one of the nerves within the sheath, or one of the nerves is stimulated with the nerve stimulator. These signs indicate that the needle is within the sheath, and after negative aspiration for blood, the local anesthetic is injected slowly.
  - If blood appears with aspiration, the needle is advanced through the posterior wall of the artery until there is no aspiration of blood. Local anesthetic is injected slowly after ensuring negative aspiration for blood.

- To promote local anesthetic spread up the sheath, gentle distal pressure should be applied while injecting. Often the patient notes a dull, achy sensation during initial injection (pressure paresthesia), which is acceptable.
- Local anesthetic injection should be stopped immediately if signs of intravascular injection occur, or if the patient complains of sharp, lancinating pain, which may indicate intraneural injection. Repeated aspiration for blood during dosing is advised. Dysrhythmias, circumoral numbness, dizziness, apprehension, agitation, tongue paresthesia, and tinnitus are manifestations of local anesthetic toxicity and may indicate intravascular injection.
- The intercostobrachial (T2) and medial brachial cutaneous (C8-T1) nerves supply the inside of the upper arm and must be blocked separately if a pneumatic tourniquet is to be used on the upper arm. Before withdrawing the needle, 5 to 10 mL of local anesthesia solution is injected subcutaneously and perpendicular to the long axis of the arm to block these nerves.
- After the needle is completely withdrawn, gentle pressure is applied, and the patient's arm is positioned at the side. This maneuver removes the mechanical obstruction (humeral head) and allows local anesthetic flow within the sheath. Gentle massage also may aid spreading local anesthetic up the perivascular sheath.

15. What are potential complications with the axillary approach?

Potential complications include intraneural injection, inadvertent intravascular injection, and local anesthetic toxicity due to the large volume of local anesthetic used. Because the axillary approach occurs distal in the brachial plexus, it avoids potential complications from neuraxial structures and the lung.

16. How can the anesthetist quickly assess adequacy of the axillary block?

The *four Ps* mnemonic for *push, pull, pinch, pinch* provides a quick assessment tool. Hold the patient's hand as if attempting to "arm wrestle," and tell the patient to push your hand away, then pull it toward him or her. This maneuver checks the radial and musculocutaneous nerves. Gently pinch the palmar side of the index finger and pinch the little finger. This maneuver checks the median and ulnar nerves. A slight modification of the mnemonic associates the respective nerves with the words *push 'er* ("r" for *radial*), *pull 'em* ("m" for *musculocutaneous*), *pinch, pinch*.

17. The block appears to be working well in all areas except the musculocutaneous distribution; can you salvage this block?

The musculocutaneous nerve exits the perivascular sheath above the axilla and enters the coracobrachialis muscle just lateral to the pectoralis minor muscle. This proximal exit of the musculocutaneous nerve from the perivascular sheath may result in occasional sparing of this nerve. If this occurs, inject the coracobrachialis muscle at the level of the axilla to provide anesthesia to the nerve. To locate the coracobrachialis muscle, identify the axillary pulse at the level of the axilla. The coracobrachialis muscle lies just above the axillary artery and runs parallel to it. The musculocutaneous nerve lies within it similar to "pencil lead within a wooden pencil." Injecting 5 mL of local anesthetic into the substance of the coracobrachialis muscle, after negative aspiration for blood, should anesthetize the nerve sufficiently.

ILIOINGUINAL NERVE BLOCK

18. Identify the indications for ilioinguinal/iliohypogastric nerve block.

Ilioinguinal/iliohypogastric nerve block provides excellent postoperative analgesia after inguinal herniorrhaphy and appendectomy. It is also useful in providing anesthesia for reducing strangulated inguinal hernias and inguinal herniorrhaphy under local anesthesia. The analgesia provided facilitates early ambulation and may be useful in the outpatient setting.

19. Describe the clinically relevant anatomy.

Originating from L1, the ilioinguinal and iliohypogastric nerves separate under the transversus abdominis muscle, piercing it near the anterior superior iliac spine. As the nerves progress, they pass through the internal and external oblique muscles to supply the skin of the suprapubic and inguinal regions. The anterior branch of the iliohypogastric nerve supplies the skin of the hypogastric region, whereas the ilioinguinal nerve supplies sensation to the skin of the groin and medial thigh (scrotum and penis in men; labia and mons pubis in women). Approximately 2 cm medial to the anterior iliac spine, both nerves lie between the transversus abdominis and internal oblique muscles. The iliohypogastric nerve immediately becomes more superficial between the internal and external oblique muscles, whereas the ilioinguinal nerve continues to run parallel to, but slightly below, the iliohypogastric nerve.

20. Describe the technique for performing the ilioinguinal block.

The patient is placed supine, and the anterior superior iliac spine is identified by palpation. The point of needle entry is on a line between the anterior superior iliac spine and the navel, 1 to 2 fingerbreadths medial to the anterior superior iliac spine. After the insertion point is identified and prepared with antiseptic solution, a 1.5- to 3.5-inch, 22-gauge to 25-gauge needle, attached to a 10-mL syringe, is introduced through the skin. The syringe is held lightly and gently advanced to the fascia (increased resistance is noted). As the tip of the needle pierces the fascia of the oblique muscle (a pop or release is detected), local anesthetic solution is infiltrated into the subfascial and muscular (external and internal oblique) tissues. Following a fan-shaped path, local anesthetic solution is injected along a line from the anterior superior iliac spine toward the navel in the subcutaneous, subfascial, and muscular tissues. The needle depth must be cautiously controlled. Placing the needle too deep may perforate the abdominal viscera. Because of the close proximity of the ilioinguinal and iliohypogastric nerves, 10 to 15 mL of local anesthetic solution usually blocks both.

LUMBAR PLEXUS BLOCK (POSTERIOR APPROACH)

21. When is the lumbar plexus block (LPB) indicated?

The lumbar plexus arises from spinal cord segments L1-4 and forms the following nerves:
- Iliohypogastric nerve
- Ilioinguinal nerve
- Genitofemoral nerve
- Lateral femoral cutaneous nerve
- Femoral nerve
- Obturator nerve

The LBP, also called the *psoas compartment block,* is indicated for procedures on one lower extremity involving the thigh or knee. Surgical candidates who may benefit from LPB anesthesia include patients undergoing patellar tendon repair, anterior cruciate reconstruction, reduction of fractures, or skin grafting. The LPB also is used to diminish intraoperative tourniquet pain and to reduce postoperative pain after total knee arthroplasty or hip surgery. Any procedure on the lower extremity may be performed when the LPB is combined with a sciatic nerve block.

22. How is the patient positioned for LPB?

The patient is placed in the lateral decubitus position with the extremity to be anesthetized, slightly bent at the knee, on top of the other extremity. In other words, the patient is lying on the side opposite the extremity to be blocked. Positioning the shoulders and hips perpendicular to the bed aids with maintaining correct needle alignment. This position also is convenient if the patient requires a sciatic nerve block for complete lower extremity anesthesia/analgesia.

23. Is special equipment required to perform the LPB?

The LPB requires a 4- to 6-inch (depending on the size of the patient), insulated, short-bevel needle attached to a peripheral nerve stimulator. Both items are specifically designed for PNB placement. The nerve stimulator's current output should be adjustable from 0 to 5 mA. Emergency airway equipment and resuscitative medications should be immediately available.

24. Describe the anatomical landmarks for LPB.

Only two landmarks are necessary for the LPB:
- A line drawn between the tip of each iliac crest (indicates the L4-5 interspace)
- A second line drawn 4 to 5 cm lateral and parallel to the spine, on the operative side, passing through the posterior superior iliac spine

The insulated short-bevel needle is inserted at the intersecting point of these two lines.

25. How is the LPB performed?

As with any PNB procedure, intravenous analgesics and sedatives are important for patient comfort. The patient's electrocardiogram, blood pressure, and oxygen saturation should be monitored closely. Supplemental oxygen is highly recommended.

After the appropriate landmarks are identified and the point of needle insertion marked, the skin is prepared with antiseptic solution. A fast-acting local anesthetic such as lidocaine is used to localize the skin, using a 25- or 30-gauge needle. A 4- to 6-inch, insulated, short-bevel needle is inserted (at the intersection of the two lines), perpendicular to the skin with a slight medial direction. Medial direction should be minimal to avoid entry into the epidural or subarachnoid space. When beyond the skin and subcutaneous tissues, the nerve stimulator output is set to 1.5 mA. The needle is advanced until either the transverse process is encountered or the lumbar plexus is stimulated. Rhythmic contraction of the quadriceps femoris muscle accompanied by twitching of the patella ("dancing patella") indicates lumbar plexus stimulation.

If the transverse process is encountered, note the depth and angle of the needle, withdraw the needle to the skin, and reinsert in a slightly caudad direction, advancing the needle until lumbar plexus stimulation occurs. If the transverse process is again encountered, walk the needle off the inferior or superior border of the transverse process until lumbar plexus stimulation occurs.

When stimulation is confirmed, the needle should be manipulated until lumbar plexus stimulation is observed at 0.5 mA or less. At this point, after careful and repeated aspiration to prevent inadvertent intravascular injection, a local anesthetic may be incrementally injected.

26. Which local anesthetic is considered appropriate for the LPB?

Local anesthetic choice should be tailored for the desired duration of the block and the degree of motor and sensory block required (see the table below). As

Local Anesthetics for Lumbar Plexus Block

Local Anesthetic	Epinephrine	Procedure Time* (hr)	Onset Time (min)
Chloroprocaine 3%	1:400,000	1–1.5	10–15
Mepivacaine 1.5%[†]	1:400,000	2–2.5	15–20
Ropivacaine 0.5%	1:400,000 (slows systemic uptake)	2.5–4	15–30

[†]Alkalinized with 1 mL sodium bicarbonate/10 ml local anesthetic.
*Time for surgical anesthesia; analgesia lasts longer.

with most PNBs, the LPB is a volume-dependent block. Most authors recommend 30 to 40 mL of local anesthetic for the average-sized adult. The approximate volume may be estimated by dividing the height in inches by 3.

27. Identify possible complications associated with LPB.

Potential complications include inadvertent epidural or subarachnoid injection, local anesthetic toxicity, or postoperative pain from lumbar paravertebral muscle spasm.

SCIATIC NERVE BLOCK (POSTERIOR APPROACH)

28. Which surgical procedures are appropriate for sciatic nerve block?

The sciatic nerve forms from spinal cord branches L4-S3 and is composed of the tibial nerve and the common peroneal nerve. The sciatic nerve innervates the posterior aspect of the thigh, the lateral aspect of the calf, most of the ankle, and all of the foot. Sciatic nerve block alone is satisfactory for procedures on the foot, such as for amputation due to peripheral vascular disease. Sciatic nerve block often is combined with a lumbar plexus block, and together this combination produces anesthesia/ analgesia of the entire lower extremity, also blunting the sympathetic response to tourniquet pain.

29. How is the patient positioned for sciatic nerve block from the posterior approach?

Positioning is the same as for a posterior approach to the LPB. The patient is placed in the lateral decubitus position on the side not to be blocked, with the extremity to be anesthetized uppermost.

30. Identify the anatomical landmarks for the sciatic nerve block.

Identify the posterior superior iliac spine and the midpoint of the greater trochanter. Connect these two points with a line, and determine the midpoint of this line. At the midpoint, draw a perpendicular line 5 cm caudomedially. The end point of this line identifies the needle insertion point.

31. How is the sciatic nerve block performed?

As with any PNB, intravenous analgesics and sedatives are important for patient comfort. The author prefers careful titration of fentanyl, 50 to 150 mcg, combined with small amounts of midazolam before needle insertion. The patient's electrocardiogram, blood pressure, and oxygen saturation should be monitored closely. Supplemental oxygen is highly recommended. After the appropriate landmarks are identified and the point of needle insertion marked, the skin is prepared with an antiseptic solution. After skin infiltration with a local anesthetic, a 4- to 6-inch, insulated, short-bevel needle, connected to a nerve stimulator, is inserted perpendicular to the skin in all planes. When beyond the skin and subcutaneous tissues, the nerve stimulator output is set to 1.5 mA. The needle is advanced into the deeper tissues until motor stimulation of the gluteal and piriformis muscles occurs. When piriformis twitches disappear, sciatic stimulation should begin as the needle is advanced. Usually, sciatic stimulation begins as twitching of the hamstring muscles. As the needle is advanced, rhythmic contractions of the foot are observed (plantar flexion with stimulation of the tibial nerve component; dorsiflexion with stimulation of the peroneal nerve). If the sciatic nerve is not identified, the needle is withdrawn to the skin and redirected toward the greater trochanter. If this fails, the needle is withdrawn to the skin and redirected toward the posterior superior iliac spine. When stimulation is confirmed, the needle is manipulated until stimulation of the foot is observed at 0.2 to 0.4 mA. The needle is immobilized, negative blood aspiration is confirmed, and the local anesthetic is incrementally injected to a total dose of 15 to 20 mL. The needle traverses near the inferior gluteal artery and vein, and repeated aspiration for blood during dosing is vital. To prevent intraneural injection, injection of local anesthetic should be avoided when stimulation of the foot is less than 0.2 mA.

32. When completed, how is the sciatic nerve block assessed?

Onset of motor blockade follows sensory blockade; diminished motor function indicates success. The patient should lose the ability to plantar flex (tibial) and dorsiflex (peroneal) the foot against resistance.

Key Points

- The axillary approach for block of the brachial plexus, axillary block, is well suited for operations distal to the elbow, especially procedures on the forearm and hand.

- The axillary block involves injecting local anesthetic within the perivascular sheath to anesthetize musculocutaneous, median, radial, and ulnar nerves.

- Common approaches to performing an axillary block include the transarterial technique, elicitation of paresthesias, four-quadrant approach, or use of a peripheral nerve stimulator and insulated needle.

- The four Ps mnemonic for "push, pull, pinch, pinch" provides a quick assessment tool for adequacy of the axillary block.

- Ilioinguinal/iliohypogastric nerve block provides excellent postoperative analgesia after inguinal herniorrhaphy and appendectomy.

- Sciatic nerve block alone is satisfactory for procedures on the foot, such as for amputation due to peripheral vascular disease. Sciatic nerve block is often combined with an LPB, and together this combination produces anesthesia or analgesia or both of the entire lower extremity, also blunting the sympathetic response to tourniquet pain.

Internet Resources

Online Regional Anesthesia Techniques: Do It Yourself!:
http://www.csen.com/blocks.htm

Virtual Anaesthesia Textbook:
http://www.virtual-anaesthesia-textbook.com/

New York School of Regional Anesthesia:
http://www.nysora.com/

Anesthesiology Info:
http://www.anesthesiologyinfo.com/

Nurse-Anesthesia.com:
http://www.nurse-anesthesia.com/

Bibliography

Brown DL: *Atlas of regional anesthesia*, ed 2, Philadelphia, 1999, WB Saunders.

Ellis WE: Regional anesthesia. In Nagelhout JJ, Zaglaniczny K, editors: *Nurse anesthesia*, ed 2, Philadelphia, 2001, WB Saunders.

Eriksson E, editor: *Illustrated handbook in local anaesthesia*, ed 2, Philadelphia, 1989, WB Saunders.

Morgan GE, Mikhail MS, Murray MJ: *Clinical anesthesiology*, ed 3, New York, 2002, Lange Medical Books/ McGraw-Hill.

Scott DB: *Techniques of regional anaesthesia*, Stamford, CT, 1989, Appleton & Lange.

Winnie AP: *Plexus anesthesia: perivascular techniques of brachial plexus block*, Philadelphia, 1983, WB Saunders.

Zenz M, et al, editors: *Regional anesthesia*, ed 2, St. Louis, 1990, Mosby-Year Book.

Pain Management

Rick Hand

1. Identify the physiological effects of pain.

The presence of pain can have a tremendous impact on all major organ systems (see the following table). These responses are mediated through the sympathetic nervous system and the neuroendocrine system.

Physiological Effects of Pain

Organ System	Physiological Effects
Respiratory Skeletal muscle tension Decreased lung compliance	Hypoxemia, hypercarbia Ventilation-perfusion mismatch Atelectasis
Endocrine Increased cortisol Increased epinephrine Increased glucagon, decreased insulin	Lipolysis, hyperglycemia, protein catabolism Inceased heart rate, increased myocardial contractility Hyperglycemia
Cardiovascular Increased myocardial work (mediated by SNS activation)	Dysrhythmias, angina, myocardial infarction, congestive heart failure
Immunological Lymphopenia Depression of reticuloenothelial system Reduced T-cell cytotoxicity	Depressed immune response
Coagulation Increased platelet activation Coagulation cascade activation Decreased fibrinolysis	Enhanced risk for thromboembolism

SNS, sympathetic nervous system.

2. What is the difference between acute and chronic pain?

Acute pain is associated with injury to body tissues that initiates the nociceptive process. Nociception often causes stimulation of the sympathetic nervous system, resulting in hypertension, tachycardia, diaphoresis, mydriasis, and pallor. The sympathetic nervous system response is proportional to the intensity of the painful stimulus. Acute pain is generally self-limiting or resolves when the underlying pathology is treated.

Chronic pain is pain lasting for 3 months after the usual course of an acute illness, pain associated with a chronic pathological process, or pain that is recurrent over months or years.

3. What is the difference between tolerance, physiological dependence, psychological dependence, and pseudoaddiction?

A fundamental barrier to effective pain management is the confusion that exists between tolerance, physiological dependence, psychological dependence, and pseudoaddiction. These misconceptions often lead practitioners to believe that their patients may be "addicted" to the analgesics.

- *Tolerance* is characterized by a change in the dose-response relationship induced by exposure to the drug and manifested as a need for a higher dose to maintain an effect. This is a normal physiological response to therapy.
- *Physiological dependence* describes the occurrence of an abstinence (withdrawal) syndrome after abrupt discontinuation of the drug or administration of an antagonist. Clinicians should assume that physiological dependence exists after repeated administration of an opioid for more than a few days. Physiological dependence with opioid analgesics is similar to physiological dependence people may have with caffeine or nicotine. Similar to tolerance, developing physiological dependence to opioids is a normal response to therapy.
- *Psychological dependence* describes a psychological and behavioral syndrome characterized by a continued craving for an opioid drug to achieve a psychic effect despite physical, psychological, and social harm to self or others.
- *Pseudoaddiction* refers to individuals who exhibit opioid-seeking behavior similar to patients who may be psychologically dependent on opioids. The cause of this behavior is not the psychic effects that opioids can produce, but rather inadequate analgesia. Patients no longer show this drug-seeking behavior when adequate analgesia is provided.

4. Define nociception.

Nociception is the process whereby chemical, thermal, mechanical, or trauma stimuli are propagated to the cerebral cortex and perceived as pain. The receptors associated with the transmission of noxious information can be grouped as: A-delta fiber mechanothermal and C fiber polymodal nociceptors.

5. Why is the use of meperidine in patient-controlled analgesia (PCA) discouraged for acute postoperative pain and chronic pain management?

One of the metabolites of meperidine metabolism is normeperidine. This metabolite is a central nervous system excitotoxin. Particularly in the elderly and patients with impaired renal function, accumulation of normeperidine can lead to anxiety, tremors, multifocal myoclonus, and ultimately generalized seizures. Meperidine has an analgesic half-life of 2 to 3 hours and an elimination half-life of 20 hours. Consequently, if the patient received meperidine every 3 to 4 hours, he or her conceivably could receive five to six doses before any of the normeperidine was eliminated. Presently the American Pain Society recommends that meperidine not be prescribed for chronic pain management. Additionally the American Pain Society recommends that if meperidine is used for management of acute pain, it should not be prescribed for longer than 48 hours and doses should not exceed 600 mg in a 24-hour period.

6. Identify, compare, and contrast the different opioid receptors.

Opioid receptor subtypes include mu (subtypes 1 and 2), kappa, and delta (see the table below). These receptors are located throughout the central nervous system, and all produce analgesia and miosis when activated. They differ in the degree to which they produce side effects in the cardiovascular, respiratory, central nervous, and genitourinary systems.

Initially, sigma receptors were identified as opioid receptors. This is no longer the case, because the effects produced by sigma receptor activation (hallucinations, dysphoria, and increased ventilatory rate) differ from the other opioid receptors and cannot be reversed with naloxone administration.

Characteristics of Opioid Receptor Subtypes

Effects	Mu_1	Mu_2	Kappa	Delta
Analgesia	Supraspinal	Spinal	Supraspinal, spinal	Supraspinal, spinal
Cardiovascular	Decreased heart rate	Decreased heart rate		
Respiratory		Depression	Depression (?)	Depression
CNS	Euphoria, sedation, hypothermia	Euphoria	Dysphoria, hallucinations, sedation	
Genitourinary	Urinary retention	Urinary retention	Diuresis (inhibits vasopressin release)	Urinary retention
Gastrointestinal		Ileus, nausea and vomiting		
Physical dependence	Low abuse potential	Yes	Low abuse potential	Yes
Pruritus		Yes		Yes

CNS, central nervous system.

7. **Explain equianalgesic dosing between different opioids and between routes of administration for the same opioid.**

Opioid analgesics do not show an analgesic "ceiling effect." That is, the amount of analgesia obtained increases as long as the dose is escalated. In the event that adequate analgesia cannot be obtained or the side effects become intolerable or unmanageable with a given opioid, it may be necessary to switch from one opioid to another. Prescribing an alternate opioid may provide effective pain management because of the large intraindividual variability between opioids.

Patients on long-term opioid therapy have an incomplete cross-tolerance between opioids. This mandates that the equianalgesic dose for the alternate opioid be calculated and the dose decreased by 50% before initiating therapy. When calculating an equianalgesic dose, the total amount of opioid received by the patient in a 24-hour period should be determined.

Example: If a patient is receiving 10 mg of morphine sulfate (MSO_4) intravenously (IV) per hour and the anesthetist wishes to switch the analgesic to hydromorphone, the practitioner would calculate that the patient receives 240 mg of MSO_4 per 24 hours. Based on an equianalgesic dosing chart, 1 mg of hydromorphone = 6.6 mg of MSO_4. MSO_4, 240 mg IV, is equianalgesic to hydromorphone, 36 mg IV, in 24 hours. This calculates to a hydromorphone dose of 1.5 mg/hr IV. Because of the incomplete cross-tolerance between opioids, this dose is decreased by 50%, and the patient's hydromorphone infusion is started at 0.75 mg/hr. Changing from one opioid to another requires strict vigilance and continual assessment of the patient. Additionally, until adequate analgesia is obtained with the new opioid, the patient should have access to additional bolus doses of opioid in the event of breakthrough pain.

When continuing with the same opioid but with a different route of administration, one formulation is converted to the other with the equianalgesic dose.

Example: MSO_4, 240 mg IV, is equianalgesic to MSO_4, 720 mg orally. This amount is divided equally for an oral dose of 240 mg every 8 hours.

8. **Describe the mechanism of action of nonsteroidal antiinflammatory drugs (NSAIDs).**

Similar to aspirin, NSAIDs inhibit the enzyme cyclooxygenase (COX) and consequently inhibit prostaglandin synthesis at peripheral sites of inflammation and injury. Prostaglandins are responsible for sensitizing and amplifying peripheral nociceptors to inflammatory mediators (substance P, bradykinin, serotonin) released when tissue is traumatized.

9. **Describe the differences between the isoforms of the COX enzymes, COX-1 and COX-2.**

COX exists in two isoforms, COX-1 and COX-2. COX-1 is located throughout the body, but especially in the kidneys, gastric mucosa, platelets, and endothelium.

Conversely, COX-2 is normally present only in minute amounts, and its synthesis is primarily induced in the presence of inflammation. Until recently, all NSAIDs were nonselective in their COX inhibition. As a result, in addition to obtaining analgesia from the inhibition of the COX-2 isoform, inhibition of COX-1 led to the detrimental side effects of gastric irritation, renal micro-vasculature constriction, and platelet inhibition. Presently, several selective COX-2 inhibiting NSAIDs are available. Their introduction has greatly reduced the incidence of side effects associated with the use of nonselective NSAIDs, without sacrificing analgesic efficacy.

10. With regard to the pathophysiology of pain transmission, what are the three classifications of pain? Therapeutically, why is it important to make a distinction between the three?

Generally, pain can be classified into three categories based on the patho-physiology of how the pain is transmitted.

Nociceptive pain is pain that is secondary to stimulation of nociceptors. This type of pain is perceived to be commensurate with the level of tissue damage. Additionally, nociceptive pain can be subdivided into two types, *somatic* and *visceral*. Superficial somatic pain (skin) can be well localized and is described as intense and sharp. In contrast, visceral somatic pain is diffuse and may be described as cramping, gnawing, aching, sharp, or throbbing. Nociceptive pain responds well to NSAIDs and opioid analgesics.

Neuropathic pain results from abnormal function in the central or peripheral nervous system or both. It is often described as burning, shooting, stabbing, and lancinating. Additionally, this type of pain may be associated with subjective numbness, loss of sensation, and weakness. Accurately diagnosing neuropathic pain is crucial because it does not generally respond well to NSAIDs or opioid analgesics alone. Adjuvant analgesics, particularly tricyclic antidepressants and some anticonvulsants, are efficacious in the treatment of neuropathic pain.

Idiopathic pain is excessive for the extent of organic pathology. In the presence of idiopathic pain, the nurse anesthetist still must rely on patient self-report to determine the amount and intensity of the pain. Recognizing pain as idiopathic mandates that the practitioner pursue other treatment alternatives—further diagnostic tests to rule out disease progression, involvement of physical/occupational therapy, or consultations with social or psychiatric workers.

11. What is meant by an adjuvant analgesic?

An *adjuvant analgesic* is a medication that is traditionally approved and used for purposes other than its analgesic properties. Several medications under select circumstances can be used as analgesics, including antidepressants (tricyclic antidepressants, selective serotonin reuptake inhibitors), anticonvulsants, antihypertensives, and glucocorticoids.

12. Why is intramuscular injection discouraged for acute pain management?

The use of intramuscular injections for acute pain management is strongly discouraged for two reasons:
- Intramuscular injection discourages patients from reporting their pain because the injections themselves are painful.
- The absorption of the medication is often unreliable.

13. Explain the advantage of using intravenous PCA versus intermittent intravenous boluses for postoperative pain management.

Intermittent intravenous bolus dosing is the most appropriate method of administration during the initial phases of acute pain management. This method provides rapid alleviation of pain, while establishing a therapeutic serum level. When the patient has initially received adequate analgesia, PCA may be an effective method of providing adequate analgesia for select patients.

PCA allows the patient to avoid the side effects associated with the peaks (sedation, respiratory depression) and troughs (pain perception) associated with intermittent bolus dosing, maintaining an adequate therapeutic serum level of opioid. PCA allows patients to retain some of their autonomy and independence.

14. Name medications that have *N*-methyl-D-aspartate (NMDA) receptor antagonist properties.

Dextromethorphan, magnesium sulfate, ketamine, and amantadine have NMDA receptor antagonist properties.

15. Where are NMDA and alpha-amino-3-hydroxy-5-methylisoxazole-4-propionic acid (AMPA) receptors located; what is their role in pain transmission?

NMDA and AMPA receptors are located throughout the brain and spinal cord. Their interaction in the transmission of pain is predominantly at the level of the dorsal horn. Both receptor subtypes are ionotropic glutamate receptors, located postsynaptically on the second-order neuron. When glutamate (an excitatory neurotransmitter that transmits nociception) is released from a primary afferent pain fiber, it binds postsynaptically to NMDA and AMPA glutamate receptors to depolarize the second-order neuron, which continues pain transmission to the central nervous system. Activation of AMPA receptors is associated with normal nociceptive pain transmission. Activation of NMDA receptors is associated with chronic pain, heightened pain sensitivity, and resistance to opioids.

16. What is meant by central sensitization and wind-up of spinal neurons and primary nerve afferents?

Central sensitization is a general term that refers to an enhanced responsiveness of primary afferent and spinal neurons to nociceptive input. Central sensitization may cause patients to sense benign stimuli (touching, pressure) as if they were painful (allodynia). *Wind-up* of spinal cord neuronal activity is part of central sensitization and occurs when pain fiber input is exceptionally frequent and protracted, resulting in the activation of NMDA receptors. This intense response is the result of repetitive pain input from nociceptive C fibers. Wind-up also is associated with increased receptive fields, which enable previously unresponsive neurons to respond to nociceptive input. Central sensitization and wind-up may explain the hyperalgesia associated with certain pain states.

17. What is dexmedetomidine, and what is the mechanism of action for the analgesic effects?

Similar to clonidine, dexmedetomidine (Precedex) is an alpha$_2$ receptor agonist. Dexmedetomidine is a second-generation formulation of the alpha$_2$ receptor agonist class of medications. Alpha$_2$ receptors are located on or near the terminals of unmyelinated peripheral nerves and on postsynaptic fibers within the dorsal horn. Dexmedetomidine inhibits nociceptive neuron firing and the release of substance P in the central nervous system by stimulating alpha$_2$ receptors. Clinically, dexmedetomidine administered during the perioperative period has shown an anesthetic and opioid-sparing effect.

Key Points

- Chronic pain is defined as pain lasting for 3 months after the usual course of an acute illness, being associated with a chronic pathologic process, or being recurrent over months or years.

- Opioid receptor subtypes include mu (subtypes 1 and 2), kappa, and delta. These receptors are located throughout the central nervous system, and all produce analgesia and miosis when activated.

- Opioid analgesics do not show an analgesic "ceiling effect." That is, the amount of analgesia obtained increases as long as the dose is escalated.

- COX exists in two isoforms, COX-1 and COX-2. COX-1 is located throughout the body, but especially in the kidneys, gastric mucosa, platelets, and endothelium. Conversely, COX-2 is normally present only in minute amounts, and its synthesis is primarily induced in the presence of inflammation.

- Pain can be classified into three categories based on the pathophysiology of how the pain is transmitted: (1) nociceptive, (2) neuropathic, and (3) idiopathic.

- The role of NMDA and AMPA receptors is in the transmission of pain predominantly at the level of the dorsal horn.

- Activation of AMPA receptors is associated with normal nociceptive pain transmission. Activation of NMDA receptors is associated with chronic pain, heightened pain sensitivity, and resistance to opioids.

- Central sensitization is a general term that refers to an enhanced responsiveness of primary afferent and spinal neurons to nociceptive input.

Internet Resources

Anaesthetists.com: Pain physiology:
http://www.anaesthetist.com/icu/pain/pain3.htm

American Medical Association: Pain management: pathophysiology of pain assessment:
http://www.ama-cmeonline.com/pain_mgmt/module01/03patho/index.htm

Virtual Anaesthesia Textbook:
http://www.virtual-anaesthesia-textbook.com/

Nurse-Anesthesia.com:
http://www.nurse-anesthesia.com/

Update in Anaesthesia Cumulative Index:
http://www.nda.ox.ac.uk/wfsa/html/pages/up_issu.htm

The International Association for the Study of Pain (IASP):
http://www.iasp-pain.org/

The American Pain Society:
http://www.ampainsoc.org/

Bibliography

American Pain Society: *Principles of analgesic use in the treatment of acute pain and cancer pain*, ed 4, Skokie, IL, 1999, American Pain Society.

Faut-Callahan M, Hand R: Pain management. In Nagelhout JJ, Zaglaniczny K, editors: *Nurse anesthesia*, ed 2, Philadelphia, 2001, WB Saunders.

Loeser JD, editor: *Bonica's management of pain*, ed 3, Philadelphia, 2001, Lippincott Williams & Wilkins.

Lubenow TR, Ivankovich AD, McCarthy RJ: Management of acute postoperative pain. In Barash PG, Cullen BF, Stoelting RK, editors: *Clinical anesthesia*, ed 3, Philadelphia, 1997, Lippincott-Raven.

Morgan GE, Mikhail MS, Murray MJ: *Clinical anesthesiology*, ed 3, New York, 2002, Lange Medical Books/McGraw-Hill.

Wall PD, Melzack R, editors: *Textbook of pain*, ed 4, Philadelphia, 1999, Churchill Livingstone.

Special Considerations

Latex Allergy

Maureen Reilly

1. What is latex?

Industrial use latex or natural rubber latex (NRL) originates from a tree, *Hevea brasiliensis,* which grows in South America and Malaysia. Latex is a milky substance containing rubber particles coated with layers of proteins, lipids, nucleotides, cofactors, and phospholipids. Some, but not all, of these proteins are removed during the manufacturing process.

2. Is the use of latex-containing products regulated in the United States?

Effective September 1998, federal regulations mandated labeling of latex content of medical supplies. The label consists of the international symbol of a circle with a diagonal slash through it containing the word latex. In addition, although not in general use by all manufacturers, some opt to label their device or product as "latex free." These regulations do not cover stocks of medical supplies that already existed in facilities, however.

3. What are the most common sources of sensitization to latex in health care workers or consumers?

Three products have caused most latex allergy reactions in health care consumers and providers: (1) rubber tips on barium enema catheters, (2) latex examination gloves, and (3) latex surgeon's gloves. The increase in latex examination glove use in health care workers has occurred as a result of the 1991 Occupational Safety and Health Administration (OSHA) mandate for the use of rubber gloves. The seriousness of the incidences of barium enema catheter sensitizations prompted the U.S. Food and Drug Administration (FDA) to recall rubber-tipped barium enema catheters and issue a medical device warning alert.

4. Identify additional factors that have contributed to the increased incidence of latex allergy.

With the advent of the Centers for Disease Control and Prevention (CDC) Guidelines for Universal Precautions in the late 1980s, glove usage increased from 1.4 billion in 1988 to 8.3 billion in 1993. The increased demand for latex products has caused the manufacturing process to be shortened, resulting in insufficient extraction of the latex protein.

5. The incidence of latex allergy is highest among which group of health care providers?

Dentists have the highest reported incidence of latex allergy (10% to 38%), followed by laboratory staff (16.9%). The incidence of latex allergy is increasing in the general health care workforce. Incidence rates in all hospital employees have been reported to be 2.9% to 30%. The incidence in physicians is 7.4% to 13.3%; in nurses, 3.3% to 10.65%; and in housekeeping staff, 8%.

6. Which patient group has the highest incidence of latex allergy?

Yassein et al described the incidence of latex allergy in several subgroups of the general population. The most frequent occurrence of latex allergy was reported in *children with neural tube defects,* such as spina bifida (67%). Children who have had three or more surgeries also have a high incidence (55%). The repeated exposure to latex products produces sensitivity. Studies of latex industry workers have revealed an overall latex allergy incidence of 11%. The incidence of latex allergy in the general population is approximately 6.6%.

7. Name the government agencies that regulate the use of latex in the workplace.

- The National Institute for Occupational Safety and Health (NIOSH) issued "Natural Rubber Latex in the Workplace Alert" (publication number 98-13). The alert provides guidelines for health care facilities to reduce worker exposure to latex and to minimize latex-related health problems.
- OSHA has no specific guidelines for latex exposure in the workplace but issued guidelines in 1991 for barrier protection to include the use of gloves.
- The FDA Final Rule on labeling of medical devices containing latex became effective in 1998. This ruling requires all medical devices containing NRL to be labeled accordingly and to include warnings of the possibility of allergic reaction. It does not cover workplace exposure risks or recommendations.
- The CDC was the first agency to make recommendations for universal precautions in 1988.

8. Are employers required to provide health care workers with known latex sensitivity appropriate barrier protection and safeguards in the work environment?

The Occupational Safety and Health Act of 1970 (OSH Act) mandates that every worker be provided with a safe workplace. Although no specific OSHA regulation exists for latex allergy as an occupational hazard, the general duty clause of the OSH Act charges every employer to abide by the responsibility to "furnish to each of his employees employment and a place of employment which are free from recognized hazards that are causing or are likely to cause death or serious physical harm."

9. **Describe known risk factors for the development of latex allergy.**

Risk factors for the development of latex allergy include persons with an atopic history, that is, persons who are diagnosed with conditions such as asthma, hay fever, or food allergies. Allergies to avocado, kiwi, banana, chestnut, and tomatoes place individuals at a higher risk for latex allergy. Specific occupations can increase an individual's chance to develop latex sensitivity. These occupations include any job that requires the use of latex gloves in everyday work situations. Higher risk occupations include health care provider, hairdresser, and mortician.

10. **List the types of physical reactions that can be produced in response to latex exposure.**

Physical reactions include:
- Irritant contact dermatitis
- Type IV (delayed) hypersensitivity
- Type I hypersensitivity

11. **What is the most common skin reaction to latex?**

The most common skin reaction to latex products is irritant contact dermatitis, which is exhibited by dry, itchy, irritated areas on the skin, usually the hands. Irritant contact dermatitis is a nonallergic dermatitis and is restricted to the area of contact. Additional causes of irritant contact dermatitis are skin abrasions; hyperhydration; and use of topical alcohols, soaps, or detergents.

12. **Define a type I allergic reaction.**

The most serious response to latex is a type I, IgE-mediated, hypersensitivity reaction. A type I reaction is the result of prior latex exposure that initiates formation of systemic antibodies in response to cutaneous, mucosal, hematogenous, or aerosolized contact with latex proteins. Exposure is not limited to medical devices. Environmental exposure can range from condoms for birth control to repeated occupational exposure.

A type I reaction begins within minutes of exposure in a sensitized individual. The response is characterized by urticaria, angioedema, hypotension, and bronchospasm and can progress to cardiovascular collapse and death.

13. **Define a type IV reaction.**

A type IV hypersensitivity reaction is a delayed reaction mediated by T cells in the skin. This reaction may be similar to that seen with exposure to poison ivy, typically with a delay of several hours before development of a rash that may spread and blister. The degree of response is related to the degree of exposure. Itching, redness, and oozing vesicles in the contact area may persist for days.

A type IV reaction is not a true allergy. In the case of latex, this type of exposure and reaction is related most often to the chemical additives in the latex product.

Chemicals most commonly associated with these reactions are known as *latex accelerators,* with thiurams being the most common source of irritation.

14. Is there a relationship between asthma and latex sensitivity?

There is a high correlation between occupational asthma and the development of latex allergy.

15. Discuss some safeguards and behaviors that can minimize exposure to latex allergens in the operating room.

Because the most common cause of contamination in the operating room with latex proteins is via NRL gloves, replacement of these gloves with non–latex-containing gloves is an effective mechanism to decrease latex exposure. The most popular materials used for synthetic glove manufacturing are nitrile, chloroprene, polymers, and polyurethane. The common practice of discarding NRL gloves, by snapping them into the trash, contaminates the operating room environment with aerosolized latex proteins and should be avoided.

16. What preoperative patient information should alert the anesthetist to a possible latex allergy?

The following patient information should alert the anesthetist to a possible latex allergy:
- History of latex allergy
- Multiple food allergies, including bananas, kiwi, avocados, and chestnuts
- Reported symptoms with contact to NRL material, such as nondisposable latex gloves, condoms, balloons, carpeting, baby bottle nipples, rubber bands, erasers, and computer mouse pads.

All patients with reports of reaction to latex should be treated with latex precautions.

17. Discuss tests used to diagnose latex allergy.

It is important to differentiate any abnormal latex response as being a type IV reaction, contact irritant dermatitis, or a type I reaction. Diagnosis of latex sensitivity and latex allergy is often made by a combination of patient history, clinical findings, and laboratory tests. Patient reports of reactions when wearing NRL gloves, including the timing of the appearance of a rash and coincidental symptoms, are useful diagnostic criteria. Common laboratory diagnostic tests to detect serum IgE are the radioallergosorbent test and enzyme-linked immuno-sorbant assay. The skin prick test may be used, but is considered less predictable.

18. List potential causes, other than NRL gloves, of operating room contamination with latex proteins.

Other potential causes include the following:
- Syringes

- Medication bottle stoppers
- Stethoscopes
- Blood pressure cuffs
- Mattresses
- Nasal airways
- Foley catheters
- Wound drains

Any medical device may contain NRL, and appearances can be misleading. Package labeling, conforming with FDA guidelines, should indicate the presence of latex. If a piece of equipment is not labeled, its contents should be confirmed with the manufacturer.

19. How should the anesthetist prepare for an elective surgical procedure on a known latex-allergic patient?

Guidelines are available from several organizations, including the Association of Operating Room Nurses and the American Association of Nurse Anesthetists, on the procedures necessary to provide the safest environment for a latex-sensitive patient. See the box below for recommendations for provision of a latex-safe environment according to the American Association of Nurse Anesthetists Latex Allergy Protocol (1993). A consensus of opinion exists across organizations that an elective case for a latex-sensitive patient should be scheduled as the first case of the day because this minimizes pollution of the environment due to a maximal number of air exchanges in a specific room.

American Association of Nurse Anesthetists Latex Allergy Protocol

Operating Room
- Schedule latex-allergy and latex-risk patients as the first case in the morning. This allows latex dust (from the previous day) to be removed overnight.
- Remove all latex products from the operating room.
- Bring a latex-free cart (if available) into the room.
- Use a latex-free reservoir bag.
- Use a nonlatex circuit with plastic mask and bag.
- Ventilator bellows must be latex-free.
- Place all monitoring device cords and tubes in stockinet and secure with tape to prevent patient contact.

Intravenous Line Preparation
- Use intravenous tubing without latex ports.
- If unable to obtain intravenous tubing without latex ports, cover latex ports with tape and label as "Do not inject or withdraw fluid through the latex port."

Continued

American Association of Nurse Anesthetists Latex Allergy Protocol *continued*

Operating Room Patient Care

- Use nonlatex gloves. (Use caution when selecting nonlatex gloves; not all substitutes are equally impermeable to blood-borne pathogens.)
- Use nonlatex tourniquets.
- Draw medication directly from opened multidose vials (remove stoppers) if medications are not available in ampules.
- Draw up medications just before the beginning of the case. The rubber allergen can leach out of the plunger of the syringe causing a reaction.
- Glass syringes are an alternative.
- Use stopcocks to inject drugs rather than latex ports.
- Minimize mixing and agitating lyophilized drugs in multidose vials with rubber stoppers.
- Notify pharmacy and central supply that patient is latex sensitive so that these departments can implement the appropriate preparations for the patient.

20. What is the recommended pharmacological prophylaxis for a latex-sensitive patient?

A preoperative regimen may include diphenhydramine, prednisone, and an H_2 blocker, such as ranitidine.

21. Describe standard measures that are used to prepare an anesthesia machine for use with a latex-sensitive patient.

Preparation of the anesthesia machine should include removing all NRL components of the machine and replacing them with nonlatex alternatives. Latex-free facemasks and straps should be used. Blood pressure cuffs and stethoscopes should be replaced with nonlatex alternatives. If nonlatex alternatives are not available, stethoscopes and blood pressure cuffs should be wrapped with cotton padding to avoid direct contact with the patient. All medications should be drawn through nonlatex stoppers, and emergency drugs to treat an anaphylactic reaction should be immediately available.

 Key Points

- Effective September 1998, federal regulations mandated labeling of latex content of medical supplies.
- Three products have caused most latex allergy reactions in health care consumers and providers:
  - Rubber tips on barium enema catheters

Key Points   *continued*

- Latex examination gloves
- Latex surgeon's gloves
- The most frequent occurrence of latex allergy in subgroups of the general population was reported in children with neural tube defects, such as spina bifida (67%). Children who have had three or more surgeries also have a high incidence (55%).
- The government agencies that regulate the use of latex in the workplace are NIOSH, OSHA, FDA, and CDC.
- The OSH Act of 1970 mandates that every worker be provided with a safe workplace, including the avoidance of latex.
- Risk factors for the development of latex allergy include an atopic history; allergies to avocado, kiwi, banana, chestnut, and tomatoes place individuals at a higher risk for latex allergy.
- The types of physical reactions produced in response to latex exposure are:
  - Irritant contact dermatitis
  - Type IV (delayed hypersensitivity)
  - Type I hypersensitivity
- A pharmacological prophylaxis plan for a latex-sensitive patient may include diphenhydramine, prednisone, and an H_2 blocker such as ranitidine.

Internet Resources

CRNA: Certified Registered Nurse Anesthetists: AANA latex protocol:
http://www.aana.com/crna/prof/latex.asp

Latex allergy:
http://www.unc.edu/~rvp/RP_Anesthesia/Basics/LatexAllergy.html

How to manage a latex-allergic patient:
http://www.anesth.com/lair/latex/manage.html

Latex allergy—pretest:
http://www.anesth.com/lair/latex/pretest.html

AnesthesiaPatientSafety.com: American Association of Nurse Anesthetists warns of occupational health hazards posed by exposure to latex:
http://www.anesthesiapatientsafety.com/patients/latex/default.asp

Cardinal Health Medical Products and Services: Latex allergy management:
http://www.cardinal.com/mps/focus/latex/anesthesia.asp

Bibliography

American Association of Nurse Anesthetists: Latex allergy guidelines: AANA Infection/Environmental Control Task Force. Approved by the AANA Board of Directors, Chicago, April 1993.

Blazys D: Asthma and latex allergy, *J Emerg Nurs* 26:583-584, 2000.

Bolyard EA, Tablan OC, Williams WW, et al: Guideline for infection control in health care personnel, *Am J Infection Control* 26:289-354, 1998.

Brehler R, Kutting B: Natural rubber latex: a problem of interdisciplinary concern in medicine, *Arch Intern Med* 161:1057-1064, 2001.

Cerone E, Brosnan J, Pelletier C: Open heart surgery and the latex-sensitive patient, *AORN J* 72:105-106, 2000.

Dillard S, Kaczmarek R, Petsonk E, et al: Health effects associated with medical glove use, *AORN J* 76:88-96, 2002.

Doepke S: Identfying the risk, *Semin Periop Nurs* 7:226-238, 1998.

Eckout G: Anaphylaxis due to airborne exposure to latex in a primigravida, *Anesthesiology* 95:1034-1035, 2001.

Flaherty L, Snyder JA: From the feds: Food and Drug Administration: medical glove powder report, *J Emerg Nurs* 24:26, 1998.

Graves P, Towney C: The changing face of hand protection, *AORN J* 76:248-264, 2002.

Hourihane J, Allard J, Wade A, et al: Impact of repeated surgical procedures on the incidence and prevalence of latex allergy: a prospective study of 1263 children, *J Pediat* 140(4):479-482, 2002.

Kedas AM, Dillard S, Tomazic V: US Food and Drug Administration proposes federal regulation of labeling of latex-containing medical devices, *AORN J* 64:290-292, 1996.

Kellett PB: Latex allergy: a review, *J Emerg Nurs* 23:27-36, 1997.

Korniewicz D, McLeskey S: Latex allergy and gloving standards, *Semin Periop Nurs* 7:216-221, 1998.

Lewis L, Norgan G, Reilly M: Are nurses knowledgeable in regards to latex allergy, *Semin Periop Nurs* 7:239-251, 1998.

McLeskey S, Korniewicz D: Understanding latex allergy, *Semin Periop Nurs* 7:206-215, 1998.

Mitchell NA: Innovative informatics: latex allergy: accessing information on the Internet, *J Emerg Nurs* 23:51-52, 1997.

Nieto A, Mazon A, Pamies R, et al: Efficacy of latex avoidance for primary prevention of latex sensitization in children with spina bifida, *J Pediatr* 140:370-372, 2002.

Paquet J: Latex hypersensitivity: the IGE response, *Semin Periop Nurs* 7:203-205, 1998.

Patriarca G, Nucera E, Pollastrini E, et al: Sublingual desensitiziation: a new approach to Latex allergy problem, *Anesth Analg* 95:956-960, 2002.

Reilly M: Latex allergy update, *Semin Periop Nurs* 7:201-256, 1998.

Seivold G: Managers forum: switching to latex-free gloves, *J Emerg Nurs* 24:447-448, 1998.

Shoup AJ: Clinical issues: Guidelines for the management of latex allergies and safe use of latex in perioperative practice settings, *AORN J* 66:726, 729-731, 1997.

Trape M, Schenck P, Warren A: Latex gloves use and symptoms in health care workers 1 year after implementation of a policy restricting the use of powdered gloves, *Am J Infection Control* 28:352-358, 2000.

Wilburn S: When latex allergies limit employment: nurses may be covered under the law, *Am J Nurs* 101:88, 2001.

Worthington K: Towards a latex safe workplace, *Am J Nurs* 99:71, 1999.

Yassin MS, Lier MB, Fischer TJ, et al: Latex in hospital employees, *Ann Allergy* 72:245-249, 1994.

Temperature Disturbances

Dennis Hugh Woods, Jr.

1. Where does temperature regulation occur?

Temperature regulation occurs almost exclusively in the *hypothalamus*. The anterior preoptic hypothalamic area contains heat-sensing and cold-sensing neurons that increase their rate of firing as body temperature increases or decreases. Thermal receptors located in the skin, spinal cord, great vessels, and abdominal viscera also send temperature information to the hypothalamus. In contrast to the hypothalamus, most peripheral thermal receptors respond to a cold stimulus rather than a heat stimulus.

2. How does the body defend against cold?

There are three reflex reactions that help the body defend against cold:
* Sympathetic stimulation and skin vasoconstriction
* Piloerection
* Overall increase in heat production through shivering, sympathetic-mediated increase in basal metabolic rate, and increase in thyroxine secretion from the thyroid gland

3. What principles describe how heat loss occurs?

Heat loss occurs from the body to the environment through four processes: radiation, evaporation, convection, and conduction (see the figure below).

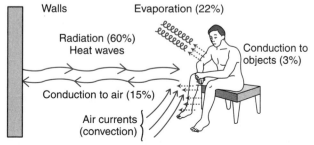

Mechanisms of heat loss from the body. *(From Guyton AC, Hall JE: Body temperature, temperature regulation, and fever. In: Textbook of medical physiology, ed 10, Philadelphia, 2000, WB Saunders, pp 911-922.)*

- *Radiation* heat loss occurs when heat is lost in the form of infrared rays. In the operating room, radiation heat loss occurs when heat from the warm patient is radiated to cooler surrounding objects. When surrounding objects are warmer than the body, heat can be gained. Radiation is the main form of heat loss in the surgical patient, accounting for 60% of the surgical patient's heat loss.
- *Evaporation* accounts for 20% of body heat loss in operating rooms. When water evaporates from the skin and mucous membranes, heat is lost. The amount of heat lost through evaporation depends on the body surface area, surgical wound exposure, and humidity of inspired gases.
- *Convection* occurs when heat is transferred from the patient to moving air currents in the operating room. It accounts for approximately 15% of total body heat loss in surgical patients. Modern operating rooms have high airflow rates, which can result in significant heat loss.
- *Conduction* accounts for approximately 5% of a surgical patient's heat loss. It occurs when warmer objects come into contact with cooler surfaces. Conductive heat loss is directly proportional to the temperature difference, thermal conductivity, and exposed body surface area.

4. **Describe differences that account for how infants and elderly patients respond to changes in temperature.**

   Infants and children have greater body surface-to-body weight ratios, which predisposes them to greater heat loss. This also accounts for why pediatric patients can be warmed more quickly. Elderly patients are more prone to hypothermia secondary to a blunted sympathetic nervous system response, decreased basal metabolic rate (decreased heat production), thin skin, slowed blood circulation, and decreased lean muscle (delayed and ineffective shivering).

5. **How do infants younger than 3 months old respond to cold?**

   Infants younger than 3 months old do not respond to cold by shivering. They respond to cold stress by increasing norepinephrine production, which increases thermogenic metabolism of brown fat.

6. **Identify the effects of hypothermia on tissue solubility of volatile anesthetics.**

   As the patient's temperature decreases, the tissue solubility increases, potentially prolonging recovery from anesthesia because larger amounts of sequestered volatile anesthetics need to be expired from the body.

7. **What effect does hypothermia have on minimal alveolar concentration (MAC) of inhalational anesthetics?**

   For every 1° C decrease in body temperature, the MAC of volatile anesthetics decreases by 5%.

8. **How does hypothermia affect the kinetics of neuromuscular blocking drugs?**

The duration of a neuromuscular blocking agent is usually increased in the presence of reduced core temperature. Vecuronium's duration of action is two times longer in patients with only a 2° C decrease in core body temperature. Atracurium's duration is increased by 60% in the presence of a 3° C reduction in temperature.

9. **How does hypothermia affect wound healing and infection rates for the surgical patient?**

Subcutaneous oxygen tension directly correlates with the incidence of wound infections. Thermoregulatory vasoconstriction, induced by hypothermia, increases the incidence of wound infection by decreasing subcutaneous oxygen tension. Immune function is impaired by mild core hypothermia.

10. **What effect does hypothermia have on coagulation?**

Blood loss is increased with mild hypothermia. Hypothermia impairs platelet function by decreasing levels of thromboxane A_2. Hypothermia also may prolong prothrombin time and partial thromboplastin time through direct inhibition of clotting factor function. Laboratory values may not accurately reflect a bleeding tendency. Tests are normally performed at 37° C, regardless of actual patient temperature. As a result, laboratory values may be normal when measured at 37° C but abnormal at actual core temperature. Fibrinolysis does not change during mild hypothermia, suggesting that hypothermia-induced coagulopathy does not result from excessive clot lysis.

11. **What are effective means of temperature monitoring during surgery?**

There are many ways to monitor patient temperature during surgery. Common monitoring sites include the tympanic membrane, rectum, esophagus, pulmonary artery, axilla, and nasopharynx. Considering the advantages and disadvantages of each monitoring site, the *esophageal* and *nasopharyngeal probes* are excellent choices based on economy, performance, and safety. Proper placement of an esophageal probe is essential to avoid the measurement of tracheal gas temperatures. Proper positioning is behind the heart into the lower one third of the esophagus.

12. **Name the most effective ways to avoid heat loss during surgery.**

The two most effective means for keeping a patient warm during surgery are maintaining a *warm ambient temperature* and *use of a forced air warming device*.

13. **Identify some beneficial central nervous system effects of hypothermia.**

The most effective means of protecting the brain after or during focal or global ischemia is hypothermia. For each 1° C reduction in temperature, cerebral oxygen consumption and cerebral blood flow decrease by 5% to 7%. Hypothermia also offers spinal cord protection during periods of ischemia.

14. **List conditions that may cause hyperthermia.**

Conditions include:
- Thyroid storm
- Pheochromocytoma
- Malignant hyperthermia
- Sepsis
- Transfusion reactions
- Alcohol withdrawal
- Neuroleptic malignant syndrome
- Impaired sweating

15. **What physiological responses occur when core body temperature increases?**

The body attempts to decrease temperature by three main mechanisms (see the table below):
- Vasodilation of the skin blood vessels can increase the rate of heat loss eight times over basal heat loss.
- Sweating increases heat loss through evaporation.
- Mechanisms that normally increase heat production, such as shivering and chemical thermogenesis, are inhibited.

Physiological Responses to Hypothermia and Hyperthermia		
	Hypothermia	**Hyperthermia**
Respiratory	Left shift in oxyhemoglobin curve, decreased arterial oxygen saturation, decreased respiratory rate	Decreased tidal volume, increased respiratory rate, increased ventilatory response to hypoxemia, increased hypoxic pulmonary vasoconstriction
Cardiovascular	Vasoconstriction, increased metabolic oxygen consumption secondary to shivering, increased systemic vascular resistance, dysrhythmias, myocardial depression, decreased cardiac output	Vasodilation, decreased systemic vascular resistance and venous return, increased heart rate (10-beat increase for each 1° C increase in temperature), increased stroke volume
Renal	Diabetes insipidus, decreased renal blood flow secondary to vasoconstriction, decreased oxygen consumption	Decreased renal blood flow secondary to dehydration, temperature-induced tubular damage

Physiological Responses to Hypothermia and Hyperthermia   *continued*

	Hypothermia	Hyperthermia
Metabolic/ endocrine	Decreased metabolic rate and oxygen consumption 5–7% per 1° C decrease in temperature, decreased tissue perfusion may lead to metabolic acidosis	Metabolic rate and oxygen consumption increase 5–7% for each 1° C increase in temperature, metabolic acidosis, electrolyte imbalance secondary to sweating and dehydration, hyperkalemia
Hematological	Increased blood viscosity, impaired coagulation, and thrombocytopenia	Coagulopathy may be a result of direct inactivation of clotting factors and platelets
Central nervous system	Decreased cerebral blood flow and metabolic consumption, increased cerebrovascular resistance, decreased MAC, prolonged emergence from general anesthesia	Seizures, delirium, coma, and death as a result of temperature toxcity on neuronal cells

MAC, minimal alveolar concentration.

 Key Points

- Temperature regulation occurs primarily in the anterior preoptic area of the hypothalamus.
- The body loses heat from radiation, evaporation, convection, and conduction.
- Infants, children, and elderly are predisposed to greater heat loss.
- Hypothermia increases the tissue solubility of inhalational anesthetics, resulting in prolonged recovery.
- For every 1° C decrease in body temperature, the MAC of volatile anesthetics decreases by 5%.
- A neuromuscular blocking agent's duration is usually increased in the presence of reduced core temperature.
- Thermoregulatory vasoconstriction, induced by hypothermia, increases the incidence of wound infection by decreasing the subcutaneous oxygen tension. Immune function is impaired by mild core hypothermia.
- Hypothermia increases blood loss, impairs platelet function, and prolongs prothrombin time and partial thromboplastin time.
- Common temperature monitoring sites include tympanic membrane, rectum, esophagus, pulmonary artery, axilla, and nasopharynx.

Continued

Key Points   *continued*

- The two most effective means for keeping a patient warm during surgery are maintaining a warm ambient temperature and use of a forced air warming device.

- Hypothermia is the most effective means of protecting the brain and spinal cord during or after focal or global ischemia is suspected.

Internet Resources

Anesthesia issues related to hypothermia:
http://www.anesthesia.org.cn/asa2002/rcl_source/222_Schwartz.pdf

Less core hypothermia when anesthesia is induced with inhaled sevoflurane than with intravenous propofol, Anesth Analg 88:291, 1999:
http://www.anesthesia-analgesia.org/cgi/content/abstract/88/4/921

References for prevention and treatment of hypothermia:
http://www.or.org/Reviews/three/refs.html

Virtual Anaesthesia Textbook:
http://www.virtual-anaesthesia-textbook.com/

GASNet Video Library:
http://www.gasnet.org/videos/index.php

Bibliography

Fielder MA: Thermoregulation: anesthetic and perioperative concerns, *AANA J* 69:485-499, 2001.

Guyton AC, Hall JE: Body temperature, temperature regulation, and fever. In: *Textbook of medical physiology,* ed 10, Philadelphia, 2000, WB Saunders, pp 911-922.

Hemmings H, Hopkins P: *Foundations of anesthesia: basic and clinical sciences,* New York, 2000, Harcourt.

Leo J, Huether SE: Pain, temperature regulation, sleep, and sensory function. In McCance KL, Huether SE, editors: *Pathophysiology,* ed 3, St. Louis, 2002, Mosby, pp 422-459.

Morgan EG, Mikhail MS, Murray MJ: Patient monitors. In: *Clinical anesthesiology,* ed 3, Stamford, CT, 2002, Appleton & Lange, pp 73-106.

Rice LJ, Cravero JP: Pediatric anesthesia. In: *Clinical anesthesia,* ed 4, Philadelphia, 2001, Lippincott Williams & Wilkins, pp 1195-1204.

Sessler DI: Complications and treatment of mild hypothermia, *Anesthesiology* 75:531-543, 2001.

Winkler M, et al: Aggressive warming reduces blood loss during hip arthroplasty, *Anesth Analg* 91:978-984, 2000.

Cardiopulmonary Resuscitation

William Hartland, Jr.

1. What are the most common resuscitation medications that can be given via the endotracheal tube (ETT)?

The most common resuscitation drugs that can be given through the ETT are *atropine, lidocaine,* and *epinephrine.* Naloxone (Narcan) also can be administered by this route. If these drugs are administered through the ETT, a lower serum concentration results than if an equal amount of the same drug were administered via the intravenous (IV) route. Tracheal doses of these drugs should be two to four times greater than IV doses. For example, the recommended tracheal dose of epinephrine is 2 to 2.5 times the peripheral intravenous dose.

2. What is the most common cause of airway obstruction in the unresponsive patient, and how is it initially treated?

When a patient is unresponsive, decreased muscle tone may result in obstruction of the pharynx by the tongue. Because the tongue is attached to the lower jaw, the tongue can be lifted away from the back of the throat by moving the lower jaw forward, relieving the obstruction. This can be accomplished by using the head tilt–chin lift maneuver or, in the case of trauma and suspected cervical spine injury, the jaw thrust maneuver.

3. Identify the most important determinant of survival for an adult patient in ventricular fibrillation (VF).

The most important determinant of survival for a patient in VF is rapid defibrillation. The probability of a successful defibrillation in this situation diminishes rapidly over time. With every minute that defibrillation is delayed, survival rates decrease 7% to 10%. This means that with delayed defibrillation, patient survival rate decreases to 50% after 5 minutes, to 30% after 7 minutes, and to about 5% beyond 12 minutes.

4. Halfway through a seemingly uneventful surgical case, the CRNA looks at the electrocardiogram monitor and immediately notices that the waveform has changed to a "flat line." What is the first action the CRNA should take?

Asystole is a specific diagnosis, but a flat line is not. A flat line is nonspecific and could apply to several conditions besides asystole. The first action the CRNA should take is to evaluate the patient rapidly by checking arterial pulses, pulse oximeter waveform, and blood pressure. When the CRNA is satisfied that the patient has not had a cardiac arrest, other causes for the flat line can be explored, such as lead disconnect, monitor failure, and insufficient gain. Changing lead selection may assist the CRNA in identifying a disconnected lead.

5. **During cardiopulmonary resuscitation (CPR), what are the ventilation rates, compression rates, compression depths, and compression-to-ventilation ratios for a child, infant, and newborn?**

The following table shows the ventilation rates, compression rates, compression depths, and compression-to-ventilation ratios for a child, infant, and newborn.

Cardiopulmonary Resuscitation

	Child	Infant	Newborn
Ventilations/min (approx.)	20	20	30–60
Compressions/min (approx.)	100	100 (at least)	90 compressions/ 30 ventilations
Compression depth (approx.)	$1/3$ to $1/2$ the depth of the chest (1 to 1.5 inches	$1/3$ to $1/2$ the depth of the chest (0.5 to 1 inch)	$1/3$ the depth of the chest
Compression-to-Ventilation ratio (1 or 2 rescuers)	5:1	5:1	3:1

6. **Is establishing IV access in a patient in cardiac arrest a high priority; which vein(s) should a rescuer first attempt to cannulate?**

Although IV access is important, it does not take precedence over basic CPR, proper airway management, chest compressions, or defibrillation as indicated. The first-choice site for cannulation is a peripheral vein, such as the antecubital or external jugular. Central lines provide direct drug access to the circulation, but they require interruption of chest compression and are associated with a higher incidence of complications. Because drugs administered through peripheral lines have a longer circulation time, it is recommended that medications administered via this route be given as rapidly as possible, followed by a bolus of IV fluid (20 mL for an adult) and elevation of the extremity for 10 to 20 seconds.

7. **Describe the basic CPR life support techniques for an adult patient when one or two rescuers are present.**

ONE RESCUER
When performing CPR on an adult patient, a single rescuer should deliver approximately 12 breaths/min. Chest compressions, on the lower half of the

sternum, should be administered at a rate of approximately 100/min. The depth of these compressions should be 1.5 to 2 inches. The rescuer should deliver a compression-to-ventilation ratio of 15:2 to a patient with an unprotected airway.

TWO RESCUERS

When two rescuers are present, the compression-to-ventilation ratio should remain the same for a patient with an unprotected airway. Research indicates that perfusion pressure increases with sequential compressions. It has been shown that after each pause for ventilation, it takes several compressions to reestablish previous levels of perfusion. As such, 15 uninterrupted compressions are recommended before a short pause is taken for ventilation. If the patient's airway is protected with a cuffed ETT, compressions may be continuous and ventilations may be asynchronous, with a ratio of five compressions to one ventilation.

8. **Summarize the universal steps to operate all automated external defibrillators (AEDs).**

The following table shows the universal steps for operation of AEDs.

Universal Steps to Operate Automated External Defibrillators

Step	Description
1. Power on	This initiates the voice prompts. Some AEDs are turned on by pushing the power button; some by lifting the monitor cover or screen to the up position
2. Attach electrode pads	Pads with elctrodes should be attached directly to the patient's skin. One designated pad is attached on the upper right sternal border directly below the clavicle. The other is positioned lateral to the left nipple with the top margin a few inches below the axilla
3. Analyze the rhythm	To avoid artifact errors during analysis, the patient should not be moved or be in contact with another individual
4. Clear the victim and press the shock button	If a shock is recommended, ensure that no one is touching or in indirect contact with the patient. When everyone is clear, the shock should be delivered

9. **The CRNA has attached an AED to a patient who is pulseless and not breathing. The AED advises "no shock indicated." What should the CRNA do?**

The first thing the CRNA should do is check again for signs of circulation quickly by checking the patient's carotid pulse. If signs of circulation are present, the CRNA should check for breathing. If respirations are adequate, the patient may be placed in the recovery position and monitored carefully. If respirations are inadequate, rescue breathing should begin at a rate of 1 ventilation every 5 seconds. If no signs of circulation are present, CPR should commence, with reanalysis of the rhythm after 1 minute.

10. A patient has no detectable pulses, but electrical activity other than ventricular tachycardia (VT) or VF is detected; a diagnosis of pulseless electrical activity (PEA) is made. What are the most frequent causes of PEA?

The 10 most frequent reversible causes of PEA can be remembered as the *5 Hs* and the *5 Ts*.
- Five Hs
  - Hypoxemia
  - Hypoxia
  - Hydrogen ion—acidosis
  - Hyperkalemia and hypokalemia
  - Hypothermia
- Five Ts
  - Tablets—drug overdose
  - Tamponade—cardiac
  - Tension pneumothorax
  - Thrombosis—coronary
  - Thrombosis—pulmonary embolism

If reversible causes are not addressed, successful treatment is severely hindered.

11. An adult patient remains in VF after three initial progressive shocks. CPR is continued. What two agents are recommended to optimize cardiac output and blood pressure?

Epinephrine and vasopressin are recommended. *Epinephrine* may be given in a dose of 1 mg, IV bolus, and repeated every 3 to 5 minutes as appropriate. The appropriate dose of *vasopressin* is 40 international units, as a single IV dose. If after 10 to 20 minutes there is no clinical response to the single dose of vasopressin, it is acceptable to return to 1 mg of epinephrine every 3 to 5 minutes.

12. Identify some appropriate interventions if VF or pulseless VT is shock-refractory.

According to the American Heart Association:
- Amiodarone, 300 mg IV bolus, may be administered for cardiac arrest due to VF/VT that persists after multiple shocks.
- Lidocaine, 1 to 1.5 mg/kg IV bolus, may be tried. Lidocaine may be repeated in 3 to 5 minutes to a maximal dose of 3 mg/kg.
- Procainamide, 30 mg/min, may be given to a maximal dose of 17 mg/kg for patients who respond to shocks with intermittent return of a pulse or non-VF rhythm.

- Magnesium sulfate, 1 to 2 g intravenously, may be used in the presence of torsades de pointes or when it is suspected that the arrhythmia may be caused by hypomagnesium.
- Sodium bicarbonate, 1 mEq/kg intravenously, may be helpful for several conditions associated with VF arrest, such as hyperkalemia, bicarbonate-responsive acidosis, and tricyclic antidepressant overdose. Sodium bicarbonate may be harmful in the presence of hypercarbic acidosis.

13. **If a patient converts to a perfusing rhythm only to revert to VF/pulseless VT, a continuous infusion of an antiarrhythmic may be warranted. For recurrent VF/VT, which antiarrhythmic agents should be considered?**

Antiarrhythmic agents are presented in the following table.

Antiarrhythmic Agents for Recurrent Ventricular Fibrillation/Ventricular Tachycardia	
Amiodarone	Initial: rapid infusion, 150 mg IV over 10 min (15 mg/min), followed by 360 mg over the next 6 hr (1 mg/min) Maintenance infusion: 540 mg IV over the next 18 hr (0.5 mg/min) Maximum cumulative dose: 2.2 g over 24 hr Monitor for hypotension and bradycardia
Procainamide	20 mg/min IV until arrhythmia is suppressed, hyotension develops, QRS is prolonged by 50% from baseline, or a maximal dose of 17 mg/kg is reached Maintenance infusion: 1-4 mg/min
Lidocaine	Loading dose: 1-1.5 mg/kg to a total of 3 mg/kg if the patient has not received any during the arrest Maintenance infusion: 1-4 mg/min

14. **Name some "red flag" bradycardias that are likely to deteriorate, even if they are presently asymptomatic.**

Two red flag bradycardias are:
- Second-degree atrioventricular block, type II
- Third-degree atrioventricular heart block (complete heart block)

CONTROVERSY

15. **Should the CRNA shock a patient who is in confirmed asystole?**

Some practitioners argue that shocks for confirmed asystole do not hurt and may help. At this time, however, there do not seem to be any valid data in human adults that support this rationale. During asystole, shocks may be harmful by producing a "stunned heart" and profound parasympathetic nervous system discharge. In this situation, shocks could be counterproductive to promoting spontaneous cardiac activity. The American Heart Association considers the practice of empirical shocking of patients in asystole potentially harmful and without support.

Key Points

- The most common resuscitation drugs that can be given through the ETT are atropine, lidocaine, epinephrine, and naloxone.
- The most common cause of airway obstruction in an unresponsive patient is the tongue resting against the back of the pharynx.
- The 10 most frequent reversible causes of PEA are hypoxemia, hypoxia, acidosis, hyperkalemia and hypokalemia, hypothermia, drug overdose, cardiac tamponade, tension pneumothorax, coronary thrombosis, and pulmonary embolism.
- Bradycardias that are likely to deteriorate, even if they are asymptomatic, are:
  - Second-degree atrioventricular block, type II
  - Third-degree atrioventricular block (complete heart block)
- The American Heart Association considers the practice of empirical shocking of patients in asystole potentially harmful and without support.

Internet Resources

ACLS megacode simulator:
http://www.mdchoice.com/Cyberpt/acls/aclsbody.asp

New York Emergency Room RN: Advanced cardiac life support—ACLS:
http://www.nyerrn.com/er/acls.htm

Bibliography

American Heart Association in collaboration with the International Liaison Committee on Resuscitation (ILCOR): Guidelines 2000 for cardiopulmonary resuscitation and emergency care, *Circulation* 102(suppl):8, 2000.

Cummins RO: *ACLS provider manual,* Dallas, 2001, American Heart Association.

Eisenburg MS, et al: Cardiac arrest and resuscitation: a tale of 29 cities, *Ann Emerg Med* 19:179-186, 1990.

Emerman CL, et al: Effect of injection site on circulation times during cardiac arrest, *Crit Care Med* 16:1138-1141, 1988.

Hazinski MF, et al: Instructor update to ECC Guidelines 2000, *Currents Emerg Cardiovasc Care* 12:1, 2001.

Hazinski MF, et al: *PALS provider manual,* Dallas, 2002, American Heart Association.

Kern KB, et al: Efficacy of chest compression-only BLS CPR in the presence of an occluded airway, *Resuscitation* 39:179-188, 1998.

Larson MP, et al: Predicting survival from out-of-hospital cardiac arrest: a graphic model, *Ann Emerg Med* 22:1652-1658, 1993.

Losek JD, et al: Prehospital countershock treatment of pediatric asystole, *Am J Med* 7:571-575, 1989.

Devices for Managing Cardiac Arrhythmias

Elizabeth Monti Seibert

1. What types of devices are available for treating cardiac arrhythmias?

Two types of implanted, battery-powered, computerized electronic devices are used to control heart rate and rhythm:
- Pacemakers
- Internal cardioverter-defibrillators (ICDs)

The difference between a pacemaker and an ICD is that the ICD incorporates cardioversion and defibrillation capabilities in addition to pacing modalities. Both devices include circuitry to assess spontaneous cardiac activity (sense) and modulate current output and rate (pace).

2. Discuss the components of pacemakers and ICDs.

Pacemakers and ICDs are composed of a generator and electrodes. Pacemaker and ICD generators typically are placed in an infraclavicular pocket that is either subcutaneous or beneath the pectoral muscle. Alternatively, generators can be implanted in the anterior abdominal wall. Intracardiac electrodes are placed transvenously through the subclavian or cephalic vein. The generator includes electronic circuitry for sensing and analyzing arrhythmias, a telemetry device for communi-cating with programmers, and a battery. The pulse generator casing is either titanium or stainless steel to shield the device from electromagnetic interference (EMI).

Modern pacemakers are powered by lithium-iodide batteries that have an expected life of 5 to 12 years. These batteries have a distinct advantage over older mercury-zinc batteries in that power is lost gradually so that failure does not occur suddenly. ICDs are powered by lithium-silver-vanadium oxide batteries that last 5 to 9 years. The incorporation of telemetry into cardiac rhythm management devices allows evaluation of remaining battery life.

Current is conducted from the generator to the myocardium by electrodes or leads placed within the cardiac chambers. Although leads typically are placed in one or both right-sided chambers, innovations in pacemaker technology make left heart pacing possible through coronary sinus leads. Either single (unipolar) or dual (bipolar) electrodes are used. The anode and cathode are located in close proximity on the single wire of a bipolar electrode, reducing the susceptibility of the electrodes to EMI. If a unipolar electrode is used, the generator case acts as the cathode.

3. What types of pacemakers are available?

Pacemakers are designed to pace either one (single-chamber) or two (dual-chamber or physiological pacing) cardiac chambers. Although single-chamber devices that pace either the atrium or the ventricle were the norm for many years, dual-chamber pacemakers are currently the favored treatment option. *Dual-chamber pacemakers* allow the heart to respond to increases in sinus rhythm due to exercise and preserve atrioventricular synchrony. Studies have shown improved quality of life for patients with dual-chamber pacemakers, a reduced incidence of pacemaker syndrome, and a decrease in atrial fibrillation and emboli.

Rate-adaptive pacemakers are prescribed for individuals whose heart rate does not increase in response to demand, a condition termed *chronotropic incompetence*. Rate-adaptive pacemakers use sensors that detect changes in body motion or other physiological parameters to increase activity. Changes in body movement, minute ventilation, respiratory rate, blood temperature, pH, oxygen saturation, right ventricular pressure, or electrocardiogram (ECG) intervals can be used as the basis for rate adaptation. The most common type of rate-adaptive sensor detects changes in body movement. Rate adaptation is indicated by an "R" in the five-letter pacemaker code.

Rate adaptation is only one of the many programmable features of permanent pacemakers and ICDs. All modern pacemakers have multiple modes that can be evaluated and reprogrammed via the communication devices. The following functions of pacemakers can be modified by programmers:
- Pacing mode (chambers sensed and paced)
- Output (voltage, current, and pulse duration)
- Sensitivity
- Rate
- Refractory period

Current estimates are that 60% of implanted pacemakers are dual chamber, 83% are rate adaptive, and 30% include both functions.

4. Discuss the indications for insertion of a permanent pacemaker or ICD.

The American College of Cardiology, American Heart Association, and North American Society for Pacing and Electrophysiology (NASPE) jointly developed extensive guidelines for insertion of pacemakers and ICDs. The indications are grouped into three classes based on research evidence or expert opinions. Class I indications are conditions for which there is general agreement that the device is useful and effective. Class II indications are conditions for which the device is often used, but evidence to support use is conflicting. Conditions for which the device is not effective, useful, and potentially harmful are categorized as class III. A complete listing of the guidelines is available on the websites of each association (i.e., www.americanheart.org, http://www.naspe.org/).

With pacemaker technology advances, indications for insertion of pacemaker and arrhythmia detection devices have expanded beyond heart block. General indications for pacemaker implantation are for bradycardias due to third-degree and some second-degree atrioventricular conduction abnormalities, sinus node dysfunction, post–acute myocardial infarction in select patients, and autonomic nervous system disorders. Newer indications include neuromuscular diseases with underlying cardiac disease, syncope from hypersensitive carotid sinus or vasovagal causes, and dilated and hypertrophic obstructive cardiomyopathies. Pacemakers also are useful in treating some tachyarrhythmias and atrial fibrillation.

ICDs are implanted for prevention of sudden death due to ventricular fibrillation and tachycardia. The use of ICDs in patients with ejection fractions of less than 30% after myocardial infarction can reduce the risk of sudden death by 31%. Other patients with indications for ICDs include patients with a family history of sudden cardiac death and patients awaiting cardiac transplantation.

5. How are pacemakers classified?

The NASPE and British Pacing and Electrophysiology Group (NASPE/BPEG) have developed a coding system to describe pacemaker and defibrillator capabilities. The following table describes the 2001 revised pacemaker code. A similar coding classification is available for ICDs.

2001 Revised Pacemaker Code

I — Chamber(s) Paced	II — Chamber(s) Sensed	III — Response to Sensing	IV — Rate Modulation	V — Multisite Pacing
0 = none	0 = none	0 = none	0 = none	0 = none
A = atrium	A = atrium	T = triggered	R = rate modulation	A = atrium
V = ventricle	V = ventricle	I = inhibited		V = ventricle
D = dual (A + V)	D = dual (A + V)	D = dual (T + I)		D = dual (A + V)

Using the code allows interpretation of pacemaker modes. A device that is labeled VOOOO provides only asynchronous ventricular pacing with no sensing, rate modulation, or multisite pacing. A DDDR pacemaker is a dual-chamber paced, dual-chamber sensed, dual response, rate modulated device. A DDDOV pacemaker dual paces, dual senses, and is inhibited by the atrium and ventricle but does not include rate modulation. The "V" indicates that the device paces both ventricles or has more than one pacing site in one ventricle or both.

6. How should patients with pacemakers or ICDs be assessed preoperatively?

In addition to optimizing the patient's condition, the goal of preoperative assessment and perioperative management of patients with cardiac rhythm management devices is to reduce the risk of device malfunction and any subsequent complications. The technology of pacemakers and ICDs is changing rapidly, and devices have become increasingly sophisticated and complex. As a result, cardiology consultation is strongly recommended.

Cardiology consultation should be obtained before the day of surgery to avoid potential surgical delays and perioperative problems. The cardiologist should assess the patient's underlying disease state and evaluate the functional status of the pacemaker or ICD. Most importantly, the patient's dependency on the pacemaker should be determined because lack of an intrinsic cardiac rhythm places the patient at risk in the event that intraoperative events interfere with pacemaker function. Information that should be relayed to the anesthetist includes the pacemaker mode and type of leads, the manufacturer, and the date the device was last evaluated. If the device is an ICD, it is important to know the date that the last shock was administered. The cardiologist should determine the effect of a magnet placed over the device, suggest whether the pacemaker should be reprogrammed to a temporary mode for the duration of the surgical procedure, and verify the availability of personnel and devices to reprogram the pacemaker.

A thorough preoperative evaluation and medication history should be obtained. The patient should be questioned as to the reason for implantation of the pacemaker or ICD and the type of symptoms experienced at the time. The presence of associated cardiac disease, such as congestive heart failure, ischemia, or valvular disease, must be ascertained, and the presence of common coexisting diseases, such as diabetes and hypertension, must be determined. Compliance with medications that may affect pacing or defibrillation thresholds should be evaluated. The patient should be asked when the pacemaker was last checked. If a cardiology consultation has not been obtained and the patient is unaware of specifics about the pacemaker, the identification card given to the patient at the time of device implantation can provide important information about the manufacturer and type of pacemaker. Many manufacturers maintain websites or 24-hour emergency services. The anesthetist should not hesitate to contact the manufacturer for assistance in identifying devices and for recommendations for managing the unit.

7. What diagnostic studies should be ordered preoperatively?

Preoperative diagnostic studies include a *12-lead ECG, chest x-ray,* and *appropriate blood work*. A chest x-ray can identify the presence of a pacemaker or ICD and the location and continuity of leads. A radiopaque code facilitates identification of the manufacturer and type of device. Electrolyte abnormalities, particularly of potassium, should be identified and corrected because these predispose patients to conduction abnormalities that may interfere with pacemaker function.

Previous ECG recordings can be compared with current tracings to evaluate rate, rhythm, pacing, and ischemic changes. Functioning of the pacemaker can be grossly evaluated if the patient's heart rate is less than that of the programmed rate and pacing spikes are evident. If the pacing mode is known, pacemaker function can be evaluated by examining the location of pacing spikes on the ECG in relationship to the chambers being paced. Interpretation of ECG tracings of paced rhythms is, however, difficult and confusing. Because most anesthesia providers are not familiar with the intricacies of pacemakers and ICDs, cardiology consultation is recommended to obtain a more definitive evaluation of the functional status.

8. Define pacemaker syndrome.

Pacemaker syndrome is a diffuse constellation of signs and symptoms that is thought to result from atrioventricular asynchrony in patients with single-chamber ventricular pacemakers. Symptoms include weakness, fatigue, headache, syncope, confusion, and shortness of breath. Retrograde impulse conduction and contraction of the atria against closed mitral and tricuspid valves are postulated to cause loss of the atrial "kick," decreased cardiac output, and hypotension. Because atrial filling contributes approximately 20% to ventricular filling, cardiac output may decline substantially with its loss. Additionally, failure of the atria to empty completely or contraction against close valves can lead to atrial distention and activation of atrial stretch receptors with a reflex decrease in systemic vascular resistance. Atrial enlargement as a result of chronic atrial distention can lead to the development of atrial fibrillation. Pacemaker syndrome has been reported during anesthesia. Diagnosis is facilitated by the observation of hypotension concurrent with pacing that resolves when the patient's intrinsic rhythm returns. Physiological or dual-chamber pacing is the definitive treatment for pacemaker syndrome.

9. Do any surgical procedures pose particular risks for patients with a pacemaker or ICD?

Procedures that are minimally invasive, such as surgeries on the eye or an extremity, may pose little risk to patients with pacemakers or ICDs. Because possible sources of interference with these devices are not always recognized or known, however, a cautious approach should be adopted, and a contingency plan should always be ready.

Procedures involving use of electrosurgical units (ESUs) or other types of electromagnetic radiation, orthopedic drills and saws (vibration sources), and peripheral nerve stimulation can have serious consequences on the functional status of these devices. Mechanical ventilation, position changes, postoperative shivering, or succinylcholine-induced muscle contractions may trigger pacing by sensors that detect body motion. Fixed rate pacing is recommended for patients undergoing electroconvulsive therapy. Unexplained tachycardia and pacemaker failure have been reported as a result of extracorporeal shock wave lithotripsy. Lithotripsy does not present a hazard to patients with a pacemaker as long as the target is more than 2 inches away from the generator. Magnetic resonance imaging is generally contraindicated in patients with pacemakers and ICDs. Diagnostic and gamma radiation do not affect pulse generators, but therapeutic, ionizing radiation can adversely affect device functions in an inconsistent manner.

10. Which anesthetic drugs and techniques are best for a patient with a permanent pacemaker?

There is no one best anesthetic technique for patients with a permanent pacemaker or ICD. The selection of monitors and anesthetic techniques should be governed by the patient's condition and the planned procedure, rather than the presence of a pacemaker. General and regional anesthesia can be administered.

Most anesthetic agents and drugs do not interfere with pacemaker function. Defasciculation is recommended before succinylcholine administration because muscle potentials can inhibit some rate-adaptive pacemakers. Diffusion of nitrous oxide into the pocket of a newly implanted pacemaker has been reported as a cause of intermittent pacemaker malfunction. Inhalational agents and propofol do not affect pacing or defibrillation thresholds. Some antiarrhythmic drugs can raise the defibrillation threshold (DFT); as a result, more energy is required to terminate arrhythmia episodes. Drugs that are known to increase the DFT are lidocaine, phenytoin, mexiletine, flecainide, propranolol, and amiodarone. Administration of lidocaine to reduce the pain of injection of propofol may raise the DFT substantially. Prophylactic antibiotics are not required for patients with a pacemaker or ICD.

Alternative methods of monitoring cardiac rhythm should be available in the event that electrocautery devices interfere with ECG signals. Pulse oximetry, precordial or esophageal stethoscopes, or a finger on the pulse may be sufficient in many instances. For other procedures, an arterial line or pulmonary artery catheter can provide information about cardiac rate and rhythm during periods of interference with the ECG. The presence of pacemakers or ICDs is not a contraindication to placement of a pulmonary artery catheter.

11. Discuss possible sources of EMI with pacemakers and ICDs.

Electromagnetic radiation has a spectrum of frequencies and wavelengths that includes x-rays; gamma rays; ultraviolet, visible, and infrared light; microwaves; and radio waves. Bipolar leads, shielding, and filters reduce the risk of EMI with pacemakers and ICDs; however, EMI of 5 to 100 Hz is not filtered because this is the range of cardiac activity. Diagnostic radiation and gamma radiation do not affect pacemakers or ICDs, but ionizing (therapeutic) radiation can damage the devices. In the operating room, electrosurgical units (ESUs), such as cauteries or Bovies, pose the greatest source of EMI.

Pacemaker and ICD pulse generators and leads can act as direct conductors of EMI or can act as antennae. Current can damage pulse generators or cause a burn if current is conducted directly to the myocardium. Devices may be triggered, inhibited, reprogrammed, or placed in an asynchronous mode. Ventricular fibrillation can be induced by stimulation of the myocardium. Because the ICD may discharge in this situation, the defibrillation mode should be disabled preoperatively, and appropriate monitoring and backup emergency drugs and defibrillation equipment should be readily available.

Several steps can be taken to minimize or avoid ESU interference with a pacemaker, as follows:
- Substitution of a bipolar cautery for a monopolar device is preferable because current flows only between the tips of the bipolar forceps.
- If monopolar cautery must be used, the following steps are recommended:
  - Place the grounding or dispersion pad as close to the surgical site and as far from the pulse generator as possible. The generator should not be between the dispersion pad and the surgical site.
  - Use as low a setting as possible.
  - Use the cautery only for short periods.
  - Do not use monopolar cautery within 5 inches of the device.

12. What precautions should be taken and what emergency equipment should be available when caring for a patient with a pacemaker or ICD?

Pacemakers should be programmed to the asynchronous (fixed rate) mode before surgery, and unnecessary, programmable features should be rendered inoperative. In particular, rate-adaptive features should be disabled because intraoperative events may cause the pacemaker to switch modes abruptly. ICDs should have defibrillation and tachyarrhythmia detection features disabled if an ESU (Bovie) is used.

If a patient is pacemaker dependent, an alternative pacing source is necessary in the event of pacemaker failure. A temporary pacemaker, atropine, and isoproterenol should be immediately available in the event of pacemaker failure or if antiarrhythmic drugs raise DFTs excessively. Temporary pacing can be supplied by a transcutaneous pacemaker, or the surgeon can expose the pacemaker leads and connect them to a temporary pacemaker. Backup defibrillation equipment should be available if the defibrillation mode of an ICD is disabled.

13. Should a magnet be used to switch pacing modes in the event of a pacemaker malfunction?

Some sources recommend placing a magnet over a pacemaker pulse generator to place the pacemaker in the "fixed" or asynchronous mode in the event of EMI with pacemaker functioning. Magnetic stimulation of pacemakers generally is not recommended, however, because it can have unexpected and undesirable consequences. The magnet feature is programmable, and if in the "off" mode, the device does not respond to a magnet. Magnets can place the pacemaker in an asynchronous mode, disable sensing, inhibit or trigger pacing, reprogram the pacemaker, trigger test programs, and even turn the device off.

Magnets should not be placed over ICDs. Defibrillation capabilities and tachyarrhythmia detection may be disabled if a magnet is placed over an ICD, and the effect on ICD pacing modes depends on the specific device and manufacturer. Postoperatively, programming of the pacemaker or ICD should be reevaluated if the device has been exposed to a magnetic field.

14. Can advanced cardiac life support (ACLS) protocols be followed in a patient with cardiac rhythm management devices?

Standard ACLS protocols can be followed as necessary in patients with pacemakers and ICDs. Disabling an ICD is recommended during cardiopulmonary resuscitation. External defibrillation is not contraindicated. Placing the paddles as far from the generator as possible and in an anterior posterior orientation is suggested to reduce potential complications of defibrillation. Current, generated by external defibrillation, can reset the devices, damage pulse generators, or cause localized myocardial damage. After external defibrillation, pacemakers and ICDs must be evaluated and reprogrammed if necessary. Discharge of an ICD poses no risk to personnel who are touching a patient when the device discharges. The sensation is reported as similar to static electricity.

15. How should pacemakers and ICDs be managed postoperatively?

Pacemakers and ICDs should be evaluated and reprogrammed after surgery if they have been placed in an asynchronous mode, they have been exposed to an electromagnetic field, or if the device does not seem to be operating effectively. Device interrogation and reprogramming can be performed by a pacemaker service, cardiologist, or manufacturer's representative.

 Key Points

- Two types of implanted, battery-powered, computerized electronic devices are used to control heart rate and rhythm: pacemakers and ICDs.
- Pacemakers and ICDs are composed of a generator and electrodes. Pacemaker and ICD generators typically are placed subcutaneously or in an infraclavicular pocket beneath the pectoral muscle.
- Modern pacemakers are powered by lithium-iodide batteries that have an expected life of 5 to 12 years.
- Pacemakers are designed to pace either one (single-chamber) or two (dual-chamber or physiological pacing) cardiac chambers.
- Rate-adaptive pacemakers are prescribed for individuals whose heart rate does not increase in response to demand, a condition termed *chronotropic incompetence*.
- ICDs are implanted for prevention of sudden death due to ventricular fibrillation and tachycardia.

Key Points   *continued*

- Pacemaker syndrome is a diffuse constellation of signs and symptoms that is thought to result from atrioventricular asynchrony in patients with single-chamber ventricular pacemakers.
- Procedures involving use of ESUs or other types of electromagnetic radiation, orthopedic drills and saws (vibration sources), and even peripheral nerve stimulation can have serious consequences on the functional status of these devices.
- Magnetic resonance imaging generally is contraindicated in patients with pacemakers and ICDs.
- Most anesthetic agents and drugs do not interfere with pacemaker function.
- Pacemakers should be programmed to the asynchronous (fixed rate) mode before surgery, and unnecessary, programmable features should be rendered inoperative.
- If the patient is pacemaker dependent, an alternative pacing source is necessary in the event of pacemaker failure.
- Disabling an ICD is recommended during cardiopulmonary resuscitation.

Internet Resources

University of Mobile Faculty Notes—Handouts for Class: Pacemakers:
http://www.umobile.edu/main/notes/pacemakers.pdf

The Anaesthetics Department, University of Sydney lectures and papers listing: Pacemakers:
http://www.usyd.edu.au/anaes/lectures/ppm_rozner/ppm_rozner.html

Association of Veterans Affairs Anesthesiologists (AVAA): Pacemakers:
http://www.vaanes.org/FORUMS/pacemakers.pdf

American Society of Anesthesologists: What's new in perioperative pacemaker-ICD management, Newsletter, Volume 66, Number 5, May 2002:
http://www.asahq.org/Newsletters/2002/5_02/whatsnew_502.htm

Virtual Anaesthesia Textbook:
http://www.virtual-anaesthesia-textbook.com/

Bibliography

Andersen C, Madsen GM: Rate-responsive pacemakers and anaesthesia: a consideration of possible implications, *Anaesthesia* 45:472-476, 1990.

Atlee JL, Bernstein AD: Cardiac rhythm management devices (part I): indications, device selection, and function, *Anesthesiology* 95:1265-1280, 2001.

Atlee JL, Bernstein AD: Cardiac rhythm management devices (part II): perioperative management, *Anesthesiology* 95:1492-1506, 2001.

Baller MR, Kirsner KM: Anesthetic implications of implanted pacemakers: a case study, *AANA J* 63:209-216, 1995.

Bourke ME, Healey JS: Pacemakers, recent directions and developments, *Curr Opin Anaesthesiol* 15:681-686, 2002.

Cardall TY, Brady WJ, Chan TC, et al: Permanent cardiac pacemakers: issues relevant to the emergency physician, part II, *J Emerg Med* 17:697-709, 1999.

Cardall TY, Chan TC, Brady WJ, et al: Permanent cardiac pacemakers: issues relevant to the emergency physician, part I, *J Emerg Med* 17:479-489, 1999.

LeVasseur JG, Kennard CD, Finley EM, et al: Dermatologic electrosurgery in patients with implantable cardioverter-defibrillators and pacemakers, *Dermatol Surg* 24:233-240, 1998.

Madsen GM, Andersen C: Rate-responsive pacemakers and extracorporeal shock wave lithotripsy: a dangerous combination? [letter], *Anesth Analg* 76:917, 1993.

Pinski SL, Fahy GJ: Implantable cardioverter-defibrillators, *Am J Med* 106:446-458, 1999.

History and Organizational Structure of the Nurse Anesthesia Profession

Lynn L. Lebeck

1. How long have nurses been administering anesthesia?

Nurse anesthesia is considered the oldest nursing specialty. There is an uncorroborated claim in the autobiography of Catherine S. Lawrence that she administered chloroform at the Second Battle of Bull Run. The first documented nurse anesthetist was Sister Mary Bernard in 1877. A chapter entitled "Administration of Anesthetics" appeared in an 1893 basic nursing textbook by the noted pioneer nurse educator, Isabel Adams Hampton Robb.

2. Who was the "mother of anesthesia"?

Alice Magaw is known as the "mother of anesthesia." Magaw initiated the development of the modern nurse anesthetist role. She successfully completed more than 14,000 anesthetics, testing different methods of delivering anesthesia and different mixes of anesthetic agents.

3. Briefly describe the evolution of nurse anesthesia education.

During the early 20th century, the education of nurse anesthetists was primarily through on-the-job training in hospitals. The period immediately before World War I saw the establishment of more formalized post–nursing school programs. Many programs contained a 3-month curriculum consisting of clinical and theoretical components.

With the establishment of a professional organization that eventually would be the American Association of Nurse Anesthetists (AANA) in 1931 came requirements for nurse anesthesia education. These standards included a minimum of 75 hours of instructional class hours and performance of 250 anesthetic cases. Within 3 years, the requirements were increased to a minimal length of 6 months (but suggested length of 1 year), 113 instructional hours, and 325 cases. Requirements that included specific types of cases and techniques were established.

In 1933, the need for accreditation of nurse anesthesia programs was recognized. An Education Department was established within the AANA in 1940, with the purpose of standardizing and elevating educational programs. The AANA accreditation program for schools was initiated in 1952. Nurse anesthesia educational programs moved into more university-based settings in the 1970s and 1980s, some granting certificates and others granting baccalaureate degrees. Rapid development of the scientific base and technology involved in the practice of anesthesia prompted an increase in minimum program length to 24 months. Graduate-level education as an entry to practice was mandated in 1998.

4. Discuss some of the early legal challenges to nurse anesthesia practice.

Dr. Francis McMechan was a physician practicing anesthesia in the early 1900s. In 1913, he presented a paper entitled "The Medical-Legal Status of Anesthesia." He advocated that State Medical Protocol Acts should abolish nurse anesthetists and that the ethics of surgeons using them be questioned.

A sentinel case regarding the legal basis for nurse anesthesia practice was *Frank v. South,* a case in which the courts found that Margaret Hatfield was not engaged in the practice of medicine when administering anesthetics for surgeon Dr. Louis Frank. In 1934, a nurse anesthetist, Dagmar Nelson, was charged with practicing medicine without a license. The courts ruled that in the practice of administering an anesthetic Dagmar Nelson was not engaged in the practice of medicine. *Frank v. South* and the Dagmar Nelson case are viewed as the legal foundation for the practice of nurse anesthetists.

5. The AANA Award for Outstanding Accomplishment in Nurse Anesthesia is named for Agatha Hodgins; what was her contribution to the profession?

Agatha Hodgins provided nursing leadership to practicing nurse anesthetists when the profession was in its infancy. Hodgins was a vocal advocate for the rights and responsibilities of the nurse anesthetist. In 1931, she helped establish the first organization of nurse anesthetists for the purpose of professional recognition and collective bargaining. In addition to being founder, Hodgins was president of the organization from 1931 to 1933. In 1939, the professional organization was named the *American Association of Nurse Anesthetists.*

6. The AANA Award for Outstanding Educator is named for Helen Lamb; what was her contribution to the profession?

Helen Lamb was a nurse anesthetist and the founder and Director of the School of Anesthesia at Barnes Hospital, St. Louis, from 1929 to 1951. As a nurse anesthetist, she pioneered techniques of endotracheal anesthesia for lung procedures and performed the first anesthetic for successful pneumonectomy. She was actively involved in the fledgling national organization, and her vision for the future of nurse anesthesia included plans for accreditation of schools and a national certification examination. She served as Chairman of the Education Committee from 1931 to 1939 and President of the AANA from 1940 to 1942.

7. **When was the first administration of the National Certification Examination (NCE), and how has the examination evolved since then?**

In 1942, the AANA established a special committee to organize the process of certification for nurse anesthetists and adopted a resolution inaugurating certification by examination. The first national qualifying examination was administered in 1945 to 92 candidates. Questions for the examination were obtained from workshops conducted by the AANA and from nurse anesthesia education programs. The NCE was administered biannually from 1945 to 1995, at which time the use of a computer adaptive test allowed multiple testing dates.

The current form of the NCE is a computer adaptive test. The NCE is composed of multiple-choice questions with a stem and four possible answer choices. There are a minimum of 90 questions and a maximum of 140 questions, with 20 items being pretested for future use. The candidate has a maximum of 3 hours to complete the test.

8. **Who was the first president of the AANA? The first black president? The first male president?**

- Agatha Hodgins was the first president of the AANA (1931-1933).
- Goldie Brangman was the first black president of the AANA (1973-1974).
- John F. Garde was the first male president of the AANA (1972-1973).

9. **Summarize are the functions of the four independent councils of the AANA?**

- Council on Accreditation of Nurse Anesthesia Educational Programs
  - Formulate standards, guidelines, and criteria for the accreditation of nurse anesthesia programs
  - Accredit nurse anesthesia educational programs
- Council on Certification of Nurse Anesthetists
  - Formulate and adopt requirements for certification
  - Formulate and adopt requirements for eligibility to take certifying examination
  - Formulate and administer the certifying examination
  - Evaluate candidate performance on the national certifying examination
- Council for Public Interest in Anesthesia
  - Make recommendations to the AANA on safety, quality of care, health care cost, and other issues
  - Facilitate education to the public on issues regarding anesthesia care
  - Facilitate communication among the public, health care professionals and nurse anesthesia profession
- Council on Recertification of Nurse Anesthetists
  - Formulate and adopt criteria for eligibility for recertification
  - Formulate and adopt criteria for approval of continuing education programs
  - Formulate and adopt criteria for delegating approval authority to nationally recognized continuing education agencies

- Develop and maintain mechanism for determination of charges and allegations against CRNAs.

10. List AANA membership classifications.

Membership classifications are as follows:
- Active—certified, recertification, nonrecertified life, and emeritus
- Inactive
- Conditional
- Honorary
- Associate—student and graduate
- International

11. List major duties of the AANA Executive Director.

The duties of the Executive Director include:
- Manage and direct the activities of the Executive Office
- Keep minutes of all meetings of the AANA
- Hire, fire, and promote employees of the AANA
- Represent the AANA to outside organizations
- Speak on behalf of the AANA on issues and policies about which the Board of Directors have made decisions

12. Who composes the AANA Board of Directors?

The Board of Directors is composed of the President, President-elect, Vice President, Treasurer, and seven Directors.

13. Describe the qualifications for and the process to become a member of the Board of Directors.

- Officers (President, President-elect, Vice President and Treasurer)
  - Member of the Board of Directors within the last 7 years.
- Directors
  - Active certified or recertified member
  - Serve at least one term as an officer or director of a State Association.

Qualified candidates are nominated by their state association or requested to run by the nominating committee of the AANA. A written ballot is conducted, with the candidate receiving the highest number of votes for each position elected.

14. What is the Assembly of School Faculty?

The Assembly of School Faculty is composed of program directors, assistant directors, faculty, medical and educational advisors, students, and other interested individuals. The Assembly currently meets twice yearly, one meeting at the AANA Annual meeting and one other separate meeting. The purpose is to discuss affairs pertinent to nurse anesthesia educational programs and provide educational content for the development of faculty.

15. What is the Assembly of States?

The Assembly of States is composed of members of the Board of Directors, members of standing committees, officers of state organizations, and other interested individuals. The purpose of the Assembly is to disseminate information and discuss issues pertinent to the Association.

 Key Points

- Nurse anesthesia is considered the oldest nursing specialty.
- The first documented nurse anesthetist was Sister Mary Bernard in 1877.
- Alice Magaw is known as the "mother of anesthesia."
- Agatha Hodgins helped establish the first organization of nurse anesthetists for the purpose of professional recognition and collective bargaining. In addition to being founder, Hodgins was president of the organization from 1931 to 1933.
- Helen Lamb was a nurse anesthetist and the founder and Director of the School of Anesthesia at Barnes Hospital, St. Louis, from 1929 to 1951. As a nurse anesthetist she pioneered techniques of endotracheal anesthesia for lung procedures and performed the first anesthetic for successful pneumonectomy.

 Internet Resources

American Association of Nurse Anesthetists:
http://www.aana.com/

Bibliography

American Association of Nurse Anesthetists: *A brief historical context of nurse anesthesia education. National Commission on Nurse Anesthesia Education*, Park Ridge, IL, 1990, AANA.

American Association of Nurse Anesthetists: *Bylaws of the American Association of Nurse Anesthetists,* Park Ridge, IL, 2001, AANA.

Bankert M: *Watchful care: a history of America's nurse anesthetists,* New York, 1989, Continuum Publishing

Gunn IP: *The history of nurse anesthesia education: highlights and influences. National Commission on Nurse Anesthesia Education,* Park Ridge, IL, 1990, AANA.

Thatcher VS: History of anesthesia: with emphasis on the nurse specialist, Philadelphia, 1953, JB Lippincott.

Legal Terminology

Lynn H. Karlet

1. Define assault and battery.

Battery is a *tort* (a civil wrong that injures someone) resulting from (1) unconsented, (2) harmful or offensive (3) touching of one by another that (4) actually results in harm. In a medical setting, a certified registered nurse anesthetist (CRNA) who provides care to a patient without any consent or exceeds the scope of consent granted commits battery against the patient. Battery against a patient may result in malpractice or worse, criminal liability, or both. A close cousin of battery is a tort called *assault,* whereby a patient has a reasonable perception that battery is imminent.

2. What if a patient never gave consent for any treatment but was about to be given an injection by a CRNA?

If the injection is given, the CRNA commits battery. If the patient watched as the CRNA approached with a syringe in hand just before the injection, an assault has occurred. Assault on an unconscious patient cannot occur because the patient has no perception of the act, but battery against an unconscious patient could occur if the patient did not grant consent or the CRNA exceeded the scope of any consent granted.

3. How does a patient grant consent?

A patient's *consent* allows medical staff to perform all manner of "harmful or offensive" touching, such as cutting, injecting, shocking, cauterizing, drilling, freezing, amputating, extracting, poking, radiating, and prodding, but none of this is battery with a patient's informed consent. The operative principle of consent involves the following:
- The scope of the consent granted
- Whether or not a CRNA remains within the contours of the scope of consent granted

People routinely consent to "harmful or offensive" touching in everyday life; for example, hockey players routinely permit physical abuse by opponents while skating on an ice rink during a game but not being punched by an opponent after the game. A patient consents to anesthesia with the expectation that the anesthetic will be administered according to the prevailing standards of the profession; that the anesthetic agents will be safe and U.S. Food and Drug

Administration approved (i.e., not experimental, unless disclosed beforehand) and in the proper dosage; and that the patient will wake up without any long-term side effects, such as paralysis, numbness, or broken teeth. If the result is otherwise, consent likely has been exceeded, and the CRNA may be exposed to professional malpractice liability.

Consent may be granted expressly, as when a patient signs a medical release or consent form, or consent may be implied, as in cases when an unconscious patient is rushed to an emergency department unaccompanied by a family member. Implied consent requires that a reasonable person under similar circumstances, if conscious and able to give consent, would have probably done so in similar circumstances.

Informed consent is a special contract that presupposes that the patient has sufficient information about the benefits and risks of treatment, side effects, possible complications, and alternative treatment options and that the patient possessed sufficient intelligence and comprehension to weigh reasonably all relevant factors in making the treatment decision. Competency is a prerequisite of all contracts, including informed consent, which demands that the signer be of the legal age of majority (i.e., not a minor, typically 18 years old, depending on state law) and is mentally competent to make the treatment decision. After all of the foregoing, the patient must make a conscious and deliberate decision to grant permission to medical staff for treatment.

4. **What about consent by the very young and the very old; how can a child of 6 or an Alzheimer's patient of 80 grant consent for medical treatment?**

In each case, the patient's lack of capacity to grant informed consent can be overcome by obtaining consent from the patient's legal guardian, who does meet the above-described criteria to provide informed consent.

5. **Define negligence.**

In lay terms, *negligence* refers to carelessness and is practically synonymous with *medical malpractice*. Legally, negligence is defined as the breach of a duty of care owed to another, as defined by the standards of the profession and appropriate under a particular set of circumstances that results in some foreseeable harm. The CRNA's negligence must result in some degree of harm to the patient for a lawsuit to move forward through the judicial system. The harm must be a foreseeable result (a natural consequence) of the CRNA's breach of duty. For example, an infected hangnail is not a foreseeable result of negligent administration of an anesthetic, but hypoxia may be a foreseeable result.

6. **How can a patient prove negligence?**

For an injured patient to succeed in suing under a negligence theory, the elements of proof can be found by dissecting the definition of negligence itself. A patient must prove:
- That the CRNA owed a duty of care to the patient

- That the CRNA breached that duty of care
- That the patient's harm was a foreseeable result of the CRNA's breach of duty
- That the CRNA's negligence actually caused the harm to the patient
- That the harm to the patient resulted in compensable damages

In many states, no case alleging medical negligence or malpractice can go to trial until a medical panel screens the facts and evidence, or unless a judge before trial first evaluates expert testimony about the case.

Sometimes, medical negligence is so obvious or witnesses are so uncooperative that the doctrine of *res ipsa loquitur* (Latin, "the thing speaks for itself") must be applied to the problem of "proving" all elements of a case in which no direct "proof" exists, so as to create a legal presumption of negligence. The presumption of negligence, under res ipsa loquitor, is rebuttable by the defendant by showing that the event was an inevitable accident having nothing to do with the CRNA's duty of care or a supervisor's responsibility to control or supervise. For example, if a power blackout caused the failure of a ventilation machine and the hospital's backup electrical system also failed causing the operating room to remain dark and powerless, after which the CRNA slipped and fell in the dark, becoming unconscious, resulting in harm to a patient because no manual ventilation was possible, this shows intervening cause of harm and will tend to rebut any CRNA negligence presumption, under res ipsa loquitor.

7. Describe the types of damages a patient can recover in a lawsuit.

Damages occur in many forms and are determined by the fact finder (a jury or a judge in a "bench trial," i.e., trial without a jury) after a verdict is rendered. *Compensatory damages* (also known as *general damages* or *actual damages*) arise from the foreseeable cost of repairing the actual harm caused by negligence. For example, the cost of capping a tooth chipped during intubation; plus the patient's time or lost wages and mileage in seeking dental treatment; plus pain, suffering, and emotional distress in connection with the harm itself; plus pain, suffering, and emotional distress incurred during and after repair all are examples of compensatory damages that could be claimed by a hypothetical patient.

Consequential damages do not arise immediately from negligent acts, but rather are a natural, but not foreseeable, consequence of such acts. For example, assume the hypothetical patient could not schedule an appointment with her dentist for several days and her appearance was so embarrassing that she could not attend a $1000 per person gala the evening after surgery. The hypothetical patient would likely have a $2000 claim for consequential damages if she and her date were unable to obtain a refund of their ticket prices. In addition, hedonistic damages could be a viable claim for the lost enjoyment of the evening.

Punitive damages serve as punishment for the defendant's acts and as a deterrent to others from committing similar acts in the future. Punitive damages sometimes are awarded as a multiple of other damages; for example, *treble damages* are a multiple of three times the other damage awards. Punitive damages are most often awarded if the defendant's conduct was found to be malicious (acts accompanied by ill will, spite, or for the purpose of injuring the patient), reckless (in disregard of the patient's rights or in complete indifference to the safety and rights of the patient), wanton, or willful. If the hypothetical patient's tooth was chipped by an intoxicated CRNA, punitive damages might be awarded.

If a CRNA's negligence results in death, survivors may sue for damages pursuant to a *wrongful death* claim payable to the patient's spouse and children, if any, or to the patient's parent(s) if the patient had no spouse or children. Wrongful death awards typically include economic support survivors would have received based on the patient's occupation, education, opportunity for advancement, and life expectancy; companionship to include loss of sexual relations with a spouse; consortium with parents and children; moral guidance for children; and in a few states, survivors' grief.

If a patient sues and proves negligence but cannot prove any damages, *nominal damages,* typically one dollar, are sometimes awarded.

Often, malpractice insurers are the parties who pay damages and provide defense counsel in medical malpractice cases. Most of these cases settle damage claims before trial without any admission of negligence through negotiation or alternative dispute resolution, such as arbitration or mediation. A high percentage of cases that do go to trial settle before a verdict is rendered. Commonly, damage awards are adjusted upward (*additur*) or downward (*remititur*) on appeal.

8. Who is responsible for a CRNA's negligence?

A patient harmed by medical negligence or malpractice typically sues everyone connected with the treatment: the hospital and its board of trustees, the surgeon, the anesthesiologist, the CRNA, the nurses, medical equipment manufacturers, drug makers, the sellers of such medical goods, and so on. Everyone in this daisy chain of treatment should have liability insurance, which is the engine that drives litigation.

Often, defendants in a lawsuit ask to be dismissed in the early stages of a case by filing a motion to dismiss because they believe that the lawsuit does not directly involve them or by summary judgment because there is considerable doubt as to the basis for their liability. For example, a hospital may assert that the anesthesia department is an independently owned medical practice or that independent contractors staff the anesthesia department, relieving the hospital of liability. Courts sometimes rule that a hospital has a nondelegable duty (i.e., they cannot "pass the buck") for anesthesia claims because anesthesia services are "bundled" with other hospital services, such as emergency department services and cannot be considered legally separate. A court also could rule that the independence of the anesthesia department is purely cosmetic because the hospital administration controlled anesthesia department practices, hiring, procedures, pay, reimbursement, and hours, even if "officially" an independent contractor. In these cases, the doctrine of *respondeat superior* (Latin, for a superior must answer for the acts or omissions of subordinates) applies, so the hospital may be compelled to defend itself from charges of vicarious liability.

Plaintiffs may try to build a case on the "captain of the ship" doctrine and assert that a physician controlled not only the surgical procedure, but also the conduct of all who participated, including CRNAs, but this theory has been widely discredited as a basis for liability. The factual issues in such cases tend to revolve around whether a duty to "control" existed, whether "control" was accepted by a team member, and whether the "control" over an anesthesia provider was negligent, if it existed at all. See *Lauro v. Knowles,* 739 A 2nd 1183 (R.I., 1999).

9. Distinguish between slander and libel.

Slander and libel are two species of defamation. A mnemonic device associating the first letter of each word with its definition can keep the two terms distinct in your mind: "*S*lander is *s*poken" refers to the oral nature of slander, and "*l*ibel is *l*etter" refers to the written nature of libel.

Slander consists of:
• A false declaration expressed in spoken words, signs, or gestures, which
• Injures the character or reputation of the person defamed, because
• The declaration is published (i.e., disseminated to one or more others), and is
• Understood by others to be defamatory, but not necessarily believed, and
• Results in damages.

Falsely stating to a non–English-speaking person that your patient is schizophrenic is not slanderous because the listener cannot understand the nature of the declaration.

Libel consists of:
• A false declaration expressed in written words or even scripts used for radio or television broadcasts (although the words are spoken), which
• Injures the character or reputation of the person defamed, because
• The declaration is published, and is
• Understood by others to be defamatory, but not necessarily believed, and
• Results in damages.

If a CRNA wrote false anesthesia notes either negligently or maliciously (i.e., the writer either knew of the falsity or recklessly disregarded the truth) in a patient's chart, and others read them and understand them to be defamatory, and as a result the patient's reputation is harmed, the CRNA's conduct is libelous. Contrast libel with a false writing in the patient's chart pertaining to dosage, which harms not the patient's reputation, but rather the patient's medical condition, in which case, the patient may have an action for medical malpractice, not libel.

The dead can be neither slandered nor libeled because although the dead leave behind "character" and "reputation," for legal purposes, actions involving defamation are reserved for the living.

The perfect defense to either slander or libel is the truth, so if a defendant can show the truth of the words uttered or written, the plaintiff's action for either slander or libel will likely be defeated. Not so for a defamation action called *public disclosure of private facts,* whereby, for example, a patient's diagnosis is released to an unauthorized third party, violating the patient's right to privacy. The newly amended Health Insurance Portability and Accountability Act of 1996 incorporates into federal statute many privacy concepts discussed here.

10. Explain the difference between statutory law and common law.

Legislatures, county commissioners, city councils, the military, the president, governors, plus federal and state regulators pass all manner of laws, rules, regulations, ordinances, statutes, acts, executive orders, treaties, and codes that we know collectively as *statutory law*—the written law.

Courts constantly interpret statutory law and use past judicial decisions, known as *precedent,* as a basis for deciding cases now before the court, a process called *stare decisis* (Latin, "to stand by that which is decided"). The resulting body of law we call *common law,* which traces its origins to many centuries of English jurisprudence, which can be traced to ancient Rome. For example, the U.S. Supreme Court decided *Roe v. Wade* (410 US 113), which has allowed abortion on demand since 1973, not from any statute, but rather from previous court decisions regarding a woman's right to privacy.

11. What does statute of limitations mean?

A law that sets a deadline for filing lawsuits within a certain period after an injury is called *statute of limitations.* Deadlines vary by state and by the cause of action to be filed. A court dismisses a lawsuit filed after expiry of the statute of limitations, subject to certain rules and exceptions.

Assume that the fictitious state of Michiana has statute of limitations of 3 years from the date of injury for medical malpractice. The patient is injured during a medical procedure on June 1, 2000. The patient must file a lawsuit before June 1, 2003 or he or she becomes time barred from seeking any relief through the courts.

Change the facts slightly: The patient is injured during a medical procedure on June 1, 2000, when a surgeon left a sponge in the patient's abdomen. On March 31, 2003, the patient was admitted to a hospital for abdominal pain, and the same sponge was found and removed, resulting in a full recovery. The patient now must file a lawsuit before March 31, 2006, because the statute of limitations in a case of latent harm is tolled (postponed) and begins to run on the day the patient discovered or should have reasonably discovered the latent harm.

Although statutes of limitation vary according to what civil wrong or crime is involved, some actions, such as a prosecution for murder, have no statute of limitations.

Key Points

- Battery is a tort (a civil wrong that injures someone) resulting from (1) unconsented, (2) harmful or offensive (3) touching of one by another that (4) actually results in harm.
- Assault occurs when a patient has a reasonable perception that battery is imminent.
- Consent can be obtained expressly via written consent or implied in an emergency situation; informed consent is usually obtained in writing.
- In the case of consent from someone who has not reached the age of majority or an adult with diminished mental capacity, the patient's parent or legal guardian can provide informed consent.
- Negligence is defined as the breach of a duty of care owed to another, as defined by the standards of the profession and appropriate under a particular set of circumstances that results in some forseeable harm.
- Slander is defamation by spoken means; libel is defamation by written means.

Internet Resources

Virtual Anaesthesia Textbook:
http://www.virtual-anaesthesia-textbook.com/

GASNet.org: Survey of Anesthesiology, April 2000:
http://www.gasnet.org/sa/2000/02/

GASNet.org: Online Journals and Newsletters Division:
http://www.gasnet.org/journals.php

Ethics in Medicine, University of Washington School of Medicine: Informed consent: in the operating room:
http://eduserv.hscer.washington.edu/bioethics/topics/infc.html

CSEN: The Global Regional Anesthesia Website: Informed consent in anesthesia:
http://www.csen.com/anesthesia/informed-consent.htm

Bibliography

American Association of Nurse Anesthetists: *Legal issues in nurse anesthesia practice*; available online: http://www.aana.com/; accessed April 24, 2003.

American Association of Nurse Anesthetists: *Informed consent in anesthesia,* Park Ridge, IL, 1991.

Blumenriech GA: Litigation too important to be entrusted to lawyers, *AANA J* 67:311-314, 1999.

Liang BA: Ulnar neuropathy following surgery: does res ipsa loquitur apply? *J Clin Anesth* 12:234-237, 2000.

Prosser W, editor: Prosser and Keaton on the law of torts (hornbook), ed 5, St. Louis, MN, 1984, West Wadsworth.

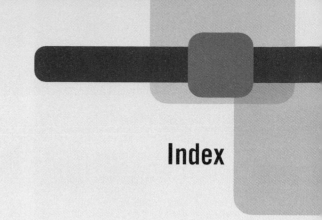

Index

Note: Page numbers followed by the letter f refer to figures and those followed by t refer to tables.

ABO blood type, 216–217
ACE inhibitor(s). *See* Angiotensin-converting enzyme inhibitor(s).
Acetaminophen, 416
Acetazolamide
  affecting anesthesia, 285t
  site of action and mechanism of action of, 137t
Acetohexamide (Dymelor)
  dosage of, 267t
  for type 2 diabetes, 266
Acetylcholine
  at neuromuscular terminal button, 103
  synthesis and metabolism of, 104
Acetylcholine receptor(s), proliferation of, 437
ACh. *See* Acetylcholine.
Acid-base balance
  maintenance of, 225
  with blood transfusion therapy, 217–218
Acid-base disorder(s), 226–233
Acid-base value(s), normal, 225
Acidosis
  causing reversion to fetal circulation, 393
  fetal, 357–358
  physiological effects of, 226
  respiratory, 230
    causes of, 226–227
Acromegaly, anesthetic considerations with, 262
ACT. *See* Activated coagulation time.
Activated coagulation time, 208
  during cardiac surgery, 307
Adamkiewicz, artery of, 329
Adenoma, pituitary, 261
Adenyl cyclase, 119
Adjustable pressure limiting valve, 22–23
Adrenergic receptor(s), classification and
    physiologic functions of, 117
Advanced cardiac life support protocols, 530
Air embolism, paradoxical, 341
Airway equipment, 287
Airway fire
  conditions for support of, 313
  with tonsillectomy, 316
Airway management, 27–35

  in ENT surgery, 317
  in tracheoesophageal fistula, 402
  in trauma patient, 419
  with rheumatoid arthritis, 291–292
Airway(s)
  assessment of, in burn injury, 436
  complications of
    in anterior cervical spine surgery, 332
    in carotid endarterectomy, 299–300
  Mallampati classification of, 30
  neonatal versus adult, 387
  obstruction of, causes of in unresponsive patient,
    515
  pathology of, in acromegaly, 262
  pediatric, 394
  preoperative evaluation criteria for, 29
Albumin
  in fluid replacement, 220
  serum level of, 251
Albuterol, preoperative, 176
Alcohol, in chronic pancreatitis, 246
Alfentanil
  physiological effects of, 94t
  potency and half-life of, 93t
Alkaline phosphatase, 253
Alkalosis
  metabolic, renal and nonrenal causes of, 229
  physiological effects of, 226
Allergic reaction
  to latex, 501–508
  to local anesthetics, 131–132
Alpha-glucosidase inhibitor(s)
  dosages of, 267t
  for type 2 diabetes, 266
Ambulatory surgery
  advantages of, 411
  anxiolytic premedication in, 414
ASA classifications as candidates for, 412
  general anesthesia for, 414–415
  laboratory tests for, 413
American Association of Nurse Anesthetists
  Award for Outstanding Accomplishment in
    Nurse Anesthesia of, 534